*Atlas of Neuropathology*

*Nathan Malamud*, M.D.

CHIEF, NEUROPATHOLOGY SERVICE, LANGLEY PORTER NEUROPSYCHIATRIC INSTITUTE;
PROFESSOR OF NEUROPATHOLOGY IN RESIDENCE, EMERITUS,
UNIVERSITY OF CALIFORNIA, SAN FRANCISCO

*Asao Hirano*, M.D.

HEAD, DIVISION OF NEUROPATHOLOGY,
DEPARTMENT OF PATHOLOGY, MONTEFIORE HOSPITAL AND MEDICAL CENTER;
PROFESSOR OF PATHOLOGY (NEUROPATHOLOGY),
ALBERT EINSTEIN COLLEGE OF MEDICINE

# Atlas of Neuropathology

SECOND, REVISED EDITION
WITH A FOREWORD BY H. M. ZIMMERMAN

*University of California Press*
*Berkeley, Los Angeles, London*

UNIVERSITY OF CALIFORNIA PRESS

BERKELEY AND LOS ANGELES, CALIFORNIA

UNIVERSITY OF CALIFORNIA PRESS, LTD.

LONDON, ENGLAND

COPYRIGHT © 1974, BY

THE REGENTS OF THE UNIVERSITY OF CALIFORNIA

FIRST EDITION PUBLISHED 1957. SECOND EDITION 1974.

ISBN: 0-520-02221-1

LIBRARY OF CONGRESS CATALOG CARD NUMBER: 78-187872

PRINTED IN THE UNITED STATES OF AMERICA

To R. K. M.

# *Foreword*

The Atlas of Neuropathology presents in superlative fashion the gross anatomic and microscopic features of an unbelievably large number of conditions, some of which are well known and others are obscure to the neurologist, neurosurgeon, and neuropathologist. The medical student, in particular, stands to benefit from a study of this work.

For all, it is a gratifying experience to find a telling illustration or two of each essential lesion in the large variety of disease states that are carefully indexed. Many are accompanied by concise clinical histories gleaned from the large experience of the author.

The first edition of this work well deserved its popularity. In the second, revised edition the author has further enhanced its usefulness by incorporating elegant electron micrographs. These are by Dr. Asao Hirano, whose usual great skill and selectivity are in evidence.

It must be kept in mind that this volume is an atlas and not a textbook. As such, it is not primarily concerned with elucidating the pathogenesis of diseases of the nervous system, nor even with the morphologic variations and details of the individual disease entities with which it deals.

Dr. Malamud has produced a work of art as well as an authoritative scientific volume. We will long remain in his debt for it.

H. M. Zimmerman, M.D.

# *Preface to the First Edition*

The need for an atlas of neuropathology has long been apparent to workers in the fields of neurology, psychiatry, neurosurgery, and pathology. Precise and detailed knowledge of the gross and microscopic changes in the nervous system is a necessary prerequisite to the understanding of nervous and mental diseases. The purpose of this book is to provide a visual approach that is not usually provided by textbooks of neuropathology.

I have attempted to illustrate the various disorders of the nervous system as comprehensively as possible. Equal space has been given to all categories, but special attention has been paid to such neglected conditions as the heredodegenerative disorders and those pertaining to geriatrics, cerebral palsy, and mental deficiency. The case presentation method was used wherever possible, to afford a correlation between lesions and symptoms and to crystallize the clinical syndromes. Owing to lack of space, theoretical discussions and references to the literature were reduced to a minimum.

The material in the atlas represents approximately five thousand specimens collected from many sources, including general and mental hospitals, and personally examined by me in the laboratory of neuropathology at the Langley Porter Clinic.

Although it is not possible to list all sources, particular acknowledgment for the use of material is made to the following: the departments of Neurosurgery, Neurology, Psychiatry, and Pathology of the University of California Medical Center, San Francisco; Letterman Army Hospital, San Francisco; United States Naval Hospital, Oakland; and Veterans Administration Hospital, Palo Alto; the state hospitals of the Department of Mental Hygiene in California; and the Armed Forces Institute of Pathology, Washington, D. C.

In reproducing illustrations and certain data, I have indicated sources in suitable places throughout the book. I want to express gratitude to the following journals for granting permission to reproduce such material: *Archives of Neurology and Psychiatry, Archives of Internal Medicine, American Journal of Diseases of Children, American Journal of Pathology, American Journal of Mental Deficiency, American Journal of Psychiatry, Archiv für Psychiatrie und Nervenkrankheiten, Journal of Nervous and Mental Diseases, Journal of Neurosurgery, Journal of Neuropathology and Experimental Neurology, Journal of Pediatrics, Neurology, Military Medicine, Transactions of the American Neurological Association*, and to Charles C. Thomas, publisher.

My special thanks are extended to: Mrs. Irene Robley, for her untiring effort and excellent technique in preparing the microscopic slides; Mrs. Marie-Jeanne Angenent, for typing the manuscript; Dr. Herbert Herzon, for reading the text.

N. M.

# *Preface to the Second Edition*

Approximately sixteen years have elapsed since the publication of the ATLAS OF NEURO-PATHOLOGY. The need for a second edition has become increasingly apparent to include new material in the light of additional experience gained following analysis of over 12,000 cases; to expand the text in order to serve more adequately as a guide to the individual case material; and to take into consideration some of the progress made in neuropathology in the past decade. An extensive revision of the first edition has thus resulted.

Although the traditional clinicopathological approach to the formulation and diagnosis of disease has retained its importance, recent advances in electron microscopy have broadened our knowledge and, in some instances, our concepts of the nature of disease processes. Towards that end we correlated the findings as revealed by light and electron microscopy, wherever possible. The second edition is thus the product of the collaboration by the two authors.

To conserve space, references were kept to a minimum, except in the case of the authors' previous publications, since illustrations from these sources had to be included. For a more extensive bibliography, the reader is referred to the General References.

In addition to acknowledgements made in the first edition, we want to express our gratitude to the following journals and book publishers for granting permission to reproduce clinical data and illustrations: Archives of Neurology, Archives of Pathology, Journal of Neurology, Neurosurgery and Psychiatry, Cancer, Journal of Ultrastructural Research, Laboratory Investigation, Plenum Publishing Corporation, C. V. Mosby Co., McGraw-Hill Book Company, Academic Press, Grune and Stratton, Charles C. Thomas, University of Chicago Press, The Rockefeller University Press, National Institutes of Health, Congress of Neurological Surgeons, and Association for Research in Nervous and Mental Disease.

It is a pleasure to acknowledge the expert services of Mrs. Irene Robley for technological work, Mr. John R. McCulloch for the preparation of the photomicrographs, and Miss Geraldine O'Keefe for the secretarial work. The authors are indebted to the publishers for the special care and attention given to the printing of the book.

N. M.
A. H.

2 February 1973

# Contents

xiii

## X DEVELOPMENTAL DISORDERS 412

*Atlas of Neuropathology*

# I$_A$

# *A Cytology and Cellular Pathology*

Pathologic processes are based ultimately on cellular pathology. The nature of a particular disorder is determined by the manner in which nerve cells and fibers are altered, the type of reaction of the supporting cells evoked, and the kind of catabolic products produced.

Different staining methods may be required to demonstrate such changes, since the various nerve structures have specific staining properties.

## STAINING METHODS

*Nissl Method.* Aniline dyes, such as thionin, toluidine blue, or cresyl violet, stain the Nissl bodies of neurons and the chromatin of all nuclei varying shades of blue to purple (Fig. 1a).

*Hematoxylin-Eosin (HE) Method.* This nonspecific method stains the cytoplasm purplish red and the nucleus blue-black. In neurons undergoing ischemic or anoxic change, the cytoplasm stains a bright red that contrasts with the deep blue pyknotic nucleus (Fig. 1b).

*Bielschowsky Method* (or its *von Braunmühl* modification). Silver nitrate stains the neurofibrils, and such argyrophilic pathologic structures as senile plaques, black against a slightly purplish background (Fig. 1c).

*Davenport Method.* Silver nitrate (similar to the Bielschowsky) stains the axis cylinders black against a purplish background (Fig. 1d).

*Weigert Method* (or any of its modifications). Iron hematoxylin, in tissue previously mordanted with chrome and copper salts, stains the myelin sheaths blue-black in contrast to the slightly yellowish color of normally unmyelinated or demyelinated areas (Fig. 1e).

*Weil Method.* A solution of iron alum and hematoxylin stains the normal myelin sheaths a bluish gray against the light gray of unmyelinated and demyelinated structures, as in a degenerating peripheral nerve (Fig. 1f).

*Laidlaw Connective Tissue Method.* A solution of lithium silver stains reticulin fibers black, as in a gumma (Fig. 1g).

*Hematoxylin-van Gieson (HVG) Method.* A solution of iron hematoxylin and picric acid-fuchsin stains collagen fibers red, and nerve tissue and hemosiderin pigment yellowish brown, as in the capsule of a brain abscess (Fig. 1h).

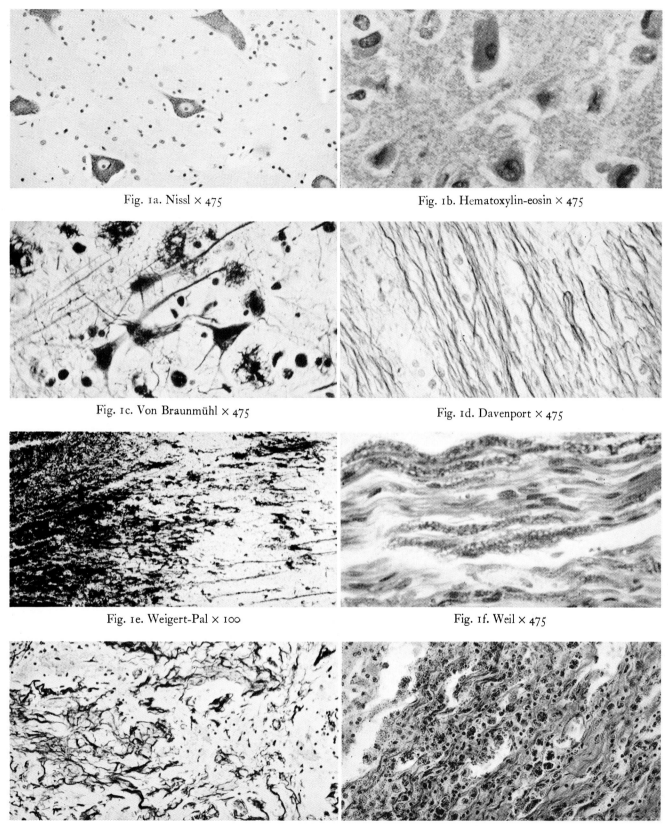

Fig. 1a. Nissl × 475

Fig. 1b. Hematoxylin-eosin × 475

Fig. 1c. Von Braunmühl × 475

Fig. 1d. Davenport × 475

Fig. 1e. Weigert-Pal × 100

Fig. 1f. Weil × 475

Fig. 1g. Laidlaw × 200

Fig. 1h. Hematoxylin-van Gieson × 200

*Hortega Silver Carbonate Method.* The microglia stain black against a purplish background (Fig. 2a).

*Cajal Gold Sublimate Method.* The astrocytes and their processes stain black against a reddish-brown background (Fig. 2b).

*Holzer Method.* Crystal violet stains the glial fibers of astrocytes a deep blue, as in a glial scar (Fig. 2c).

*Scarlet-Red Method.* Sudan III or IV, counterstained with alum hematoxylin, stains droplets of cholesterol esters and neutral fat deposited in gitter cells (macrophages) a brilliant red and the nuclei blue, as in a demyelinating lesion (Fig. 2d).

*Nile Blue Sulfate Method.* This method stains nonsudanophilic lipids varying shades of blue to violet, as in the neurons of cases of amaurotic family idiocy (Fig. 2e).

*Turnbull Blue Method.* A solution of yellow-ammonium sulphide and potassium ferri-cyanide-hydrochloric acid, counterstained with carmine, stains iron blue, and the background purplish red, as in a hemorrhagic infarct (Fig. 2f).

*Kossa Method.* Silver nitrate stains calcium black against a slightly yellowish background, as in cerebral calcification (Fig. 2g).

Other staining methods, routinely used but not illustrated, are:

*Luxol Fast Blue (LFB) Method.* Stains myelin (phospholipids) blue-green.

*McManus Periodic-acid Schiff (PAS) Method.* Stains glycolipids and mucopolysaccha-rides (mucin, colloid, amyloid, hyalin, fibrin, reticulin, most basement membranes and glycogen—latter eliminated with diastase digestion) rose to red.

*LFB-PAS Method.* A combined luxol fast blue method for myelin and PAS for myelin breakdown products.

*Kluver-Barrera Method.* A combined luxol fast blue method for myelin and cresyl violet method for neurons.

*Oil Red O Method.* Stains same lipids as the scarlet red method.

*Sudan Black B Method.* Stains phospholipids and glycolipids blue-black.

*Acetic Acid-Cresyl Violet (Nils-Peiffer) Method.* Stains sulfatides a brown metachromasia.

*Phosphotungstic Acid Hematoxylin (PTAH) Method.* A combined method staining astro-cytes and glial fibers blue and collagen reddish brown.

4

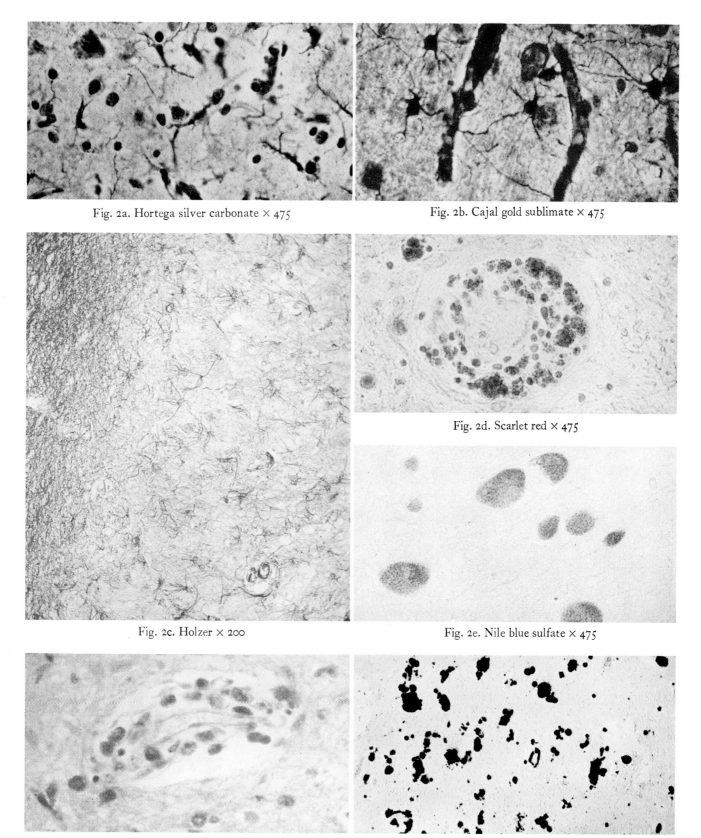

Fig. 2a. Hortega silver carbonate × 475

Fig. 2b. Cajal gold sublimate × 475

Fig. 2d. Scarlet red × 475

Fig. 2c. Holzer × 200

Fig. 2e. Nile blue sulfate × 475

Fig. 2f. Turnbull blue × 475

Fig. 2g. Kossa × 100

In Nissl preparations the normal neuron consists of Nissl bodies evenly distributed in the cell body and its dendrites, and of a clear spherical nucleus that contains a central nucleolus (Fig. 3a). In Bielschowsky preparations neurofibrils form the content of the cell (see Fig. 1c).

Under pathologic conditions various changes occur in the nerve cell that are mostly nonspecific, differing only as the underlying disease process is acute or chronic, reversible or irreversible. These changes may be classified as:

*Swelling.* Under acute injurious conditions the cell may undergo swelling of the cytoplasm and dendrites and pulverization of the Nissl bodies, but the nucleus remains intact (Fig. 3b) and the neurofibrils are generally preserved. This process is considered reversible.

*Liquefaction.* Under more intense pathologic conditions the neuron undergoes an irreversible change with ringlet and droplet formations in the cytoplasm, disintegration of the Nissl bodies and neurofibrils, pyknosis of the nucleus, dissolution of the cell membrane, and pericellular incrustations (Fig. 3c).

*Shrinkage.* Although generally found in chronic disease states, shrinkage may also accompany the previously described acute changes. It is characterized by shrinkage of the cell body, tortuosity of the dendrites, and hyperchromatosis whereby the Nissl substance and the neurofibrils fuse with the deeply staining nucleus (Fig. 3d).

*Coagulation.* Under conditions of ischemia and/or anoxia the nerve cell becomes pale, shrunken, and may be surrounded by incrustations, the cytoplasm "hyalinized," and the nucleus small and pyknotic (Fig. 3e; also Fig. 3c, large neuron at the left). This change is particularly well demonstrated in hematoxylin-eosin preparations, since the cytoplasm assumes a diffuse pinkish-red color (see Fig. 1b). As an end stage of ischemic as well as other conditions the neurons may undergo calcification (Fig. 3f).

*Fatty degeneration.* In some acute toxic disorders the cytoplasm of the neuron becomes granular as a result of deposits of sudanophilic fat droplets (Fig. 3g). In chronic "involution" states pathologic increase of the normal lipochrome pigment may result in a somewhat similar appearance, known as pigment atrophy.

*Retrograde or axonal degeneration.* After disease of, or injury to, axis cylinders, either peripheral or central, the cells of origin undergo swelling, central chromatolysis, and eccentricity of the nucleus (Fig. 3h). Such a change may or may not be reversible.

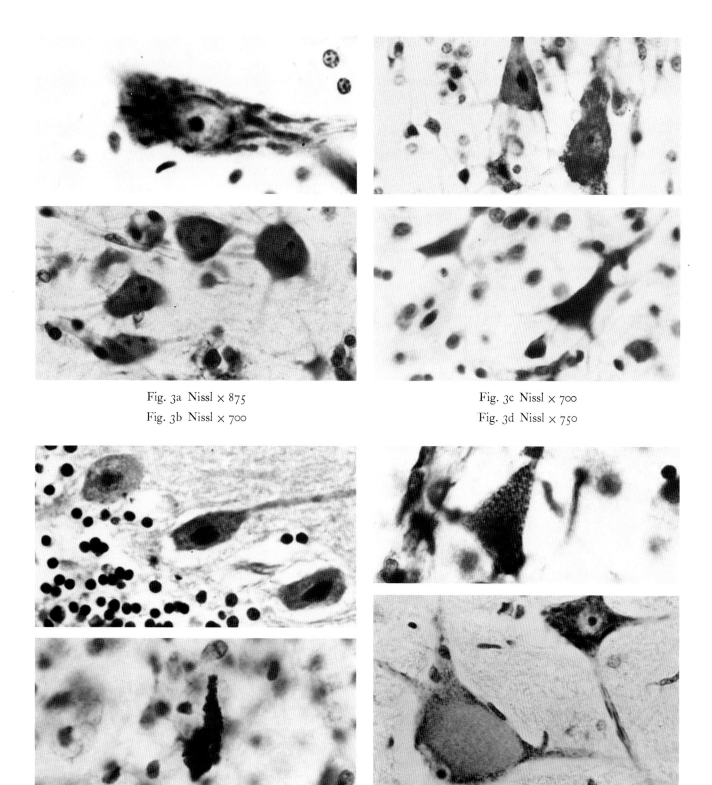

Fig. 3a Nissl × 875

Fig. 3b Nissl × 700

Fig. 3c Nissl × 700

Fig. 3d Nissl × 750

Fig. 3e HE × 725

Fig. 3f Nissl × 1050

Fig. 3g Nissl × 950

Fig. 3h Nissl × 475

The peripheral nerve fiber comprises a central axis cylinder (Fig. 4a) enclosed in a myelin sheath composed of a complex network (Fig. 4b). The myelin sheath is surrounded by the neurilemmal sheath of Schwann, which is enclosed by endoperineurial connective tissue.

Disease of the peripheral nerves causes a successive series of changes, known as Wallerian degeneration. After swelling, the result of edema, the axons and myelin sheaths fragment and disappear. The cells of the sheath of Schwann and endoperineurium react by proliferation, resulting in the formation of numerous round and fusiform cells between the degenerating myelin sheaths (Fig. 4c). The reacting elements act as phagocytes of the axon-myelin breakdown products. At the end of the first week after injury their lipid content stains black with osmic acid (Marchi stage), and at the end of the second week red with sudan for neutral fats and cholesterol esters (scarlet red stage).

The outstanding feature of lesions of the peripheral nerves is their regenerative capacity. In this process axons proliferate from the proximal end of the severed fiber to reunite with the distal end along reformed sheaths of Schwann, separated by variable amounts of connective tissue.

In the central nervous system the myelin sheath is thinner and of simpler structure, has no sheath of Schwann, and is surrounded by satellite oligodendroglia.

In central lesions, similar Wallerian degeneration takes place, but at a slower tempo, and there are only feeble or no regenerative phenomena.

Swelling, beading, fragmentation, and disappearance of myelin sheaths (Fig. 4d) are accompanied by similar changes in the axons (Fig. 4e). Phagocytic activity is carried out by microglia, which become transformed into fat-laden gitter cells or macrophages (Fig. 4f). The Marchi stage (third week) is followed by the scarlet-red stage (fourth week). Repair is a function of the astrocytes; the end stage is an astroglial scar (Fig. 4g).

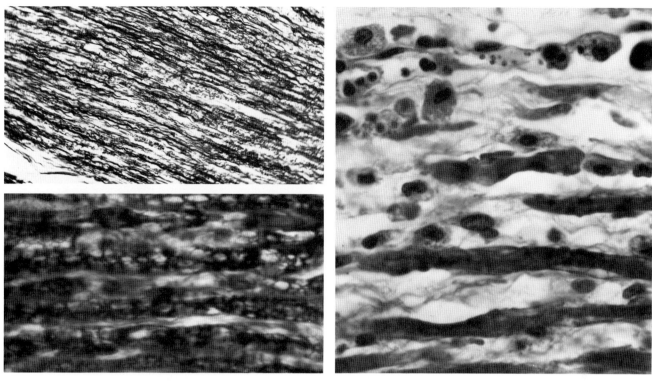

Fig. 4a Davenport × 100
Fig. 4b LFB-PAS × 560

Fig. 4c LFB-PAS × 560

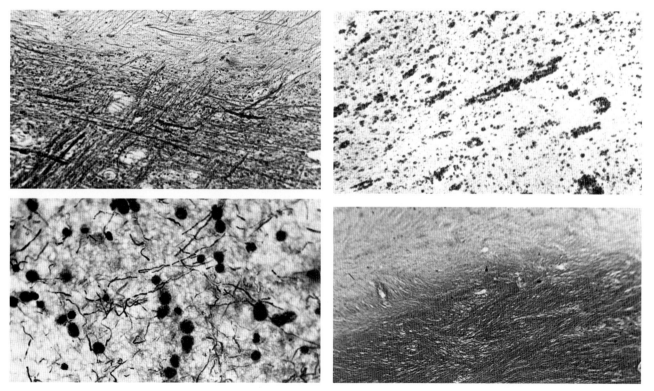

Fig. 4d Weil × 100
Fig. 4e von Braunmühl × 475

Fig. 4f Oil red O × 250
Fig. 4g Holzer × 50

The glia are the principal reacting elements to lesions of the central nervous system. Within limits of their own susceptibility to degenerate under noxious influences, they—unlike nerve cells and fibers—are capable of proliferation. There are three types of glia: microglia, astrocytes, and oligodendroglia.

## MICROGLIA

According to the generally accepted theories, the microglia are derived from mesoderm, have the ability to migrate and to act as phagocytes, and thus represent the reticulo-endothelial elements of the central nervous system.

In the resting phase the cells are sparse, small, with trabeculated unipolar or bipolar processes and oval or rodlike nuclei, which stain specifically with the silver carbonate method of Hortega (Fig. 5a).

Under acute toxidegenerative or inflammatory conditions, the cells multiply and undergo various changes. They elongate, may lose some of their trabeculae and are known as rod cells, as in general paresis (Fig. 5b), or they may be polyblastic and attach themselves to neurons that they digest in the process designated as neuronophagia, as in poliomyelitis (Fig. 5c). In various forms of encephalitis of viral origin the microglia tend to aggregate in the tissue as glial nodes or rosettes (Fig. 5d).

Under conditions of tissue necrosis, as in infarcts, the microglia undergo a change from rod forms, most of which appear to arise from the walls of proliferating blood vessels (Fig. 5e) to rounded forms known as gitter cells or macrophages (Fig. 5f).

Various phagocytosed products can be found in the cells, such as hemosiderin pigment in old hemorrhage, fat droplets (see Fig. 2d), iron (see Fig. 2f) or other catabolic elements. The microglia thus rid the tissue of waste and breakdown products, ultimately transporting these to the blood stream, where they are absorbed.

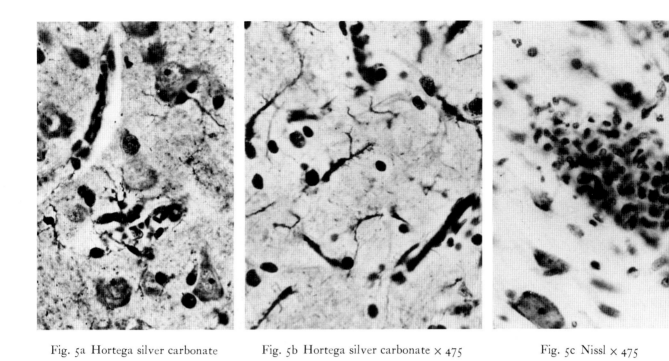

Fig. 5a Hortega silver carbonate     Fig. 5b Hortega silver carbonate × 475     Fig. 5c Nissl × 475
× 475

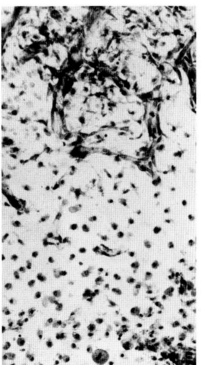

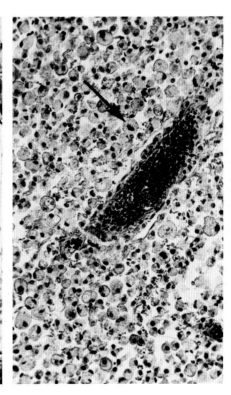

Fig. 5d Nissl × 200     Fig. 5e Nissl × 160     Fig. 5f HE × 200

Unlike microglia, the astrocytes are true ectodermal elements. Their function under pathologic conditions is that of repair.

In a resting state the astrocytes appear in Nissl preparations as vesicular naked nuclei, which are larger and paler than the small hyperchromatic oligodendroglial and microglial nuclei (see Fig. 1a). Cajal's gold sublimate stain reveals the spider-shaped cell bodies with multipolar branching processes, having single foot-plate attachments to blood vessels (see Fig. 2b). Astrocytes occur as protoplasmic and fibrillary forms, the latter because of their production of glial fibers.

Under pathologic conditions the astrocytes undergo hyperplasia and hypertrophy. The first step is the swelling of nucleus and cytoplasm, which assumes a finely granular appearance and becomes visible in Nissl preparations (Fig. 6a). In Cajal preparations the cells demonstrate an increase in their branching processes and foot plates (Fig. 6b). The second step is the multiplication of fibrillary astrocytes and the increased production of glial fibers (Fig. 6c). Finally the cells disappear as the lesions become purely fibrous scars.

Astrocytes are less resistant to toxic influences than microglia, and frequently show degenerative forms. There may be either acute ameboid glia with fragmentation of expansions or chronic gemistocytic astrocytes with hyalinization of cytoplasm and eccentricity of nucleus (Fig. 6d).

## OLIGODENDROGLIA

The oligodendroglia are small round cells that are diffusely distributed in the central nervous system as satellites of nerve cells and fibers. Their nuclei resemble lymphocytes and their cytoplasm and processes are scanty, giving the appearance of perinuclear halos. Their normal function and role in disease remain uncertain.

Under acute pathologic conditions the oligodendroglia multiply about, but do not digest, neurons—the process being known as satellitosis, which is to be distinguished from true neuronophagia by microglia.

Oligodendroglia may undergo degeneration, whereby the cytoplasm at first swells with the nucleus becoming pyknotic followed by hydropic and/or mucinous degeneration (Fig. 6e).

## PATHOLOGIC CHANGES IN CONNECTIVE TISSUE

The connective tissue of the nervous system, as found in blood vessels, meninges, and endoperineurium, reacts to pathologic conditions in much the same way as in tissues of the body. Thus, proliferation of histiocytes and macrophages takes place in inflammatory and degenerative states. In reparative processes, silver-impregnated reticulin fibers (see Fig. 1g) or fuchsinophilic collagen fibers (see Fig. 1h) are produced.

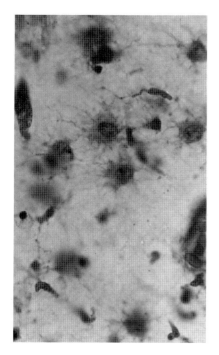

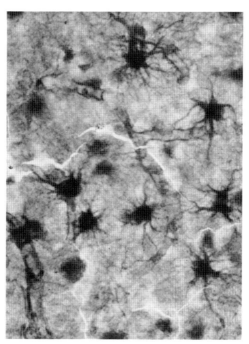

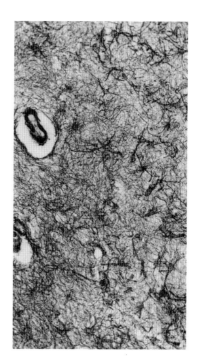

Fig. 6a Cajal gold sublimate × 475      Fig. 6b Nissl × 475      Fig. 6c Holzer × 200

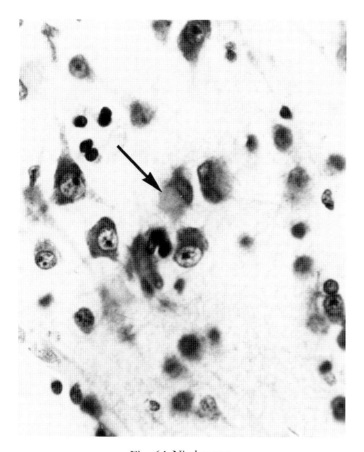

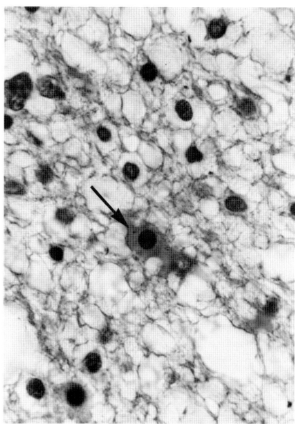

Fig. 6d Nissl × 775      Fig. 6e Hematoxylin-van Gieson × 900

# I B

# *Electron Microscopy*

## APPLICATION AND METHODS

The value of electron microscopy when applied to nervous tissue is twofold. First, it enables us to visualize very small, previously undetectable structures. In addition, the relationships among various structures, which previously could be seen only one at a time by using special staining technique in the optical microscope, can now be clearly demonstrated in a single micrograph. For example, various glial cells, neuronal processes, and myelin may all be seen in the same preparation in the accompanying micrograph (Fig. 7).

A severe limitation on the use of the electron microscope is, however, imposed by the rather rigorous conditions required for ideal fixation. These conditions are really practicable only with experimental animals. Thus, the richest source of neuropathological information, namely the formalin-fixed brains in the storerooms of hospitals and universities are the least ideal from the point of view of good preservation. In practical terms, however, the use of biopsy or even fresh autopsy material has been found to be adequate for most purposes. Furthermore, since the neuroanatomy of experimental animals has been, in many cases, well worked out using good fixation procedures, it can serve now as a yardstick by which to gauge the degree of artifact found in formalin-stored tissue and even sometimes in paraffin-embedded blocks.

Most of the human biopsy and postmortem material, illustrated by electron micrographs in this volume, was fixed in 5% glutaraldehyde in phosphate buffer at pH 7.4. The tissue was then postfixed in Dalton's chrome-osmium, dehydrated in alcohol, and embedded in Epon after two changes of propylene oxide. Thin sections were stained in uranyl and lead salts prior to examination in the electron microscope. Material from experimental animals was treated similarly except that perfusion fixation was used in most cases.

*Reference*

Hirano, A. Electron Microscopy in Neuropathology. Progress in Neuropathology, Vol. 1 (H. M. Zimmerman, ed.). Grune and Stratton (New York, 1971), p. 1.

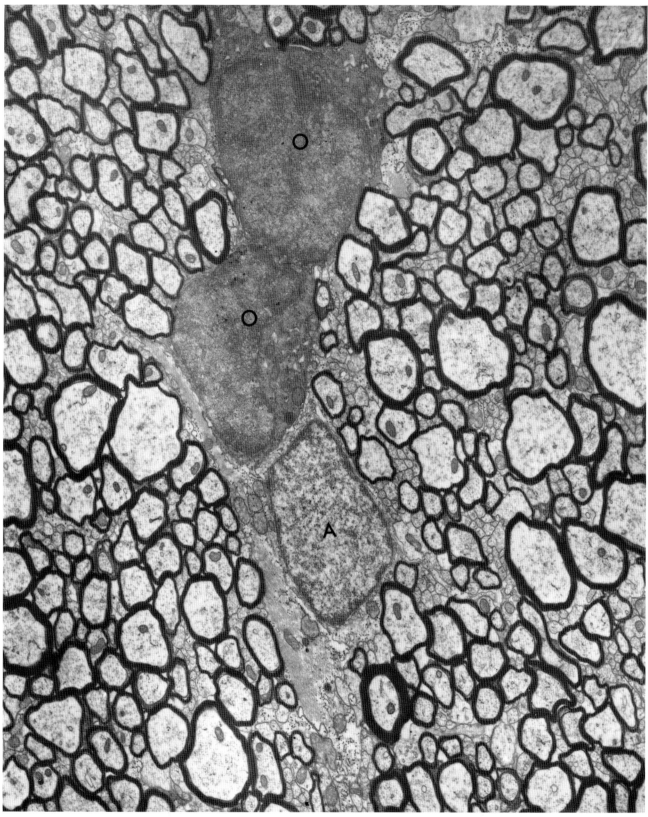

Fig. 7 A low magnification electron micrograph of the white matter of a rat. The masses of closely packed myelinated and unmyelinated processes are separated by two oligodendrocytes (O) and an astrocyte (A). × 13,000 (Hirano et al., J. Neuropath. Exper. Neurol. 24: 386, 1965).

Virtually throughout its entire length, the neuron is covered by other cells and cell processes. In most cases, these are satellite cells; glia in the central nervous system and Schwann cells in the peripheral nervous system. In addition, synaptic contacts occur at the neuronal surface which are, for the most part, either pre- or postsynaptic elements of other neurons.

The presence of numerous synapses makes each neuron unique. Unlike other tissues wherein cells are interchangeable, in nervous tissue each cell apparently fulfills a unique function by connecting a great many specific cells by virtue of its specific synaptic contacts.

The perikaryon contains a large nucleus with a prominent nucleolus (Fig. 8). In the nearby cytoplasm, many large accumulations of granular endoplasmic reticulum, known as Nissl bodies, are present. These may be found not only in the perinuclear area but also in the larger, proximal portions of the dendrites. They are not seen in axons. Scattered, free ribosomes, usually seen as polysomes, may be found in the dendrites and perikaryon. The perikaryon and the proximal portion of the apical dendrites are also rich in numerous Golgi bodies. Vesicles are occasionally seen in the neurons. Some are of the so-called "coated" variety. In certain neurons, such as in the hypothalamus, dense-core secretory granules 1200–1500 A in diameter are present. Mitochondria are common throughout the neuron. They may be found in all parts including the axon. In the processes, the mitochondria may assume a great length, sometimes up to several microns. In these instances, the cristae are usually oriented parallel to the longitudinal axis of the mitochondrion. Centrioles are rare but have been reported in certain types of neurons. Microtubules are commonly found throughout the cell. They have been called neurotubules, but are indistinguishable from the microtubules seen in other cells. They are about 240 A in diameter and their walls apparently consist of approximately 50 A globular components helically arranged around the lumen with about 13 subunits per turn. A central 50 A density may often be seen. A totally different tubular component is the so-called neurofilament, approximately 100 A in diameter, which also displays an electronlucent center. Lysosomes, multivesicular bodies, and lipid droplets are often present.

The cell surface is covered by a plasma membrane which is, for the most part, identical to other plasma membranes. However, in three regions the neurilemma displays apparently unique specializations. First, and most conspicuous, are the synapses. Second, an unusual specialization may be found at the axon hillock, initial segment, and the nodes of Ranvier of myelinated axons. Directly under the plasma membrane in these areas is an ill-defined electron-dense material which coats the inner surface of the plasma membrane. The axon hillock and initial segment are apparently the areas of impulse generation and the nodes are regions of saltatory propagation. The third area of neurilemmal specialization is in the region adjacent to the nodes of Ranvier. This specialization is described in the discussion of myelin.

*References*

Palay, S. L., and G. E. Palade. The Fine Structure of Neurons. J. Biophys. Biochem. Cytol. 1: 69, 1955.
Palay, S., C. Sotelo, A. Peters, and P. M. Orkand. The Axon Hillock and the Initial Segment. J. Cell Biol. 38: 193, 1968.
Peters, A., S. L. Palay, and H. de F. Webster. The Fine Structure of the Nervous System. The Cells and Their Processes. Hoeber (New York, 1970).

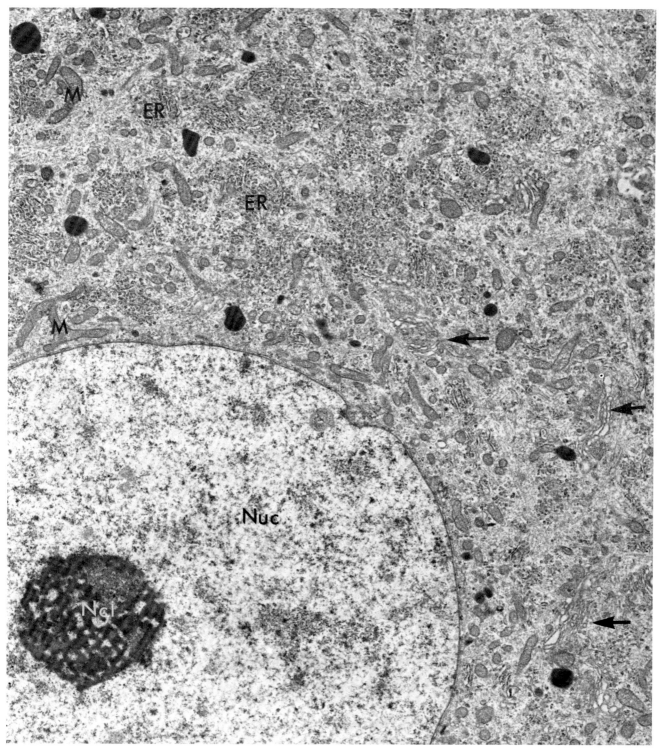

Fig. 8 An electron micrograph of the perikaryon of a neuron in the gasserian ganglion of a normal mink. The nucleus (Nuc), including the prominent nucleolus (Ncl) is at the lower left. The bulk of the cytoplasm contains scattered groups of rough endoplasmic reticulum (ER) and Golgi apparatus (arrows). Filaments, microtubules, mitochondria (M) and occasional dense bodies may be seen between them. × 10,000

A major contribution of electron microscopy to neuroanatomy has been the elucidation of the synapse. Apparently, it resolved the controversy between the neuronal and the reticular theory of nervous tissue structure. The integrity of each cell has been demonstrated by direct visualization of the synapses. Recently, however, the possibility has been raised that minute channels join two neurons in certain kinds of synapses.

Basically, the synaptic complex consists of two elements (Fig. 9). There is a presynaptic terminal derived from one neuron which transmits the impulse across the synapse to the second element, the postsynaptic terminal of a second neuron, which receives the impulse. Unlike axons, the synapse conducts in only one direction; i.e., from the pre- to the postsynaptic terminals.

Presynaptic elements are usually axonal terminals but sometimes they may be dendrites. Similarly, postsynaptic elements are usually dendrites but they may commonly be areas of the perikaryon and even, on some occasions, portions of an axon. Thus, axo-dendritic, axosomatic, and dendro-dendritic synapses all occur. Most synapses within the mammalian nervous system are so-called "chemical" synapses wherein the presynaptic elements release a neurotransmitter substance which traverses the space between synaptic elements and somehow stimulates the postsynaptic element.

Details of the structure of synaptic complexes may vary from site to site but a fundamentally similar morphology is retained. The presynaptic element contains synaptic vesicles (SV) in which the neurotransmitter substance is presumably stored. These vesicles, about 400 Å in diameter, are bounded by a unit membrane and usually display a clear interior. The plasma membrane covering the presynaptic element has a unit membrane construction but, in addition, shows characteristic specializations, some of which are observable only with special techniques. The pre- and postsynaptic membranes are separated by an intervening extracellular space which is generally somewhat wider than other nearby extracellular spaces and which contains an ill-defined electron-dense material. The postsynaptic membrane shows a conspicuous thickening in routine electron microscopic preparations (arrow). Fine filamentous material apparently arises from this thickened region, and extends back into the postsynaptic element for some distance. The entire synaptic complex is often invested by a matrix of astrocytic cytoplasm.

Variations on this basic morphology are numerous. Some of the synaptic vesicles may be larger and have a dense core. In some synapses, the vesicles may be elliptical in shape (when fixed in glutaraldehyde) rather than the more common spherical variety. The size of the cleft may be different in different synapses. Similarly, the length of the postsynaptic membranous thickening may vary depending on the synapse. Finally, more conspicuously, some cells have dendrites decorated with spines. In certain cerebral cortical neurons, these spines contain what seems to be a highly organized specialization of the endoplasmic reticulum known as the "spine apparatus."

*References*

Bloom, F. E. Correlating structure and function of synaptic ultrastructure. The Neurosciences, Second Study Program, (F. O. Schmitt, ed.). Rockefeller University Press, (New York, 1970), p. 729.
Gray, E. G. Tissue of the Central Nervous System. Electron Microscopic Anatomy, (S. M. Kurtz, ed.). Academic Press (New York, 1964), p. 369.
Pappas, G. D., and D. P. Purpura. Structure and Function of Synapses. Raven Press (New York, 1972).
Robertson, J. D. The Ultrastructure of Synapses. The Neurosciences, Second Study Program, *op.cit.*, p. 715.

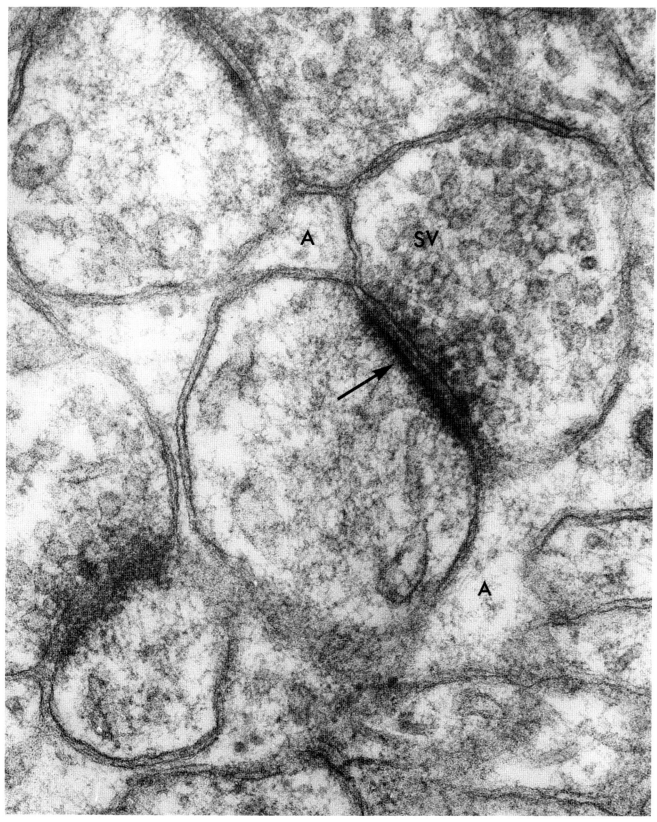

Fig. 9 An electron micrograph of several synapses in the molecular cell layer of the mouse cerebellum. Synaptic vesicles (SV) in a presynaptic element and a postsynaptic element with a prominent postmembranous thickening (arrow) are visible. The synapse is invested by astrocytic cytoplasm (A). × 128,000

Alterations in neurons can be conveniently divided into three categories. First, there may be an increase or decrease in the abundance of a normally occurring organelle. Second, some distortion of a normal cellular constituent may be present. Third, an entirely new structure may appear.

As an example of the first category of alterations, an enormous increase in 100 Å neurofilaments can occur in motor neuron disease under many other conditions. Similarly, large, abnormal accumulations of lysosomes and mitochondria occur in axons during such processes as Wallerian degeneration.

Chromatolysis is a good example of the second type of alteration. In this process, among other changes, the ribosomes within the Nissl substance dissociate from the membranes of the endoplasmic reticulum and apparently become free in the cytoplasm. Other changes, such as increased density and swelling of endoplasmic reticulum and mitochondria are often interpreted as anoxic changes reflecting early necrotic processes. However, it is often difficult to tell whether the changes are indeed antemortem or the results of improper fixation.

Probably the best known condition where totally new structures appear is Alzheimer's disease and the lipidoses (Fig. 10). The fibrils making up the Alzheimer neurofibrillary tangles are, at the fine structural level, unlike either microtubules or neurofilaments. Similarly, many of the specific lipid inclusions seen in certain lipidoses are distinctly different from the occasional dense body or lipofuscin granule sometimes encountered. In addition, the well-known neuropathological alterations, such as Lewy bodies, Lafora bodies, etc., and viral-like inclusions, must be included in this category.

Other alterations are not as easily categorized. For example, accumulations of a curious tubulo-vesicular material have been described in axons and especially in presynaptic terminals in a variety of conditions. Whether this material represents a distortion and accumulation of essentially normal organelles or a totally new structure has not yet been determined.

*References*

Andrews, J. M., and R. L. Vernand. Basic Concepts of Ultrastructural Neuroanatomy. Bull. Los Angeles Neurol. Soc. 34: 163, 1971.

Gonatas, N. K., I. Evangelista, and G. O. Walsh. Axonic and Synaptic Changes in a Case of Psychomotor Retardation: An Electron Microscopic Study. J. Neuropath. and Exper. Neurol. 26: 179, 1967.

Lampert, P. W. A Comparative Electron Microscopic Study of Reactive, Degenerating, Regenerating and Dystrophic Axons. J. Neuropath. and Exper. Neurol. 26: 345, 1967.

Odor, L., R. Janeway, L. A. Pearce, and J. R. Ravens. Progressive Myoclonus Epilepsy with Lafora Inclusion Bodies. Arch. Neurol. 16: 583, 1967.

Price, D., and K. R. Porter. The Response of Ventral Horn Neurons to Axonal Transection. J. Cell Biol. 53: 24, 1972.

Webster, H. de F. Transient, Focal Accumulation of Axonal Mitochondria during the Early Stages of Wallerian Degeneration. J. Cell Biol. 12: 361, 1962.

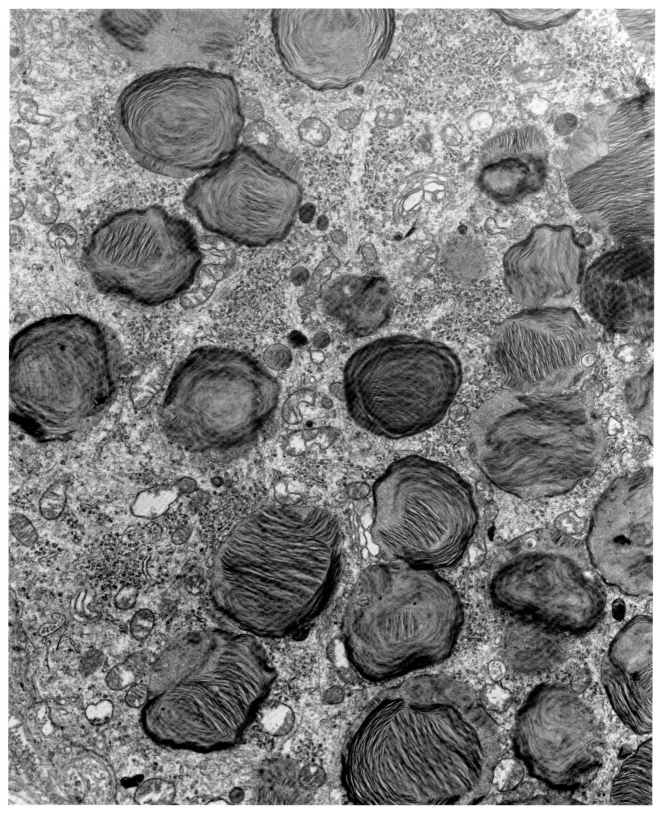

Fig. 10 A neuron in the gasserian ganglion of an Aleutian mink with wobbling showing some of the various osmiophilic inclusions. × 8,000

In the optical microscope, the myelin appears as a series of elongated beads strung closely together along the axon. The spaces between the myelin segments are called nodes of Ranvier. In cross sections of myelinated axons, the myelin sheaths appear as annuli surrounding the centrally placed axon. In similar cross sections (Fig. 11a) the electron microscope has revealed that the myelin sheath consists of a continuous spiral of myelin beginning at a small cytoplasmic tongue, the outer loop, and continuing to a similar cytoplasmic region, the inner loop, at the axonal surface. At high magnification, it can be seen that the inner leaflets of the plasma membrane of the outer loop fuse to form the so-called major dense line while the outer leaflets oppose one another and form the intraperiod line. In central myelin, the lamellae are about 120 Å thick.

In longitudinal section (Fig. 11b) the nodes of Ranvier may be seen to be regions at which the axonal surface is directly exposed to the extracellular space. The paranodal regions consist of an orderly arrangement of cytoplasmic areas, very similar to the inner and outer loops, each in contact with the axolemma and each continuous with a myelin lamella. These lateral loops are actually sections through a continuous cytoplasmic rim which winds around the axon in a helical course. Unique membrane specializations are at the interface between the lateral loops and the axon. These consist of the transverse bands which are actually differentiations of the external leaflet of the axonal plasma membrane. They appear as regularly arranged densities, about 150 Å long separated by about 150 Å, and extend within 20 Å of the external leaflet of the lateral loops. The transverse bands are seen only at the axonal-lateral loop interfaces and at all such interfaces. They are not present at the axonal surfaces between adjacent lateral loops. On three dimensional reconstruction, it has been concluded that they constitute a series of helices which wind around the axon parallel to each other and to the lateral loops (see Figs. 12 and 13; see pp. 24-25).

Peripheral myelin differs from central myelin in that the lamellae are about 10% thicker, and rather than just a single outer loop, the entire sheath is surrounded by an outer collar of Schwann cell cytoplasm. This outer cytoplasmic layer extends to the nodes of Ranvier where adjacent Schwann cells abut one another and interdigitate. Finally, the Schwann cell is, itself, covered by a basement membrane. In addition, the peripheral sheaths are characterized by regions in which the major dense lines of adjacent lamellae are split and contain cytoplasmic areas. These regularly arranged cytoplasmic areas constitute the so-called Schmidt-Lantermann clefts.

*References*

Bunge, R. P. Glial Cells and the Central Myelin Sheath. Physiol. Ref. 48: 197, 1968.

Bunge, R. P. Structure and Function of Neuroglia: Some Recent Observations in The Neurosciences, Second Study Program (F.O. Schmitt, ed.). Rockefeller University Press (New York, 1970), p.782.

Hirano, A. The Pathology of the Central Myelinated Axon. The Structure and Function of Nervous Tissue, Vol. 5 (G. H. Bourne, ed.), Academic Press (New York, 1972), p. 73.

Peters, A. The Morphology of Axons of the Central Nervous System. The Structure and Function of Nervous Tissue, Vol. 1, *op. cit.*, p. 141.

Peters, A., and J. E. Vaughn. Morphology and Development of the Myelin Sheath. Myelination. (A. N. Davison and A. Peters, eds.). Charles C Thomas (Springfield, Ill., 1970), p. 3.

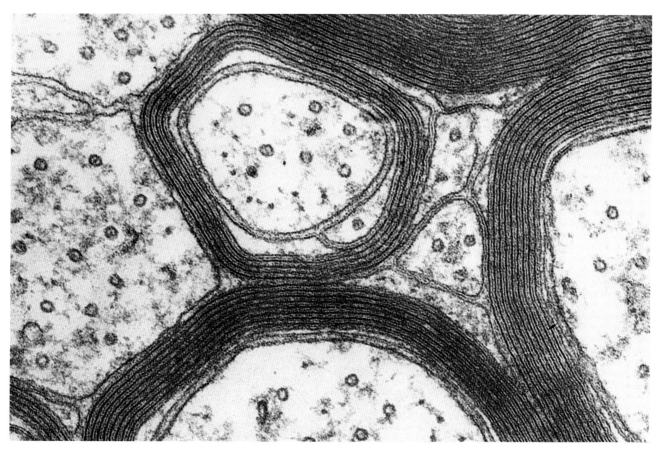

Fig. 11a High magnification electron micrograph of several myelinated axons in the white matter of a rat. × 150,000

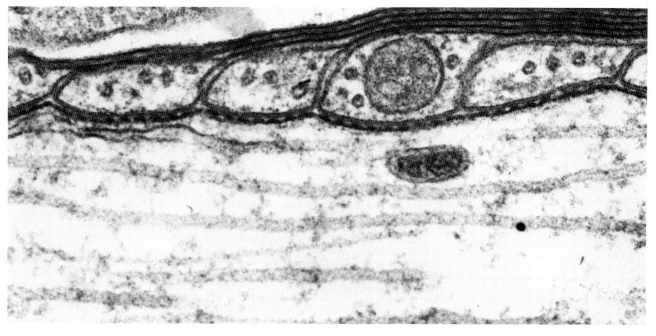

Fig. 11b High magnification electron micrograph of a longitudinal section through the paranodal region of a myelinated fiber in the white matter of a rat. × 150,000 (Hirano, J. Cell Biol. 38: 637, 1968)

Fig. 12: a. Diagram of a myelinated axon, modified after Bunge, et al. (J. Cell Biol. 10: 67, 1961). Part of the myelin is cut away to show the relationship between the lateral loops and the lamellae, between the inner loops and the axon, and between the outer loop and the connection to the myelin-forming cell. Note the periodic densities, representing sections through the transverse bands between the lateral loops and the axon. b. Diagram of the intact myelin sheath around the axon. c. Diagram of the results of partially unrolling the intact sheath from around the axon. d. Diagram of a fully unrolled myelin sheath. The resulting shovel-shaped myelin sheath is bordered on four sides by a continuous thickened rim of cytoplasm. The outer rim, when seen in section, is represented by the outer loop, and is longer than the inner rim, which is represented by the inner loop in cross-section. The lateral rims are probably of equal length and are represented by the lateral loops in longitudinal sections through the nodes of Ranvier. e. A diagram similar to Fig. 13 but showing the surface of the sheath that contacts the axon. The transverse bands are indicated by the parallel, curved lines around the axon. (Hirano and Dembitzer, J. Cell Biol. 34: 555, 1967)

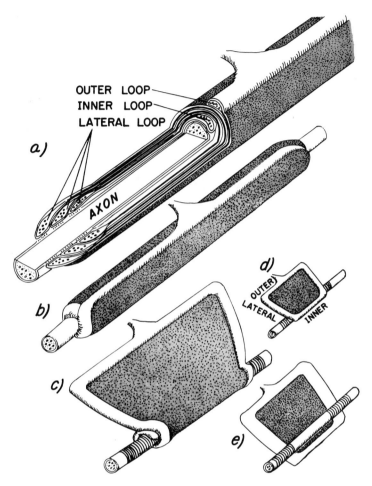

OUTER LOOP
INNER LOOP
LATERAL LOOP

a)

AXON

b)

c)

d)

OUTER)
LATERAL
INNER

e)

Fig. 12.

Fig. 13: *Upper portion*: A diagram of the normal anatomy of the mature central myelin sheath and its relationship to the axon (A). The periaxonal space is apparently sealed by the intraperiod line and, at the nodes, by the transverse bands. In this diagram, the spaces between the bands are numbered 1-4. Similarly numbered spaces are continuous and usually extend in a helical path around the axon from the extracellular space at the node to the periaxonal space.

*Middle portion*: Two possible routes of infiltration of water and solutes between the extracellular and the periaxonal spaces are schematically represented. I-Direct penetration at the level of the interperiod line. II-Various pathways all originating in the space between adjacent transverse bands.

*Lower right portion*: This diagram is designed to illustrate the relationship of the transverse bands to the hypothetically unrolled myelin sheath. The presence of the densities only at the lateral loop-axonal interfaces and at all such interfaces can be explained only by the presence of separate bands which parallel each other as well as the lateral rim. Their loci, then, may be represented as separate, parallel lines along the inner aspect of the lateral rim. The spaces adjacent to them are, as above, numbered 1-4. An extra transverse band, resulting in the extra space 3′, is included in the diagram to account for the fact that in those cases in which the lateral loop is unusually wide, one or more additional transverse bands may be observed. (Hirano and Dembitzer, J. Ultrastruct. Res. 28: 141, 1969.)

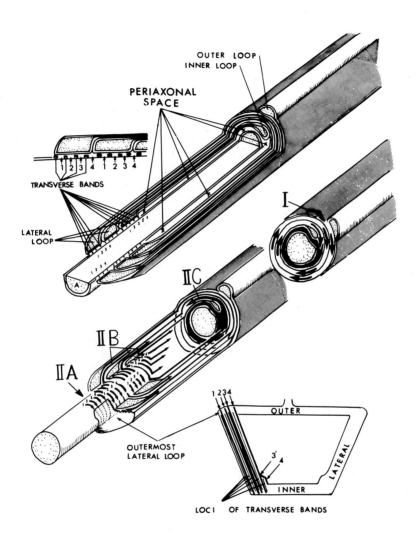

OUTER LOOP
INNER LOOP

PERIAXONAL
SPACE

TRANSVERSE BANDS

LATERAL
LOOP

I

IIC

IIB

IIA

OUTERMOST
LATERAL LOOP

1 2 3 4

OUTER

LATERAL

3'

INNER

LOCI OF TRANSVERSE BANDS

Fig. 13.

# REMYELINATION

For many years the question of remyelination in the central nervous system was in doubt. Electron microscopic evidence strongly suggests that such a process does indeed occur. The evidence consists, for the most part, of the appearance of unusual configurations of the myelin sheath seen in animals or humans some time after injury to the white matter. These configurations may be classified in several categories. First, cytoplasmic organelles such as mitochondria or dense bodies may appear in the cytoplasmic regions of the sheath. Second, isolated cytoplasmic regions may be found in regions of the lamellae where the major dense line is not fused. Third, apparently separate cell processes may appear between the innermost lamella and the axon. Finally, one or more extra myelin sheaths, each with its own inner and outer loops, may be present around the axon (Figs. 14 and 15). Most of these configurations have been explained in terms of rather simple variations on the same fundamental structure of the sheath and probably represent incomplete myelin formation by an oligodendroglial process (Fig. 15).

*References*

Hirano, A., and H. M. Dembitzer. A Structural Analysis of the Myelin Sheath in the Central Nervous System. J. Cell Biol. 34: 555, 1967.

Hirano, A., S. Levine, and H. M. Zimmerman. Remyelination in the Central Nervous System after Cyanide Intoxication. J. Neuropath. and Expt. Neurol. 27: 234, 1968.

Lampert, P. W. Demyelination and Remyelination in Experimental Allergic Encephalomyelitis. Further Electron Microscopic Observations. J. Neuropath. and Expt. Neurol. 24: 371, 1965.

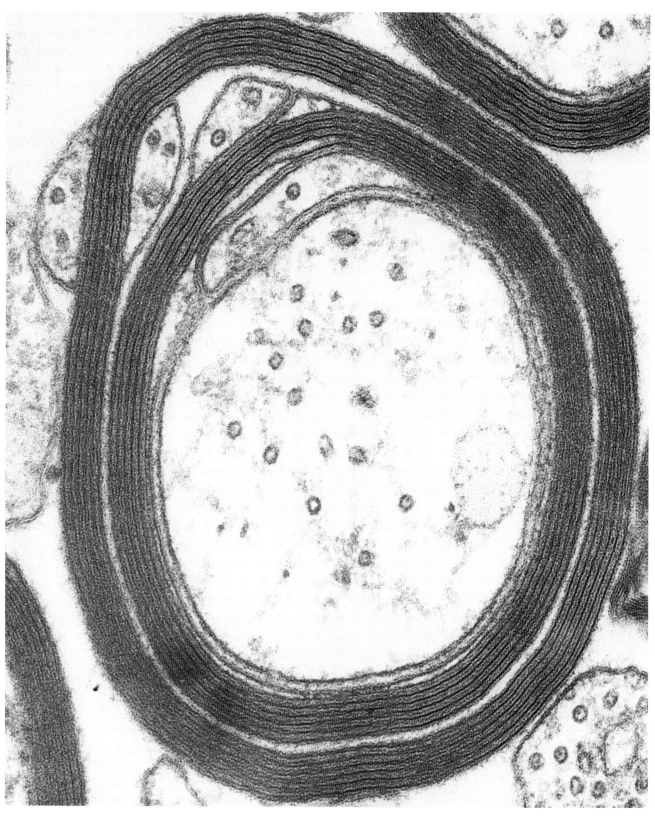

Fig. 14.  A myelinated axon surrounded by two myelin sheaths in the edematous white matter of a rat treated with cyanide gas. Since the direction of the spiral is opposite in the two sheaths depicted in this particular micrograph, their formation cannot be explained by Figure 15. × 147,000 (Hirano, in Progress in Neuropathology, Vol. I, (H. M. Zimmerman, ed.) Grune and Stratton (New York, 1971), p. 1.)

Fig. 15: A. Usual form of the myelin sheath. When rolled around an axon and sectioned in the indicated plane, we see the usual configuration of A′. B. The continuous surrounding cytoplasmic rim contains formed organelles. When rolled around an axon and sectioned in the indicated plane, we see the configuration of B′. C. An extension of the lateral cytoplasmic rim intrudes into the myelin sheath. When rolled around the axon and sectioned in the indicated plane, we see a configuration including an isolated cytoplasmic island as in C′. D. The irregularly widened inner rim is indented by a cleft of extracellular space. When rolled around an axon and sectioned in the indicated plane, we see a configuration including an apparently unconnected cell process as D′. E. The lateral rim is folded into the myelin sheath. When rolled around an axon and sectioned in the indicated plane, we see a configuration including two complete concentric myelin sheaths both spiraling in the same direction as in E′. F. A myelin sheath derived from the unrolling of a myelin sheath in the peripheral nervous system. The outer cytoplasmic rim is much wider than in the central nervous system and consists of the entire cell body of the Schwann cell, including the nucleus (N). Two thickened, vertical cytoplasmic ridges, roughly parallel to the lateral rims, are present (S-L), which give rise to the incisures of Schmidt-Lantermann when seen in longitudinal section. The outer rim is coated by a basement membrance (BM). The inner and lateral rims, of course, are devoid of a basement membrane since, in the rolled sheath, no basement membrane intervenes between the inner loop and the axon (A) or between adjacent lateral loops. When rolled around an axon and sectioned in the indicated plane, we see a typical peripheral myelin sheath as in F′. (Hirano and Dembitzer, J. Cell Biol. 34: 555, 1967)

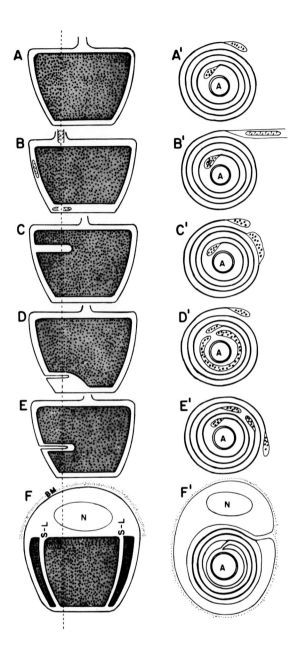

Fig. 15.

Many metallo-organic compounds are severely toxic and organic tin compounds have been used in certain proprietary preparations. The effects of triethyltin on the central nervous system have been studied in detail.

In the optical microscope, the central nervous system of animals treated with triethyltin shows extensive sponginess, especially in the white matter. Electron microscopic study revealed that the sponginess is the result of large spaces (S) that develop within the myelin sheaths (Fig. 16a). The spaces appear clear and empty and arise from an apparent split of the intraperiod line (Fig. 16b). Thus, the spaces correspond to the theoretical extracellular space but have not been shown to be in direct continuity with the parenchymal extracellular spaces. Despite the enormous size of some of the spaces, individual lamellae are of normal width and are apparently neither stretched nor compressed. To explain the phenomenon, it has been suggested that during the formation of the space, individual lamellae slip past one another in the manner in which the mainspring of a clock unwinds. Similar effects on central myelin have been produced by isonicotinic acid hydrazide and other agents.

## References

Aleu, F. P., R. Katzman, and R. D. Terry. Fine Structure and Electrolyte Analysis of Cerebral Edema Induced by Alkyl Tin Intoxication. J. Neuropath and Expt. Neurol., 22: 403, 1963.
Hirano, A., H. M. Zimmerman, and S. Levine. Intramyelinic and Extracellular Spaces in Triethyltin Intoxication. J. Neuropath. and Expt. Neurol. 27: 571, 1968.
Hirano, A., H. M. Dembitzer, N. H. Becker, and H. M. Zimmerman. The Distribution of Peroxidase in the Triethyltin-Intoxicated Rat Brain. J. Neuropath. and Expt. Neurol. 28: 507, 1969.

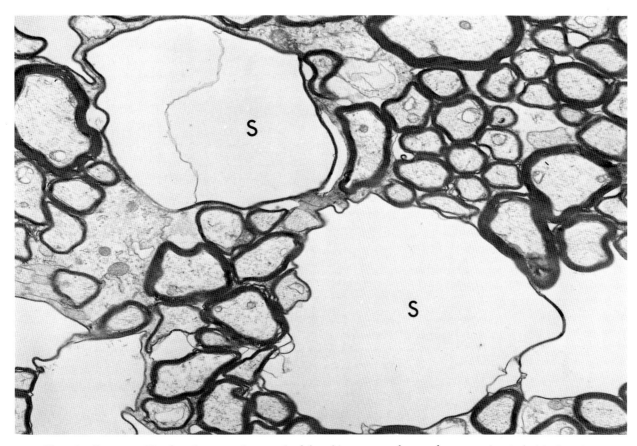

Fig. 16a. Low magnification electron micrograph of the white matter of a rat after systemic triethyltin intoxication. × 9,000 (Hirano, in The Structure and Function of Nervous Tissue, Vol. II, (G. H. Bourne, ed.). Academic Press (New York, 1969), p. 69.)

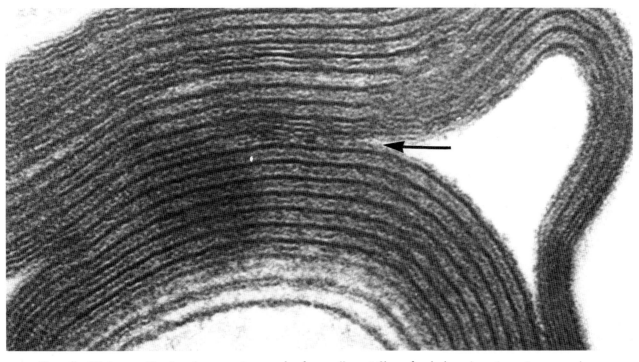

Fig. 16b. High magnification electron micrograph of a myelinated fiber of a tin-intoxicated rat demonstrating interlamellar splitting at the interperiod line (arrow). × 145,000 (Hirano, in The Structure and Function of Nervous Tissue, Vol. II, (G. H. Bourne, ed.). Academic Press (New York, 1969), p. 59.)

As in any other organ, phagocytosis is a prominent feature of nervous tissue after a variety of injuries. Occasionally, any cell in the central nervous system can exhibit some phagocytic activity but its capability in this respect is generally severely limited. The origin of the true phagocytes, which sometimes appear in large numbers, is a matter of dispute.

Traditionally, the microglia have been considered the source of the phagocytes. Electron microscopists, however, have found it difficult to differentiate between microglia and other glial cells; their reality as a separate cell type has been questioned by some authorities. Another possible origin for phagocytes within the central nervous system are the pericytes which are frequently found around blood vessels. On the basis of autoradiographic studies, it has been proposed that phagocytes can reach the interior of the central nervous system from the blood stream. Hematogenous cells are, therefore, usually considered to comprise the bulk of the brain macrophages, at least in stab wound experiments or experimental allergic encephalomyelitis.

A large variety of inclusions have been found within these macrophages (Fig. 17). The precise nature of the inclusion depends, of course, on the nature of the lesion. In a number of infections, the electron microscope has demonstrated the organism within the vacuoles of the phagocyte. In addition, the electron microscope has revealed elements of cellular debris within the lysosomal system of macrophages following cell death or injury. For example, myelin, one of the main constituents of nervous tissue is commonly found within phagocytes after some demyelinating process. These inclusions undergo a progressive disintegration often resulting in striking lamellar patterns, apparently consisting of indigestible macromolecules.

*References*

Kitamura, T., H. Hattori, and S. Fujita. Autoradiographic Studies on Histogenesis of Brain Macrophages in the Mouse. J. Neuropath. and Expt. Neurol. 31: 502, 1972.

Lampert, P. W. Fine Structural Changes of Myelin Sheaths in the Central Nervous System. The Structure and Function of Nervous Tissue, Vol. I (G. H. Bourne, ed.). Academic Press (New York, 1968), p. 187.

Vaughn, J. E., and R. P. Skoff. Neuroglia in Experimentally Altered Central Nervous System. The Structure and Function of Nervous Tissue (G. H. Bourne, ed.). Academic Press, Vol. V (New York, 1972), p. 39.

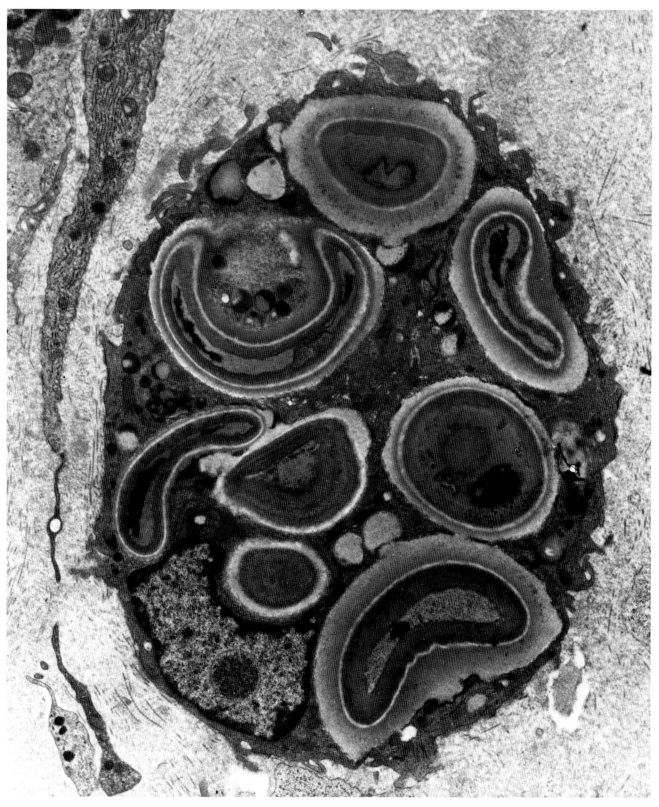

Fig. 17. An electron micrograph of a macrophage containing several engulfed cryptococci in the brain of a rat. × 14,000 (Levine et al., in Infections of the Nervous System, Res. Publ. A.R.N.M.D. Vol. XLIV. (H. M. Zimmerman, ed.). Williams and Wilkins Co. (Baltimore, 1968), p. 393.)

The electron microscope has confirmed the findings of the optical microscopists with regard to astrocytes. Astrocytes surround most of the central nervous system. They line both pial and perivascular surfaces where they are covered by a basement membrane. At these regions, also, half-desmosomes are found at the surface while adjacent astrocytic processes are joined by a junctional apparatus. Within the central nervous system, they surround neuronal perikarya, groups of axons and other neuronal processes.

Within the astrocyte, the usual organelles are found (Fig. 18). Mitochondria, rough endoplasmic reticulum, Golgi apparatus and small vesicles are present but relatively inconspicuous and scattered. The most characteristic features of the cytoplasm are the apparently hollow glial filaments, 60–90 Å in diameter, bundles of which compose the glial fibrils described by the light microscopists. Glial filaments differ from neuronal filaments in that they are somewhat smaller in diameter and tend to be distributed in bundles in contrast to the more diffusely arranged neuronal filaments. Scattered glycogen granules, 100–400 Å in diameter may also be found in the cytoplasm as may be deposits of corpora amylacea and occasional lipid droplets. Microtubules are not common in mature astrocytes but are present in small numbers.

*References*

Peters, A., S. L. Palay, and H. deF. Webster. The Fine Structure of the Nervous System. The Cells and Their Processes. Harper and Row (New York, 1970).

Wuerker, R. B. Neurofilaments and Glial Filaments. Tissue and Cell. 2: 1, 1970.

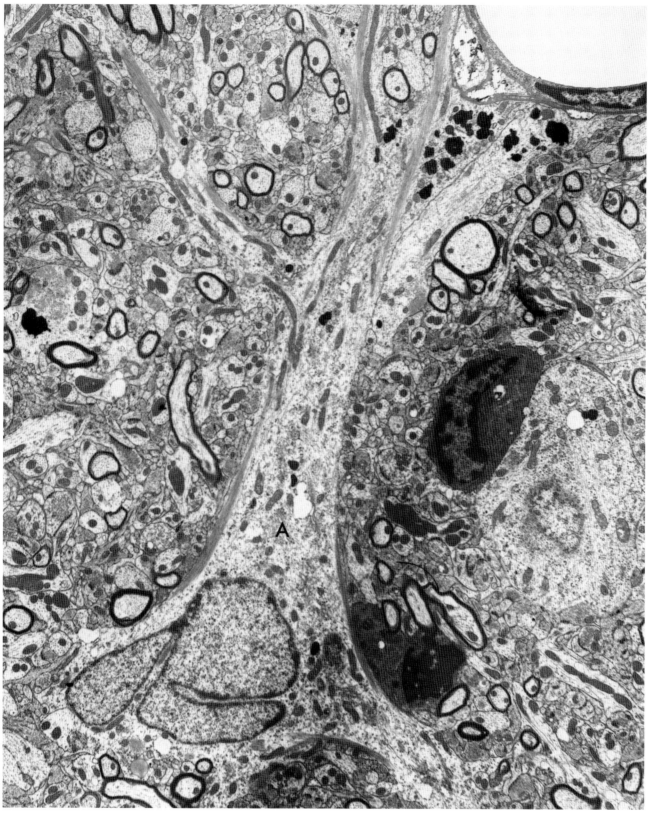

Fig. 18. An electron micrograph of an astrocyte (A) with several processes including one extending to the peri-vascular space in the brain of a rat. × 9,000

Under pathological conditions, reactive astrocytes undergo characteristic changes. Often they will show great increases in volume (Fig. 19a) while the cytoplasm fills with enormous numbers of filaments (Fig. 19b). Under other conditions, the astrocytic cytoplasm swells and becomes watery. A large accumulation of glycogen granules is also a characteristic change displayed by reactive astrocytes. Corpora amylacea deposits also increase in number under certain longstanding pathological conditions as well as in aged brain. Other specific inclusions, such as virus-like particles, have been reported in certain conditions in both the cytoplasm and the nucleus.

*References*

Hirano, A., H. M. Zimmerman, and S. Levine. Fine Structure of Cerebral Fluid Accumulation. VII. Reaction of Astrocytes to Cryptococcal Polysaccharide Implantation. J. Neuropath. and Expt. Neurol. 24: 386, 1965.
Hirano, A., and H. M. Zimmerman. Some Effects of Vinblastine Implantation in the Cerebral White Matter. Lab. Invest. 23: 358, 1970.
Ramsey, H. J. Ultrastructure of Corpora Amylacea. J. Neuropath. and Expt. Neurol. 24: 25, 1965.

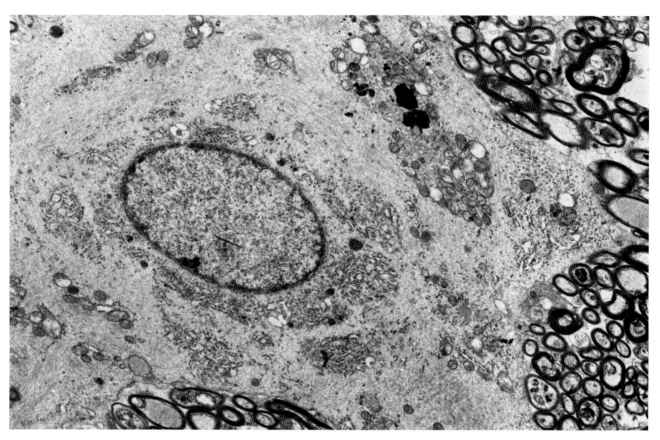

Fig. 19a. An electron micrograph of a reactive astrocyte filled with filaments in the brain of a rat after vincristine implantation. × 7,000 (Hirano and Zimmerman, Lab. Invest. 23: 358, 1970)

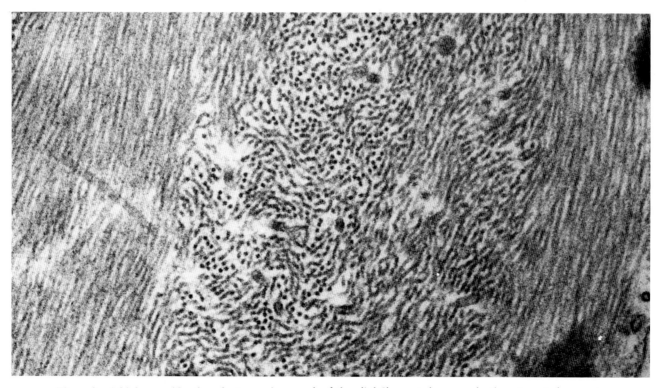

Fig. 19b. A high magnification electron micrograph of the glial filaments in a neoplastic astrocyte in an astrocytoma. × 105,000 (Hirano, in Progress in Neuropathology, Vol. I. (H. M. Zimermman, ed.). Grune and Stratton (New York, 1971), p. 1.)

# OLIGODENDROGLIA

The cellular origin of central myelin sheaths was in doubt until the advent of the electron microscope. Since that time, it has become clear that the myelin-forming cells are the oligodendroglia. The demonstration of direct communication between the outer loop of the mature myelin sheath and oligodendroglial cytoplasm has, however, proved very difficult. On this basis, some investigators have speculated that, once formed, the myelin sheaths sever connections with the myelin-forming cell. Other investigators have theorized that this difficulty is attributable to the fact that the connecting process traces a long and tortuous path which is virtually impossible to visualize in a single section. In developing animals, however, the connection is apparently shorter, and direct continuity between the sheath and the oligodendroglial cell has been shown (Bunge et al.).

In the accompanying micrograph (Fig. 20) several myelin sheaths are seen in close proximity to an oligodendroglial cell. The outer cytoplasmic region of one of these sheaths (arrow) is clearly in direct continuity with the oligodendroglial cytoplasm. This material was derived from a rat which was recovering from an experimentally induced lesion in the white matter and so probably respresents an example of remyelination. The occurrence of this process was in doubt from some time but such evidence as that presented here strongly suggests that it does, in fact, occur although it may be slow and incomplete. While it seems clear that oligodendroglial cells do form central myelin, the precise mechanism of that process remains to be clarified.

*References*

Bunge, M. B., R. P. Bunge, and G. D. Pappas. Electron Microscopic Demonstration of Connections between Glia and Myelin Sheaths in the Developing Mammalian Central Nervous System. J. Cell Biol. 12: 448, 1962.
Hirano, A. A Confirmation of the Oligodendroglial Origin of Myelin in the Adult Rat. J. Cell Biol. 38: 637, 1968.
Peters, A. Observations on the Connexion between Myelin Sheaths and Glial Cells in the Optic Nerves of Young Rats. J. Anat. 98: 125, 1964.

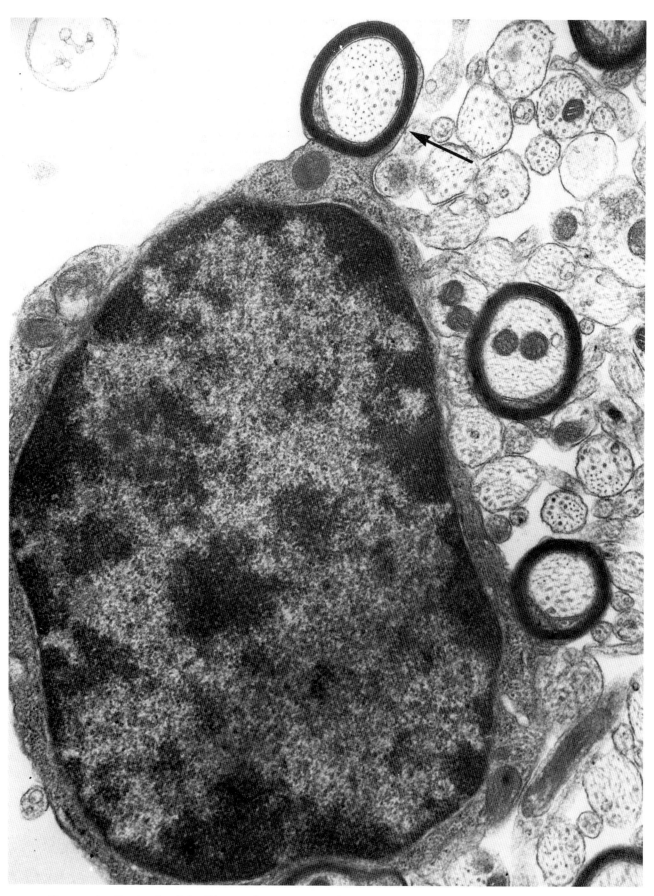

Fig. 20. An oligodendroglial cell in an enlarged extracellular space in the white matter of an adult rat. A myelin sheath surrounding an axon is in direct continuity with the oligodendroglial cytoplasm (arrow). × 30,000 (Hirano, J. Cell Biol. 38: 637, 1968)

CONNECTIVE TISSUE

Connective tissue is not a major component of the brain. Actually, its extreme paucity is a characteristic of the central nervous system. It is found, however, in the leptomeninges and within the perivascular spaces of large cerebral vessels. In addition, it is an important feature of peripheral nervous tissue and muscle.

The extracellular components are the most characteristic features of connective tissue. The components include the fibrous elements of collagen, reticulin, and elastin. Among the three, collagen is by far the most common fiber found in the nervous system. Traditionally, collagen and reticulin have been differentiated from one another on the basis of staining reactions as well as the net-like appearance of the latter. In the electron microscope, however, reticulin has been shown to be of the same basic structure as collagen and is thought to be composed of the same protein as that of collagen fibers.

Collagen is composed of individual, unbranched fibers of indeterminate length and of a constant width within a single tissue. This width is usually about 400 Å but varies widely depending on the tissue. In all tissues, however, the collagen fibers display a specific periodicity of alternating dense and less dense bands of 640 Å. This banding has been interpreted as reflecting a staggered arrangement of the tropocollagen molecules which compose the collagen fibers. Higher resolution studies have shown other periodic banding within the 640 Å spacing.

Since connective tissue within the brain is limited to the perivascular spaces and the leptomeninges, it is understandable that significant connective tissue proliferation does not usually accompany brain lesion such as gliomas. Even vascular lesions, such as infarcts or long-standing hematomas, result in relatively little connective tissue reaction.

On the other hand, certain inflammatory lesions associated with massive necrosis result in extensive connective tissue proliferation, as in an abscess wall (Fig. 21). Similarly, nongliogeneous neoplasms, especially sarcomas, produce large accumulations of collagenous tissue. In such conditions, most of the collagen fibers are indistinguishable from those of normal tissue. Occasionally, however, abnormal forms appear, such as the Luse body seen in neurilemmoma, among other conditions, and a particularly wide form of collagen seen in meningiomas and other conditions.

*References*

Ham, A. W. Histology, 6th edition. J. B. Lippincott (Philadelphia, 1969).
Luse, S. A. Electron Microscopic Studies of Brain Tumors. Neurology. 10: 881, 1960.

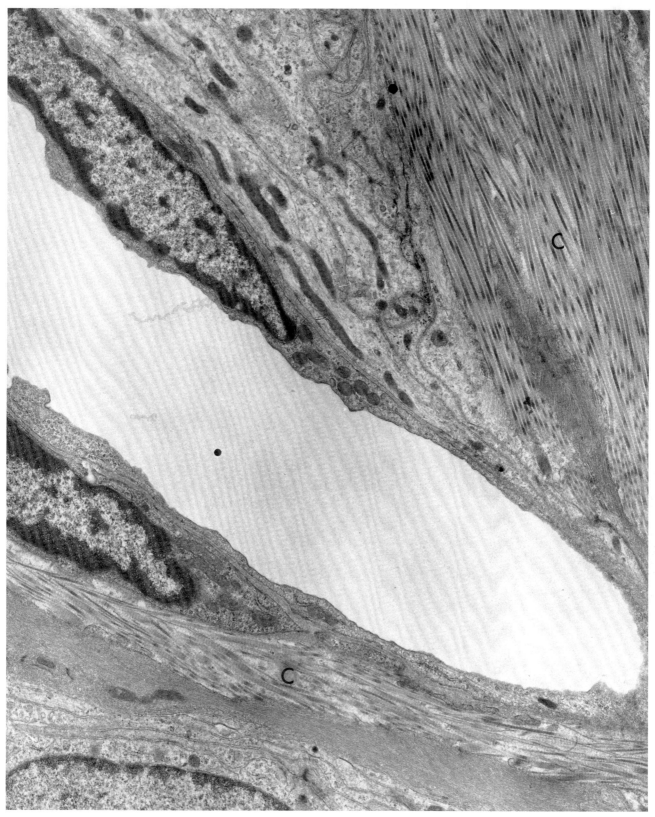

Fig. 21. An electron micrograph of a blood vessel in the wall of an abscess in the brain of a rat subjected to experimental injury. Prominent collagen fibers (C) surround the vessel. × 30,000 (Hirano, in Progress in Neuropathology (H. M. Zimmerman, ed.) Grune and Stratton (New York, 1971), p. 1.)

In most organs of the body, abnormal infiltration of hematogenous edema fluid results in the distension of the extracellular spaces and the separation of some of the parenchymal cells. The site of accumulation of edema fluid depends on the nature of the intercellular bonds; so that large amounts of fluid are found in loose connective tissue spaces while other areas, where the cells are firmly knit together, resist the infiltration of the fluid and only moderate expansions of the extracellular spaces occur.

Similar processes occur in the brain but with an important qualification. Unlike other organs, the brain is enclosed in a rigid structure so that infiltration of fluid results in increased intracranial pressure which may often reach dangerous limits. The edema fluid penetrates the vascular wall and permeates the extracellular spaces (E) (Compare Figs. 22a and b). The process is much more obvious in the white matter owing to the lack of adhesion between bundles of white matter and less prominent in the gray matter where numerous intercellular adhesive devices, including synapses, as well as the intertwining processes, resist the infiltration of edema fluid.

Several studies have been devoted to the fine structural alterations of the small vessels in in the brain under edematous conditions. Cerebral capillaries are surrounded by a basement membrane and a narrow collagen-free perivascular space, which is itself invested by a continuous layer of astrocytic processes. It is, however, the cerebral endothelium which is considered to be the seat of the blood-brain barrier under normal conditions. It differs from most other nonfenestrated endothelium in that the junctions between endothelial cells are of the so-called tight junction variety and do not normally permit the passage of such tracers as horseradish peroxidase, ferritin, or lanthanum. In addition, and in distinct contrast to other endothelial cells such as those within striated muscle, pinocytotic vesicles are rare in cerebral endothelium.

However, under edematous conditions, induced by a variety of experimental methods, these morphological features are no longer present. The intercellular junctions apparently open, permitting the passage of tracer molecules. Increased pinocytotic activity may also play a role. In addition, the luminal surface of the endothelium becomes infolded and more irregular so that "tunnel" formation may be an important feature of the endothelium in edema. Finally, sometimes entire endothelial cells are diffusely infiltrated by the tracer and conceivably, therefore, direct diffusion may play a role.

*References*

Brightman, M. W., I. Klatzo, Y. Olsson, and T. S. Reese. The Blood-Brain Barrier to Proteins under Normal and Pathological Conditions. J. Neurol. Sci. 10: 215, 1970.
Hirano, A., The Fine Structure of Brain in Edema. The Structure and Function of Nervous Tissue, Vol. 2 (G. H. Bourne, ed.). Academic Press (New York, 1969), p. 69.
Hirano, A., N. H. Becker, and H. M. Zimmerman. Pathological Alterations in the Cerebral Endothelial Cell Barrier to Peroxidase. Arch. Neurol. 20: 300, 1969.
Hirano, A., N. H. Becker, and H. M. Zimmerman. The Use of Peroxidase As a Tracer in Studies of Alterations in the Blood-Brain Barrier. J. Neurol. Sci. 10: 205, 1970.
Hirano, A., H. M. Dembitzer, N. H. Becker, S. Levine, and H. M. Zimmerman. Fine Structural Alterations of the Blood-Brain Barrier in Experimental Allergic Encephalomyelitis. J. Neuropath. and Expt. Neurol. 29: 432, 1970.

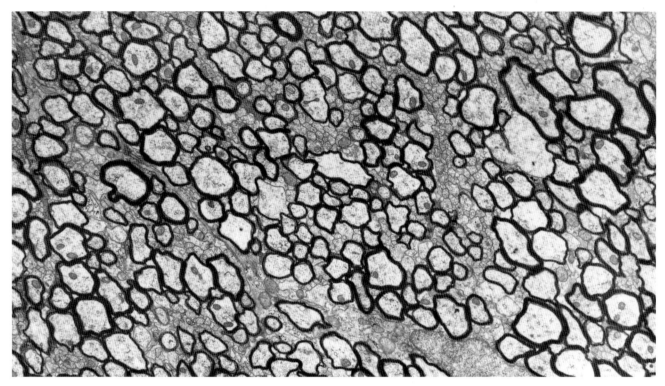

Fig. 22a. An electron micrograph of a section through the callosal radiation of a normal rat. × 11,000 (Hirano et al., J. Cell Biol. 31: 397, 1966)

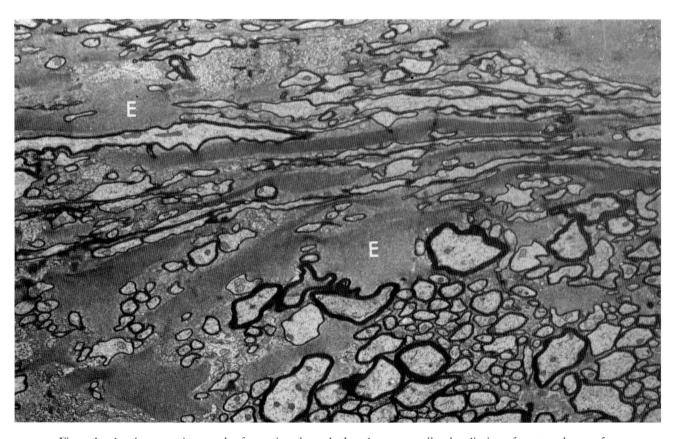

Fig. 22b. An electron micrograph of a section through the edematous callosal radiation of a rat 24 hours after experimental injury. Widened extracellular spaces (E) are obvious. × 5,000 (Hirano et al., Am. J. Pathol. 45, 1, 1964)

# II

## *Inflammatory Disorders*

Infectious diseases manifest themselves by an inflammatory reaction characterized by primary hematogenous and mesodermal tissue response to invading microörganisms. This inflammatory reaction is to be distinguished from "symptomatic" inflammation secondarily provoked by tissue damage as in infarcts and neoplasms.

Diseases caused by microörganisms may be classified, according to the type of inflammatory reaction, as: purulent, granulomatous, and nonpurulent.

### Purulent Infections

Pyogenic microörganisms, most commonly hemophilus influenzae, pneumococcus and meningococcus, induce a reaction characterized principally by exudation of polymorphonuclear leucocytes in the formation of pus.

### Purulent Meningitis

Inflammation of the dura mater—or pachymeningitis—usually develops as a direct extension from infection of adjacent tissues, as for example an osteomyelitis or leptomeningitis.

Inflammation of the pia-arachnoid membrane—or leptomeningitis—is an independent infection caused by a great variety of pyogenic microörganisms that gain entrance into the subarachnoid space either from adjacent infection, such as otitis media, or by way of the blood stream.

Grossly, the exudate consists of grayish-green pus that fills the subarachnoid space and obscures the underlying nervous and vascular structures. The exudate does not differ in appearance in accordance with the specific etiologic agent, but may vary in location. Thus such organisms as the meningococcus induce primarily a basilar meningitis (Fig. 23a), whereas other organisms may affect principally the convexities of the hemispheres, either unilaterally or bilaterally.

Microscopically, in the acute phase of the meningitis, polymorphonuclear leucocytes predominate, accompanied by scattered histiocytes and lymphocytes (Figs. 23b and c).

If the exudate is not absorbed, it becomes organized. At first a central zone of disintegrating polymorphonuclear leucocytes separates from a peripheral zone, adjacent to the nervous tissue, that consists of lymphocytes, plasma cells, and histiocytes. Later, if the exudate becomes organized, an adhesive arachnoiditis results by laying down of dense reticulin and collagen fibers.

If this is located at the base of the brain (Fig. 23d), the adhesions will tend to obstruct the cisterns and the foramina of Luschka and Magendie, resulting in hydrocephalus, which is visible externally by ballooning of the cerebral tissue.

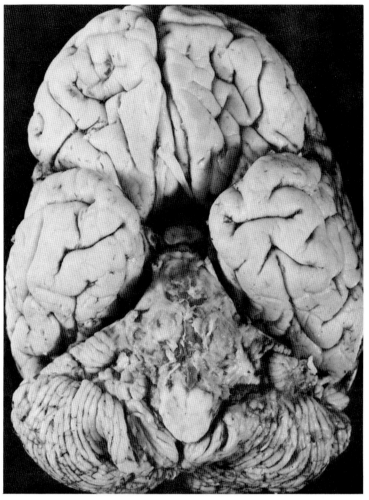

Fig. 23a. Acute basilar purulent leptomeningitis

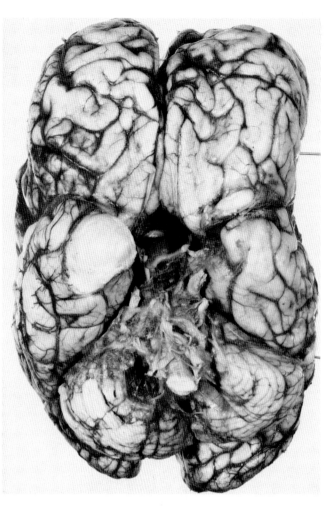

Fig. 23d. Chronic arachnoiditis

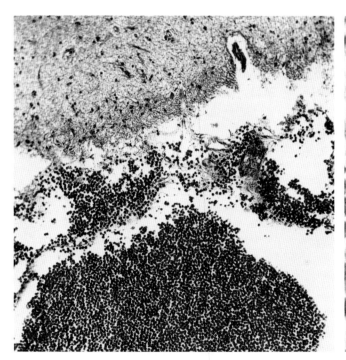

Fig. 23b. HE × 100

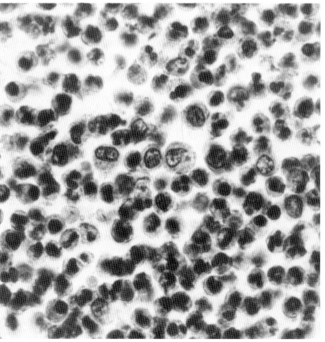

Fig. 23c. HE × 950

Leptomeningitis is usually accompanied by an ependymitis, because of direct communication of the subarachnoid spaces with the ventricles. In some cases the ependyma may be the predominant site of infection, as for example, in neonatal infections with enteric bacilli.

In the acute stage, polymorphonuclear leucocytes accumulate in the ventricles, choroid plexus, ependymal and subependymal layers. In the chronic stage lymphocytes and plasma cells supervene associated with subependymal gliosis.

The gliosis may be so marked as to occlude the narrowest parts of the ventricular system, particularly the aqueduct of Sylvius and the fourth ventricle, resulting in obstructive hydrocephalus.

*Case:* A female infant developed, on the third day following a normal birth, recurrent convulsive attacks, opisthotonus, and fever. Initially a blood calcium level of 7.6 mg per 100 cc led to a diagnosis of hypocalcemic tetany of the newborn. Later, with increasing evidence of hydrocephalus, despite specific treatment, meningitis was suspected. A ventricular tap revealed 5,000 cells per cmm, predominantly polymorphonuclear leucocytes, total protein of 480 mg per 100 cc and glucose of 22 mg per 100 cc. The fluid cultured *E. coli.* After treatment with sulfonamides and penicillin, the culture became sterile. A ventriculogram disclosed enlarged lateral ventricles. The condition progressed further, and by the age of two months the child showed marked hydrocephalus, spasticity of all extremities, and mental retardation. Death occurred at the age of four months.

The significant findings were chronic arachnoiditis occluding the cisterna magna (A), enlargement of the foramina of Luschka (B) and atresia of the fourth ventricle (C) (Fig. 24a); atresia of the third ventricle (D), enlargement of the lateral ventricles (E), dissolution from pressure atrophy of the corpus callosum, septum pellucidum and fornix, and cysts (F) in the cerebral white matter, presumably due to loculation of edematous fluid (Fig. 24b).

Microscopically, lymphocytes and glial fibers filled and surrounded the stenosed fourth ventricle (Fig. 24c).

*Reference*

Groover, R. B., J. M. Sutherland, and B. H. Landing. Purulent Meningitis of Newborn Infants. New Eng J. Med. 264: 1115, 1961.

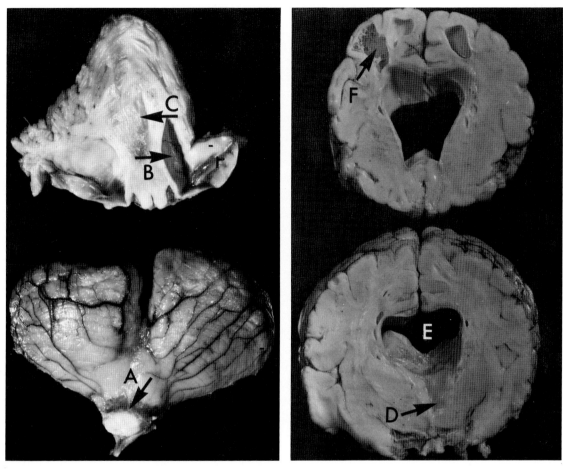

Fig. 24a. Atresia of 4th ventricle (above) and cisterna magna (below)

Fig. 24b. Atresia of 3rd ventricle (below); internal hydrocephalus (above)

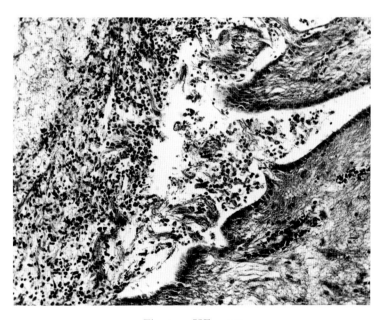

Fig. 24c. HE × 150

Meningitis usually does not extend into the underlying nervous tissue, which undergoes diffuse edematous and toxic changes that are often reversible. In some cases, however, toxic or circulatory factors may give rise to extensive noninflammatory malacia, presumably from an associated vasculitis involving basal arteries (Fig. 25a).

In a subacute phase, although the meningitis is subsiding, the underlying cortex is undergoing infarction with characteristic reactive proliferation of astrocytes in the superficial layers and of capillaries and macrophages in the deeper layers (Fig. 25b).

In a chronic stage, a condition of hemiatrophy may result.

*Case:* A 13-year-old girl developed at the age of eight months hemophilus influenzal meningitis. She was hospitalized for two months and was left with a residual right-sided hemiparesis and mental retardation. At the age of six years she was admitted to a State hospital where on examination she could not speak and showed a right hemiparesis with atrophy of the right extremities and equinovarus deformity of the right foot. She experienced infrequent grand mal seizures and expired of a virus pneumonitis.

Grossly, the brain showed atrophy of the left cerebral hemisphere, in an apparent distribution within the vascular territory of the left internal carotid artery, associated with mild fibrosis of the overlying meninges (Fig. 25c).

Microscopically, the superficial layers of the cortex were completely replaced by a dense fibrous gliosis in which nuclei of glial cells were embedded, contrasting with the relative preservation of the neurons in the deeper layers (Fig. 25d).

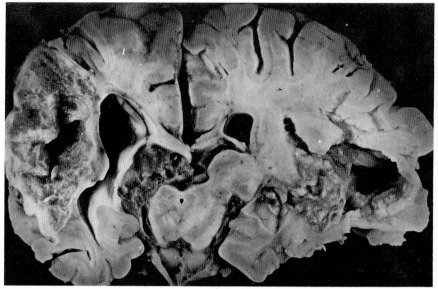

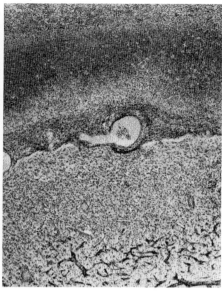

Fig. 25a. Subacute leptomeningitis and
encephalomalacia

Fig. 25b. Nissl × 30

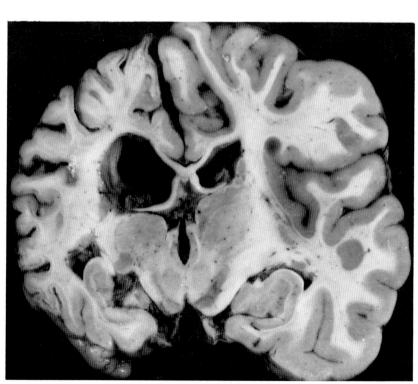

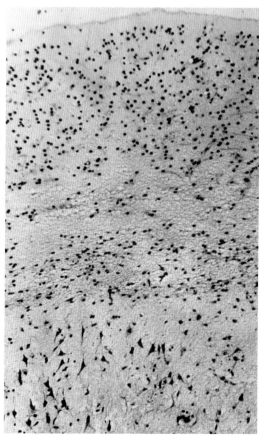

Fig. 25c. Left cerebral hemiatrophy following
meningitis

Fig. 25d. Nissl × 120

An abscess is a localized necrotizing purulent encephalitis. It develops when microörganisms gain entrance to the central nervous system either from adjacent focal infections (sinusitis, mastoiditis), through the blood stream (bacterial endocarditis, congenital cyanotic heart disease) or through penetrating open wounds. At times the source remains unknown.

Abscesses may be solitary or metastatic. Their location depends on the source. Thus adjacent abscesses are more common in the temporal lobe or cerebellum while hematogenous lesions occur more frequently in the frontal lobes. Although the incidence of brain abscesses has not been reduced with the advent of antibiotic treatment, the types of organisms have changed from hemolytic strepto-, staphylo- and pneumococci to nonhemolytic and anaerobic streptococci.

In the acute phase, the abscess appears grossly as a pus-containing cavity surrounded by extensive edema, that acts as a space-consuming mass causing displacement of ventricles, and herniation from complications of increased intracranial pressure, that may prove fatal (Fig. 26a). Microscopically, the necrotic center is filled with polymorphonuclear leucocytes (A) and is surrounded by a zone of edema (B) containing proliferated blood vessels and microglia (Fig. 26b).

In its further course, the abscess undergoes encapsulation, that generally begins after two to three weeks, depending on virulence of bacteria and resistance of host. The process of encapsulation depends on proliferation of fibroblasts from blood vessel walls that produce reticulin and collagen.

> *Case*: A 36-year-old woman was admitted to a mental hospital with symptoms of a manic-depressive psychosis. Seven years later bilateral prefrontal lobotomy was performed. Postoperatively she ran a spiking temperature, and developed nuchal rigidity, right hemiparesis, and generalized convulsions. Examination of the cerebrospinal fluid revealed 18,000 cells/cmm with 99% polymorphonuclear leucocytes. In spite of treatment she died on the forty-first postoperative day.

An encapsulated abscess (A) was located in the left frontal lobe, just behind the site of the lobotomy, associated with local meningitis, and ependymitis (B) of the ipsilateral ventricle (Fig. 26c).

Microscopically, the abscess consisted of three distinct zones, from its center: A. a zone of polymorphonuclear leucocytes undergoing lysis; B. a layer of macrophages containing sudanophilic granules intermingled with scattered capillaries; and C. a layer of fibroblasts, macrophages, lymphocytes, and plasma cells intermingled with reticulin and collagen fibers (Fig. 26d). Outside the capsule, a zone of fibrillary astrocytes associated with sparse inflammatory cells merged with the adjacent nervous tissue.

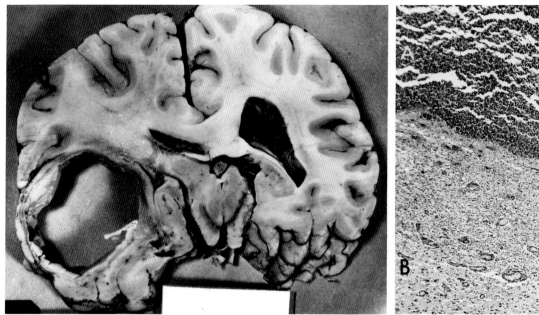

Fig. 26a. Abscess of left temporal lobe

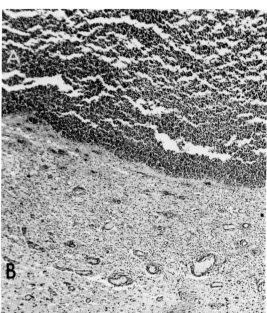

Fig. 26b. Hematoxylin-van Gieson × 38

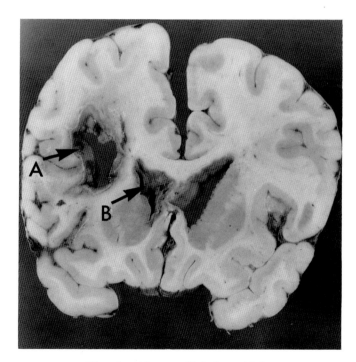

Fig. 26c. Abscess of left frontal lobe

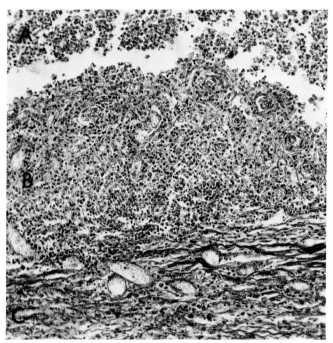

Fig. 26d. Hematoxylin-van Gieson × 100

## Granulomatous Infections

Granulomatous infections are characterized by local or diffuse infiltration of lymphocytes, epithelioid and giant cells, accompanied by variable caseation necrosis, with or without proliferation of connective tissue fibers. This type of inflammatory reaction forms the fundamental lesion in tuberculous, syphilitic, mycotic, and some protozoan infections.

### TUBERCULOSIS

Tuberculosis involves the central nervous system in the form of either meningitis or tuberculoma.

## Tuberculous Meningitis

Tuberculous meningitis is caused in the majority of instances by the human tubercle bacillus, in a few by the bovine form. The most common mode of infection is through disintegration of a local tubercle in the central nervous system that had originated from systemic tuberculous foci with discharge of the bacilli into the subarachnoid space. It may also arise from dissemination of bacilli via the blood stream in cases of miliary tuberculosis.

Pathologically, the meningitis shows the features of a granulomatous infection with predilection for the basal meninges, accompanied by involvement of the ependyma and limited extension into the adjacent parenchyma.

> *Case 1:* A 32-year-old woman developed two weeks following an upper respiratory infection headaches, stiffness of neck and vomiting of increasing severity. A chest x-ray and blood cultures were said to be negative. On admission to the hospital she was stuporous; reflexes were hyperactive associated with Babinski signs. A lumbar puncture revealed a cerebrospinal fluid pressure of 130 mm of $H_2O$, a total protein of 1130 mg%, chlorides of 580 mg%, sugar of 10 mg%, and 38 lymphocytes. She died shortly following admission to the hospital before a specific diagnosis could be established.

The general autopsy findings were miliary pulmonary tuberculosis. The base of the brain showed grossly thickened meninges, studded with grayish nodules (Fig. 27a).

Microscopically, the meninges were infiltrated with cells separated by pale areas of caseation necrosis (Fig. 27b). The infiltrations appeared both diffuse and perivascular, consisting of lymphocytes and histiocytes (Fig. 27c). Where the tubercles were well developed, an inner zone of epithelioid cells with pale nuclei (A), intermingled with scattered multinucleated giant cells of the Langhans type (B), was surrounded by an outer zone of lymphocytes (C) (Fig. 27d).

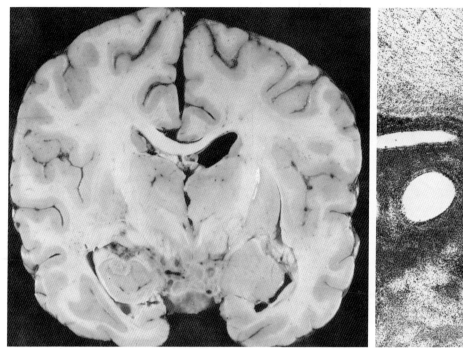

Fig. 27a. Tuberculous meningitis

Fig. 27b. Nissl × 30

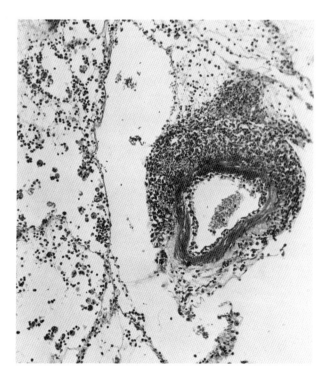

Fig. 27c. HE × 100

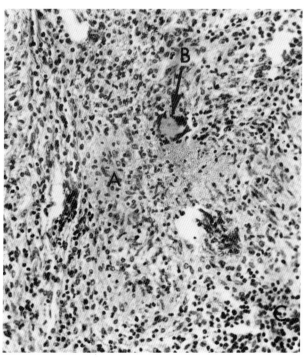

Fig. 27d. Hematoxylin-van Gieson × 200

## Tuberculous Meningitis (continued)

Vascular changes in the form of a panarteritis may be complicated by thrombosis, resulting in infarcts with corresponding neurologic symptoms.

*Case 2:* A 2-year-old girl developed fever, vomiting, and convulsions five days before admission. In the hospital she was semistuporous, and exhibited purposeless movements and spasticity of limbs. The cerebro-spinal fluid contained 220 cells/cmm, of which 13% were polymorphonuclear leucocytes and 87% were lymphocytes, 26 mg per 100 cc of sugar and 252 mg per 100 cc of protein. Treatment, with intrathecal and intramuscular streptomycin and promizole, was without effect on the progressively downhill course. Severe spastic quadriplegia developed, and death occurred on the twenty third hospital day.

The brain showed basilar leptomeningitis, which extended into both Sylvian fissures. On section, symmetrical areas of encephalomalacia involved the cerebral tissue including the basal ganglia in the territories of vascular supply by the middle cerebral arteries (Fig. 28a).

In the necrotic areas, while the leptomeninges contained only scattered tubercles (A), there was massive noninflammatory necrosis of the underlying cortex (B), which was filled with macrophages (Fig. 28b).

## Tuberculoma

Tuberculomas represent a conglomeration of tubercles that may be solitary and large or multiple and small. Their pathology is essentially similar to the tubercles in tuberculous meningitis.

*Case:* A 40-year-old woman was undergoing treatment for pulmonary tuberculosis when she became increasingly disturbed and mentally confused. She expressed auditory and visual hallucinations, and was committed to a mental hospital. There she became comatose, and died two days after admission.

The brain contained multiple discrete grayish-white nodules of uniform size, chiefly in the cortex of the right hemisphere, accompanied by an acute basilar leptomeningitis (Fig. 28c).

Microscopically, central areas of caseation necrosis were surrounded by a zone of epithelioid and giant cells and lymphocytes intermingled with sparse reticulin and collagen fibers on the periphery (Fig. 28d).

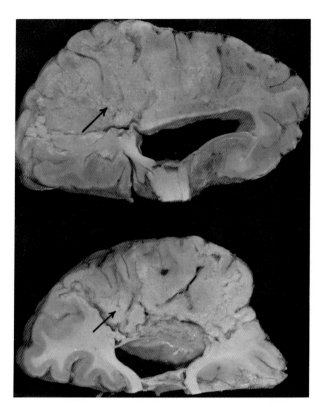

Fig. 28a.  Tuberculous meningitis and
encephalomalacia

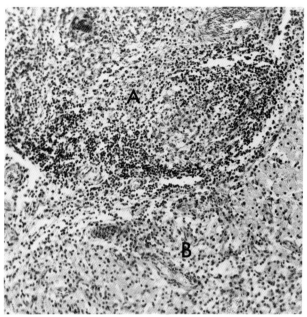

Fig. 28b.  Hematoxylin-van Gieson × 100

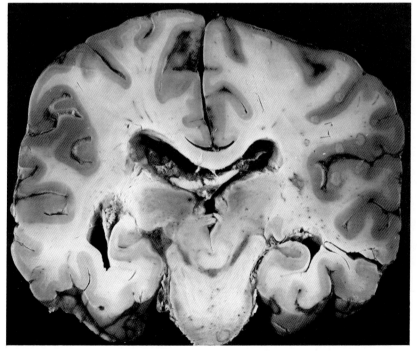

Fig. 28c.  Multiple tuberculomas

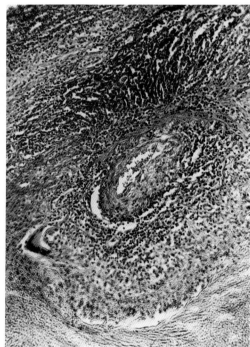

Fig. 28d.  Hematoxylin-van Gieson × 75

Sarcoidosis (Boeck's sarcoid) is a rare chronic progressive, at times remitting, disorder with systemic and central nervous system symptoms. It generally affects young adults especially blacks, tends to be self-limited but may be fatal. Although of tuberculoid nature, its etiologic relationship to tuberculosis has been questioned. It has been regarded by some as a state of hypersensitivity.

In the central nervous system its most common location is in the basal meninges, where it infiltrates the roots of the cranial nerves, especially the optic nerves, and whence it may extend into the overlying parenchyma, particularly in the region of the floor of the third ventricle.

Symptoms of optic neuritis, of other cranial nerve palsies and of disturbance of hypothalamic functions are prominent. The cerebrospinal fluid generally shows elevation of total protein and a mild to moderate increase in lymphocytes. A positive Kveim test is diagnostic as are biopsies of lymph nodes.

The lesions are characterized by a noncaseating granulomatous inflammation, associated with abundant reticulin fibers, by contrast with tuberculous lesions.

*Case:* A 32-year-old black man was admitted to a hospital on several occasions during a period of two years with symptoms of generalized weakness, weight loss, polydipsia and polyuria, headaches, convulsions, and episodes of mental confusion. Blood serology and repeated spinal fluid examinations for lues were negative. On his final admission the optic disk margins were indistinct, and there were retinal hemorrhages. The spinal fluid was under a pressure of 370 mm H$_2$O with 42 white cells per cmm, 37 of which were lymphocytes and 5 were polymorphonuclear leucocytes; the total protein was 140 mg per 100 cc, and the colloidal gold curve showed a mid-zone rise. Urinary output averaged 9,000 cc per day. Blood studies indicated signs of altered liver function. PPD skin tests were negative. A biopsy of a lymph node was diagnosed as Boeck's sarcoid. In the following weeks improvement was noted, but he died suddenly following several seizures.

Grossly, the basal meninges in the floor of the third ventricle and adjacent to the hippocampal formation, as well as in the roof of the aqueduct of Sylvius, were infiltrated by grayish nodular tissue (Fig. 29a).

Microscopically, discrete and coalescing noncaseating nodules extended from the meninges and ependyma into the floor and walls of the third ventricle (Fig. 29b). They consisted of central areas of epithelioid cells and peripheral zones of lymphocytes and multinucleated giant cells (Fig. 29c). Some of the lesions contained characteristic hematoxylin-staining Schaumann bodies (Fig. 29d).

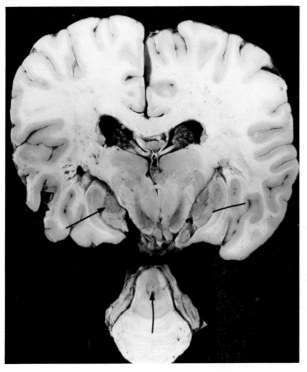

Fig. 29a. Sarcoidosis

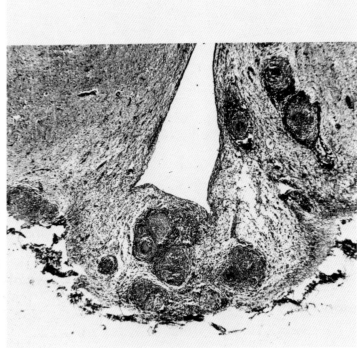

Fig. 29b. HE × 32

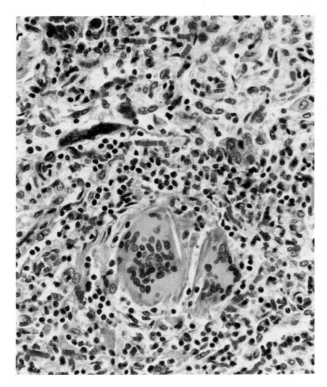

Fig. 29c. HE × 250

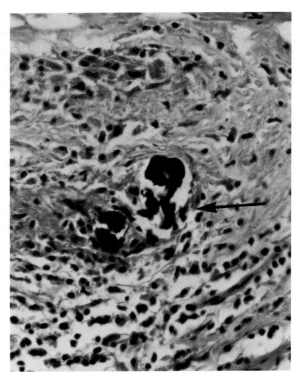

Fig. 29d. HE × 350

Syphilis involves the nervous system during the tertiary stage in a variety of ways, as meningitis, gumma, arteritis (see Vascular Disorders), general paresis and tabes dorsalis.

## Syphilitic Meningitis

Syphilitic meningitis may develop as an acute or subacute disorder during the tertiary period. It most often affects the optochiasmatic region resulting in optic and other cranial nerve palsies. It may be associated with vascular syphilis.

Pathologically, the basal meninges are grossly thickened and fibrotic (Fig. 30a) and microscopically show a granulomatous inflammatory reaction in which epithelioid and lymphocytic cells are intermingled with less frequent plasma and giant cells, with fairly abundant reticulin fibers, while necrosis is less prominent than in tuberculous meningitis (Fig. 30b).

## Gumma

Gumma is a syphilitic granuloma that may occur either as a large solitary lesion or as multiple microgummas.

The latter is illustrated by the following case:

*Case:* A 52-year-old black woman was admitted to a hospital because of episodes of mental confusion. There was a history of syphilitic infection and antiluetic treatment. Examination revealed her to be lethargic and confused. She had a shuffling gait, absent knee jerks, weakness of legs, and poor coordination. The Kahn reaction of the blood and spinal fluid was positive, and the colloidal gold curve was 5555532000. Three days before death a seizure occurred, followed by bilateral Babinski signs and coma.

The optic chiasm and walls and floor of the third ventricle were diffusely infiltrated, resulting in partial occlusion of the third ventricle and moderate dilatation of the lateral ventricles (Fig. 30c).

Microscopically, discrete and coalescing granulomatous lesions, with central fibrosis and peripheral lymphocytes and giant cells, were scattered through the floor and walls of the third ventricle (Fig. 30d).

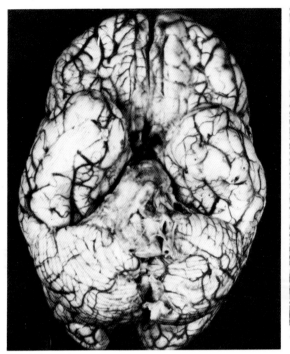

Fig. 30a. Syphilitic meningitis

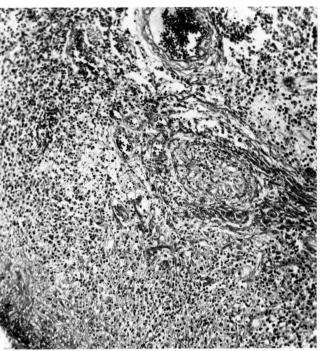

Fig. 30b. Heidenhain's aniline blue × 100

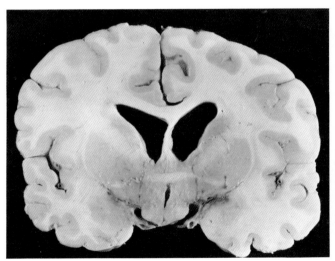

Fig. 30c. Syphilitic microgumma

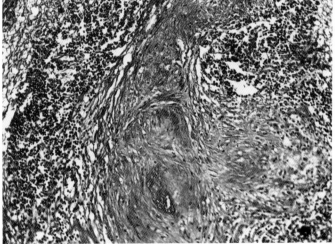

Fig. 30d. HE × 100

## General Paresis

General paresis is a meningoencephalitis with predominant involvement of the cerebral cortex and gradual decrease of the inflammatory process in subortical structures. In the more typical form, the anterior parts of the cortex are more severely affected with corresponding clinical signs of changes in personality and impairment of intellect. In the less common Lissauer's form, the posterior parts are the sites of maximal involvement, giving rise to focal seizures, hemiplegia, hemianopsia and aphasia. The histopathology is that of a nonpurulent, nongranulomatous inflammation combined with degenerative changes in the parenchyma.

> *Case:* A 46-year-old man had a sudden onset of convulsions a week before commitment to a mental hospital, followed by disorientation and violent behavior. On admission he exhibited signs of intellectual impairment and reacted to auditory hallucinations. Blood and spinal fluid Wassermann tests were positive; the spinal fluid contained 50 lymphocytes per cmm, and showed a positive Pandy reaction and a first-zone rise in the colloidal gold curve. He died suddenly of acute pancreatitis, one month after admission and before treatment was begun.

Grossly, the brain showed diffuse thickening and "milky" opacity of the leptomeninges—particularly on the lateral and mesial surfaces of the frontal lobes—diffuse atrophy of the gyri and ependymal granulations in the walls of the dilated ventricles (Fig. 31a).

Microscopically, the cerebral cortex was disorganized and the small blood vessels throughout the gray matter were infiltrated with round cells, the leptomeninges being similarly involved. The cortex exhibited disturbance of cytoarchitecture, with disappearance of the normal lamination, dropping out of neurons, and abnormal polarity of the remaining nerve cells (Fig. 31b).

The infiltrations in the perivascular spaces and the pia-arachnoid membrane were composed of lymphocytes and plasma cells, the latter identified by eccentric nuclei and central clear areas (Fig. 31c).

Microglial activity in the form of hypertrophied and greatly elongated "rod" cells was demonstrated with the silver carbonate method (Fig. 31d). With specific stains, granules of iron pigment were found in microglia and in the adventitia of blood vessels.

The activity of the macroglia was manifested by proliferating protoplasmic and fibrous astrocytes that formed a network throughout the entire width of the cortex (Fig. 31e).

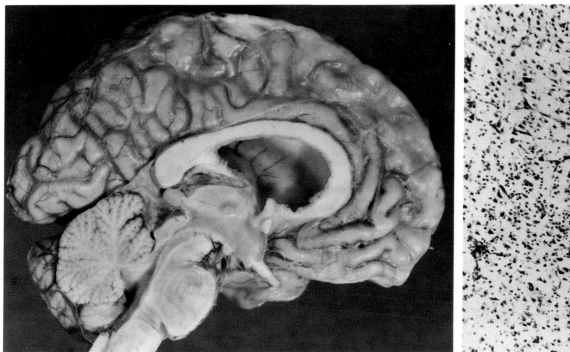

Fig. 31a. General paresis

Fig. 31b. Nissl × 100

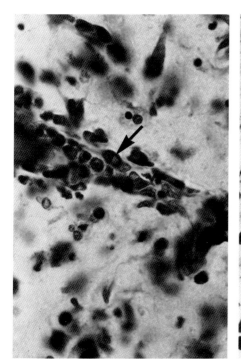

Fig. 31c. Nissl × 475

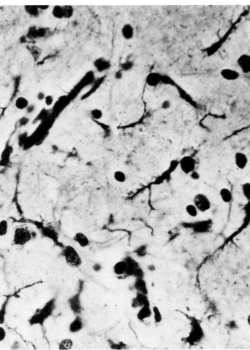

Fig. 31d. Hortega silver carbonate × 475

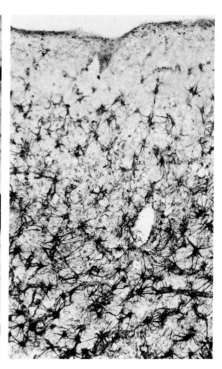

Fig. 31e. Cajal gold sublimate × 100

General Paresis (continued)

The ependymal granulations were composed of glial nuclei and fibers occurring in nests beneath the partly denuded and disorganized ependymal lining, as in the walls of the aqueduct of Sylvius (Fig. 32a).

With special stains for spirochetes, the treponema pallidum can be demonstrated in the central nervous system in some cases of general paresis. These occur either singly or in "swarms" within the nervous parenchyma, the walls of blood vessels, and the leptomeninges (Fig. 32b).

In juvenile paresis, the cerebellum and basal ganglia are apt to be as severely involved as the cerebral cortex, with corresponding symptoms of ataxia and athetosis. The atrophic cerebellum shows a diffuse reduction of neurons, especially of the granule layer, and the Purkinje cells are often binucleate.

## Tabes Dorsalis

The lesions of tabes dorsalis are found in the dorsal columns of the spinal cord and the dorsal roots. Various opinions have been advanced as to the pathogenesis and site of origin of the lesion. The generally accepted theory is that a pachyleptomeningitis at the distal end of the dorsal roots causes by constriction secondary degeneration of the roots and of the posterior columns.

*Case:* An 82-year-old man had had treatment for syphilis in his thirties. He was well until six years before his death, when he developed severe shooting pains in the legs, enlargement of the knee joints, and difficulty in walking. On admission to a hospital, examination disclosed Argyll Robertson pupils, Charcot type of knee joints, loss of muscle tonus in the legs with absent deep reflexes, generalized hypalgesia, and a "cord bladder."

Bilateral demyelinization was severe in the fasciculus gracilis, and mild in the fasciculus cuneatus; the other tracts of the spinal cord appeared normal (Fig. 32c).

A corresponding gliosis involved the tracts of the posterior columns, accompanied by fibrosis of the leptomeninges about the dorsal roots and columns (Fig. 32d); there was no trace of inflammatory reaction.

The dorsal roots showed diffuse loss of myelin, which was replaced by endoperineurial connective tissue.

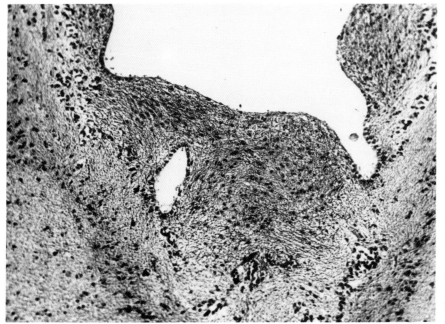

Fig. 32a. HE × 100

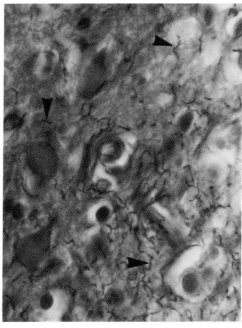

Fig. 32b. Jahnel stain for spirochetes × 200

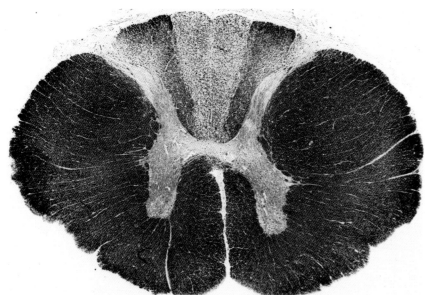

Fig. 32c. Marchi stain

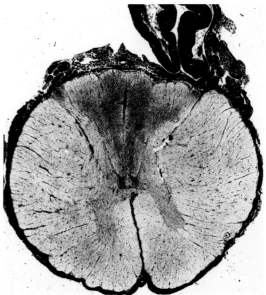

Fig. 32d. Holzer stain

A great variety of fungus infections have been known for a long time to affect the central nervous system, however, they have assumed increasing importance in recent times since the advent of antibiotic and steroid treatment because of their tendency to act as opportunistic invaders in the presence of immunosuppression.

Clinically, while most of the mycotic infections are associated with systemic manifestations, especially pulmonary, the clinical course and outcome may be determined by involvement of the central nervous system.

Pathologically, the lesions are most often characterized by granulomatous inflammation, although some may also induce either abscesses or nonpurulent inflammatory reactions similar to virus diseases.

### CRYPTOCOCCOSIS (TORULOSIS)

Cryptococcosis, caused by the fungus *C. neoformans*, or torula histolytica, is probably the most common of the fungus infections of the central nervous system for which it shows special predilection. Its source is in the soil and its mode of infection is through respiratory tract, skin, lymph nodes and muscles, whence it spreads to the central nervous system. It may develop in the course of such disorders as Hodgkin's disease, leukemia and sarcoidosis. The fungus is a spherical yeast organism, of 5-20 $\mu$, that proliferates by budding. It possesses a thick wall, surrounded by a gelatinous polysaccharide capsule, and can be demonstrated in the cerebrospinal fluid with India ink preparations.

Pathologically, the meninges and the parenchyma of the brain show as a rule noninflammatory microcystic changes although on occasion a basal granulomatous meningitis or a local solitary granuloma may develop.

> *Case:* A 44-year-old man complained of headaches and forgetfulness over a period of a month, followed by the sudden onset of a right hemiparesis associated with choreiform movements, ataxia and nuchal rigidity. In the hospital his condition progressed further to a complete right hemiplegia with bilateral papilledema and clouded sensorium. A ventriculogram was normal. The spinal fluid was found to be under a pressure of 660 mm $H_2O$, was turbid, and revealed torula histolytica organisms on direct smear. He died forty days following the onset of his illness.

Macroscopically, myriads of small cysts, having the appearance of "soap suds," were disseminated through the brain tissue, particularly the basal ganglia (Fig. 33a).

The cysts containing the organisms were aggregated in masses that for the most part showed noninflammatory reaction, the organisms staining deeply with PAS or thionin and showing budding and spinous processes, the latter due to partial fixation-shrinkage of the surrounding capsules (Fig. 33b).

In some areas, a granulomatous meningitis supervened characterized by infiltration of the pia-arachnoid with lymphocytes, epithelioid cells and giant cells (Fig. 33c) intermingled with organisms (Fig. 33d).

*Reference*

Fetter, B. F., G. K. Klintworth and W. S. Hendry. Mycoses of the Central Nervous System. Williams and Wilkins (Baltimore, 1967).

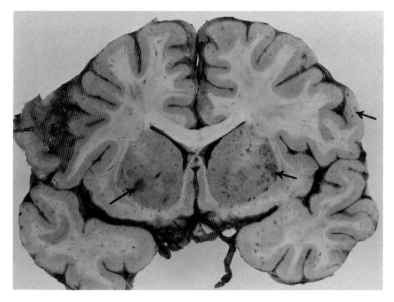

Fig. 33a. Cryptococcosis

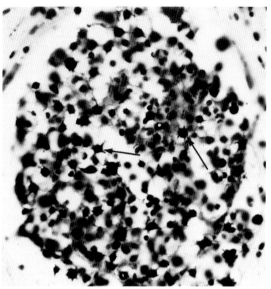

Fig. 33b. Nissl × 250

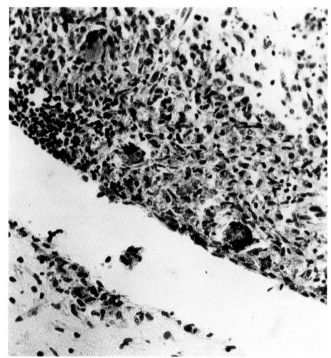

Fig. 33c. Nissl × 200

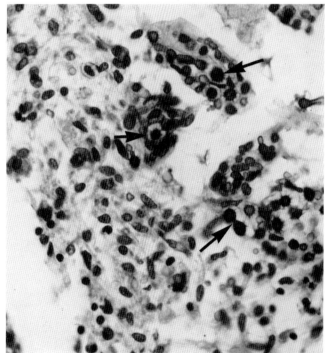

Fig. 33d. Nissl × 475

When examined in the electron microscope, *Cryptococcus* displays a characteristic fungal morphology. The cell is surrounded by a plasma membrane which infolds in places around the periphery resulting in a mesosome-like structure. Within the plasma membrane, the densely granular cytoplasm contains the usual organelles. Outside the plasma membrane, a laminated cell wall of variable thickness is present. External to the cell wall, there is a narrow electron-lucent zone which separates the cell wall from the polysaccharide capsule which is composed of a finely reticulated material.

In contrast to protein implantation, very little inflammatory reaction occurs when capsular material is implanted into the brain of experimental animals. Although edema results, only few hematogenous cells enter the parenchyma. Instead, the capsular polysaccharide spreads through the extracellular spaces and is gradually absorbed by the glial cells. The material is apparently indigestible since it can be found, with no obvious alteration, within glial cells up to 100 days after implantation.

Apparently, it is the capsular polysaccharide within the brain which prevents the parasite from eliciting a leucocyte reaction, especially polymorphonuclear leucocytes. This, no doubt, contributes to the relatively meager inflammatory reaction of the brain to cryptococcal infection which is found in many instances. This conclusion is borne out by the fact that when lyophilized cryptococci (Fig. 34) are implanted so that intracellular material is exposed, the inflammatory response is severe, resulting in abscess formation.

*References*

Edwards, M. R., M. A. Gordon, E. W. Lapa, and W. C. Ghiorse. Micromorphology of Cryptococcus neoformans. J. Bact. 94: 766, 1967.

Hirano, A., H. M. Zimmerman, and S. Levine. Fine Structure of Cerebral Fluid Accumulation: IV. On Nature and Origin of Extracellular Fluids Following Cryptococcal Polysaccharide Implantation. Amer. J. Path. 45: 195, 1964.

Hirano, A., H. M. Zimmerman, and S. Levine. Fine Structure of Cerebral Fluid Accumulation: V. Transfer of Fluid from Extracellular to Intracellular Compartments in Acute Phase of Cryptococcal Polysaccharide Lesions. Arch. Neurol. 11: 632, 1964.

Hirano, A., H. M. Zimmerman, and S. Levine. Fine Structure of Cerebral Fluid Accumulation: VI. Intracellular Accumulation of Fluid and Cryptococcal Polysaccharide in Oligodendroglia. Arch. Neurol. 12: 189, 1965.

Hirano, A., H. M. Zimmerman, and S. Levine. The Fine Structure of Cerebral Fluid Accumulation: Reactions of Ependyma to Implantation of Cryptococcal Polysaccharide. J. Path. & Bact. 91: 149, 1966.

Levine, S., A. Hirano, and H. M. Zimmerman. The Reaction of the Nervous System to Cryptococcal Infection: An Experimental Study with Light and Electron Microscopy. Infections of the Nervous System (H. M. Zimmerman, ed.), Williams and Wilkins (Baltimore, 1968), p. 393.

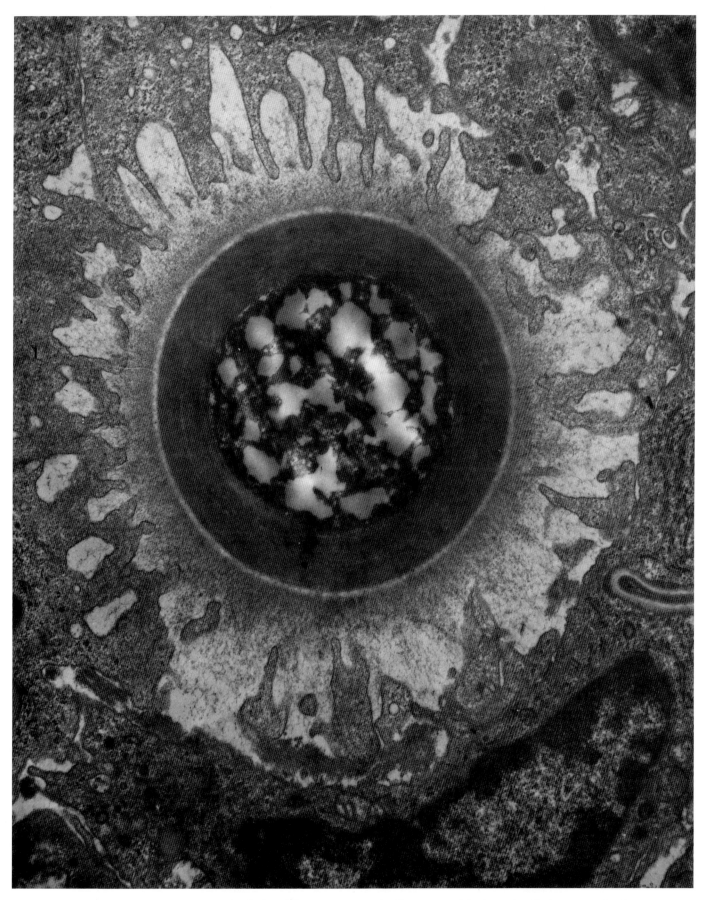

Fig. 34. An electron micrograph of a lyophilized cryptococcal cell surrounded by inward radiating macrophagic processes in a rat brain five days after implantation. × 17,000 (Levine et al., in Inflections of the Nervous System, Res. Pub. A.R.N.M.D., Vol. XLIV, (H. M. Zimmerman, ed.). Williams and Wilkins (Baltimore, 1968), p. 393.)

Coccidioidomycosis, caused by the fungus *Coccidioides immitis*, is endemic in Southwestern U.S.A. The source is in the soil and the mode of infection is through the respiratory tract and skin. The disseminated form that develops months to years following the primary infection is characterized by a progressive and malignant clinical course, invariably involving the meninges. The organism is a spherical nonbudding cyst of about 20–60 $\mu$, filled with endospores and lined by a double contoured wall. Diagnosis is based on increasing titers of complement-fixing antibodies, cultures, skin tests and the finding of spherules in the cerebrospinal fluid. Pathologically, the changes are similar to those of tuberculous meningitis.

> *Case:* A 19-year-old, black soldier, who had frequently driven through the San Joaquin Valley, became ill with systemic coccidioidomycosis, proved two months before hospitalization by biopsies of cervical lymph node and skin. On entry to the hospital he showed marked weight loss, generalized lymphadenopathy, and disseminated skin lesions. His course was progressively downhill, with daily spiking temperatures and progressive mental confusion. Examination of the cerebrospinal fluid revealed 200 white cells per cmm, 95% of which were lymphocytes, total protein of 45 mg per 100 cc, sugar of 32 mg per 100 cc, and a colloidal gold curve of 5554321000. He died eight weeks after admission.

A diffuse exudate, studded with discrete grayish nodules, infiltrated the basal meninges, particularly about the optic chiasm and in the Sylvian fissures, resulting in moderate internal hydrocephalus (Fig. 35a).

Microscopically, the meninges contained coalescing granulomas composed of lymphocytes, polymorphonuclear leucocytes, epithelioid and giant cells. The organisms were usually found within the giant cells, and consisted of double-walled spherical cysts containing numerous spores (Fig. 35b).

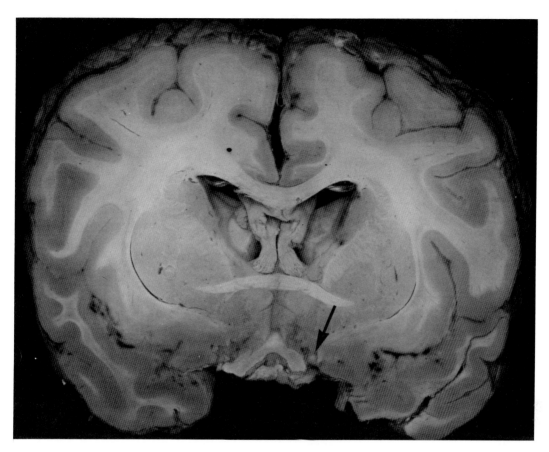

Fig. 35a. Coccidioidomycosis

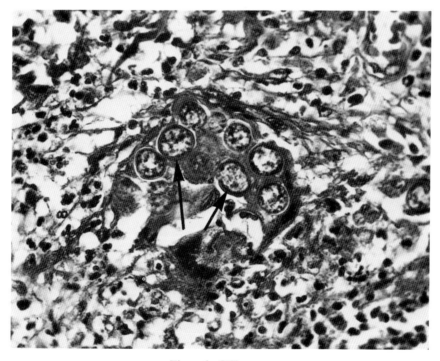

Fig. 35b. HE × 475

The fungus *Histoplasma capsulatum* is a rare infection of the central nervous system. It is endemic in the Central Mississippi Valley, Ohio, and the Appalachians. The source is in the soil. It causes either a benign acute pulmonary disease or a malignant chronic progressive disorder. The organism has an oval body of about 1–5 $\mu$, occurring within large mononuclear cells, surrounded by a PAS-positive staining capsule and stains best with Grocott's methenamine silver. Diagnosis depends on demonstration of complement-fixing antibodies, cultures, skin tests, and the presence of the fungi in smears from peripheral blood or sputum.

The pathology is either a basal granulomatous meningitis or an intracerebral granuloma.

*Case:* A 67-year-old man developed over a period of two months headaches, dizziness, ataxia, vomiting, and visual disturbance. Examination disclosed a Horner syndrome and cerebellar signs on the left, a crossed hypalgesia involving the forehead on the left and the trunk and extremities on the right, and a Babinski sign on the right. The cerebrospinal fluid showed a positive Pandy reaction and a total protein of 214 mg per 100 cc. A month later he became semicomatose, the temperature was elevated to 39.4° C, and he died four months after the onset of his symptoms.

Autopsy revealed coalescing necrotic granulomas within the vermis of the cerebellum and the fourth ventricle (Fig. 36a). Miliary granulomas were also found in the subependymal regions of all ventricles, apparently caused by seeding.

Microscopically, the lesions were composed of caseating centers surrounded by walls of epithelioid, giant, and lymphocytic cells. There were numerous large mononuclear forms that contained colonies of *Histoplasma capsulatum*, each with a round, deeply stained central mass surrounded by a clear zone and refractile capsule (Fig. 36b), that stained positively with PAS and methenamine silver methods.

## NOCARDIOSIS

*Nocardia asteroides*, an aerobic form of actinomyces, usually develops in the presence of debilitating disorders or in cases receiving corticosteroid or cytotoxic agents. It is a filamentous organism with delicate branching hyphae, staining with hematoxylin-eosin, gram, or methenamine silver methods. It usually spreads to the central nervous system from lung infection by hematogenous route and produces small unencapsulated abscesses, less commonly granulomas.

*Case:* A 60-year-old woman was hospitalized after a ten-month period of fever, cough, and hemoptysis. On admission, x-rays showed lung infiltrations. Cultures of sputum and pleural fluid, from a pleural effusion, revealed *Nocardia asteroides*. One month later she developed nuchal rigidity, increased tendon reflexes, and a Babinski sign on the left. Antibiotics had no effect on her course; she lapsed into semistupor, and died four months after admission.

Multiple discrete, small, grayish, partly necrotic foci were disseminated throughout the brain tissue (Fig. 36c).

Microscopically, the lesions were small granulomas with central necrosis and peripheral infiltrations by lymphocytes, epithelioid and giant cells. The organisms were branching filamentous mycelia contained in the granulomas (Fig. 36d).

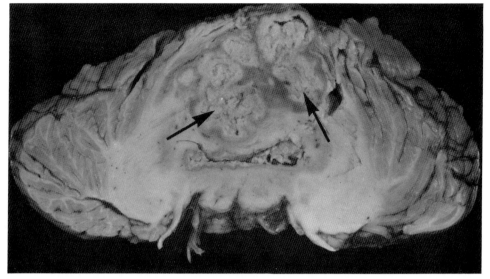

Fig. 36a. Histoplasmosis

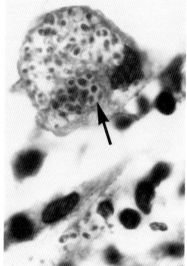

Fig. 36b. HE × 1500

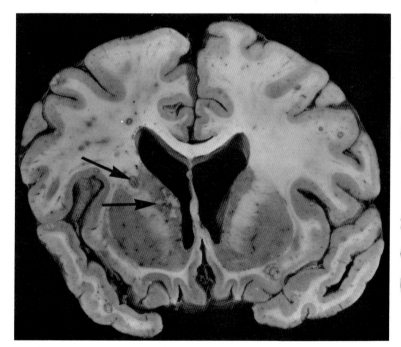

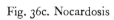

Fig. 36c. Nocardosis

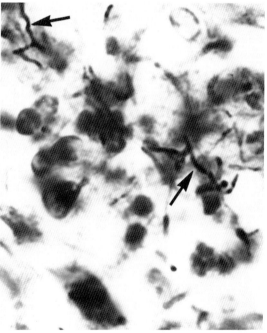

Fig. 36d. Bacterial stain × 1800

Aspergillosis is caused by an opportunistic fungus that becomes pathogenic in the presence of debilitating states, with increased use of steroid and antibiotic therapy.

*Aspergillus fumigatus* is a branching organism with septate hyphae, of about 3–6 $\mu$ in diameter, staining positively with Grocott's methenamine silver. It is identified by smear or culture. The lesions evoked in the central nervous system are either in the form of infarcts due to thrombosis caused by fungus invasion of the walls of blood vessels and/or abscesses or granulomas, miliary or large.

> *Case:* A 23-year-old woman had several admissions to the hospital because of systemic lupus erythematosus of five years' duration for which she was treated with Prednisone, Chlorambucil and Allopurinol. On June 22, 1969 she began having grand mal seizures, thought to be due to cerebral vasculitis. A lumbar puncture revealed only a total protein of 55 mg per 100 cc. She later developed thrombocytopenia and received transfusions. Drug treatment, consisting of various antibiotics was continued. Her course was marked by repeated seizures and she expired eleven days following the onset of neurologic symptoms.

Grossly, the brain showed multiple large and small discrete hemorrhagic infarcts that were bilateral but more extensive on the right side, causing displacement of the obliterated ventricles to the left (Fig. 37a).

Microscopically, the lesions were characterized by ischemic and hemorrhagic necrosis and infiltration with polymorph leucocytes. Many regional blood vessels were thrombosed. Within the necrotic foci there were collections of branching organisms with septate hyphae that stained with methenamine silver (Fig. 37b).

## CANDIDIASIS

*Candida albicans,* a gram-positive fungus, found in normal flora, may invade the nervous system under somewhat similar circumstances as aspergillus. It is an oval budding fungus producing narrow, nonseptate pseudomycelia, that stain positively with methenamine silver and PAS and can be identified in smears and cultures.

The lesions in candidiasis are either microglial nodules, small granulomas, or microinfarcts.

> *Case:* A 27-year-old man had a long history of chronic ulcerative colitis, pericholangitis and obstructive liver disease for which he was treated with azulfidine, steroids, and cholysteramine. Towards the end he lapsed into coma which persisted for several days until his demise.

The general autopsy revealed multiple abscesses in heart, liver and kidneys caused by *Candida albicans.*

The brain showed grossly scattered petechial hemorrhages.

Microscopically, miliary abscesses and hemorrhagic infarcts were noted in the cortex, basal ganglia, and cerebellum. The abscesses consisted of necrotic foci containing polymorphonuclear leucocytes and slender nonseptate pseudomycelia that stained positively with cresyl violet (Fig. 37c) and methenamine silver (Fig. 37d).

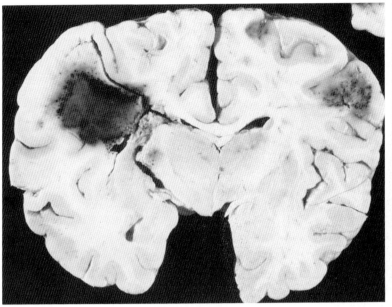

Fig. 37a. Aspergillosis

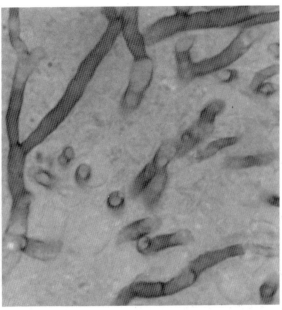

Fig. 37b. Silver methenamine × 680

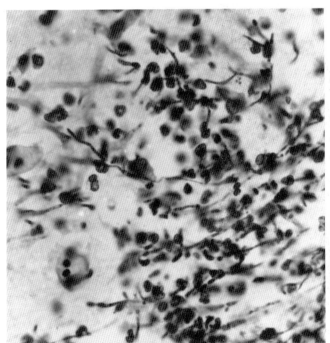

Fig. 37c. Candidiasis: Nissl × 375

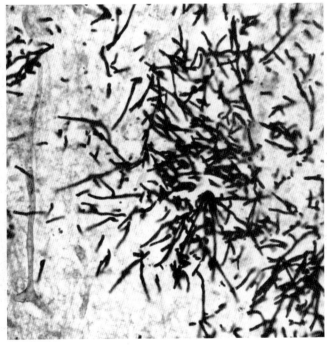

Fig. 37d. Silver methenamine × 300

Mucormycosis, caused by a fungus of the genus Mucor, may cause infection of the nervous system under the same conditions as some of the other mycoses but especially in the presence of diabetes. The sources are soil, manure, and bread mold. The organism is characterized by branching nonseptate hyphae of about 6–50 $\mu$ in diameter, and stains best with silver methenamine and PAS.

It invades the nervous system either directly from orbital or sinus infections or indirectly via ophthalmic and internal carotid arteries or through embolism from pulmonary infection. The lesions are primarily infarcts brought about by thromboembolism but occasionally may be in the nature of abscesses or granulomas.

*Case:* A 59-year-old woman with a long history of chronic alcoholism, cirrhosis, and diabetes, developed inflammation in the left eye four weeks prior to hospitalization for which she was treated with Penicillin and steroids. On admission she was described as obtunded: the left corneal reflex was absent and the left pupil was nonreactive. Examination of the cerebrospinal fluid revealed 17 lymphocytes/cmm, a total protein of 62 mg per 100 cc, and chlorides of 109 mEq. A biopsy from the left middle turbinate bone was diagnostic of mucormycosis, and she was started on 60 mg of Amphotericin-B with 20 mg of Solucortef intravenously, and 25 mg of Amphotericin-B intrathecally. At the same time treatment was instituted for her diabetes. She continued to be obtunded. On the fifth hospital day, she lost the pupillary response in the right eye as well and became completely blind. A seventh nerve palsy developed on the left, followed by a right hemiparesis and generalized seizures. She expired approximately two weeks following admission.

Grossly, the brain showed an acute hemorrhagic infarct in the territory of the left posterior cerebral artery and thrombi in branches of the posterior and middle cerebral arteries on the same side.

Microscopically, thrombi were present in many meningeal blood vessels, both veins and arteries, the underlying nervous tissue showing acute ischemic and hemorrhagic infarcts (Fig. 38a), in which there were variable numbers of polymorphonuclear leucocytes, lymphocytes, and macrophages. In the lumens of many blood vessels nonseptate branching wrinkled hyphae were visible (Fig. 38b).

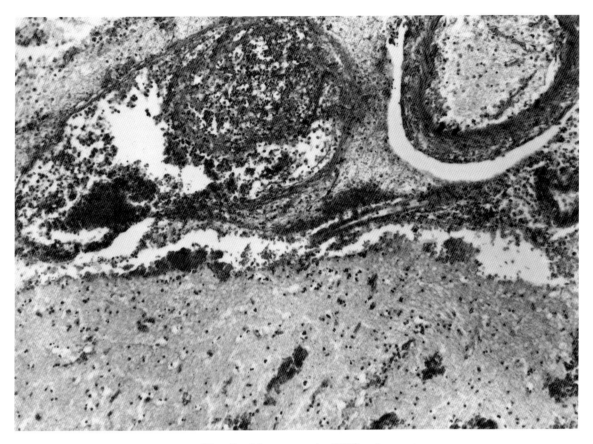

Fig. 38a. Mucormycosis: HVG × 90

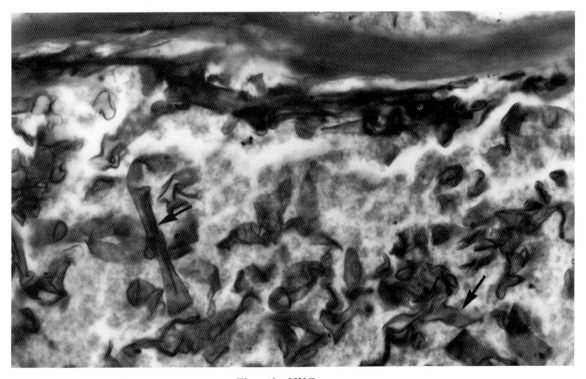

Fig. 38b. HVG × 400

## CYSTICERCOSIS

Of the various parasitic infections of the nervous system, cysticercosis is probably the most common, being endemic in Mexico and other Latin-American countries.

The ova of the Taenia solium (pork tapeworm) are ingested by man and invade principally the brain and less commonly the muscles, skin, and retina. The developing larval form (*Cysticercus cellulosae*) lodges within the meninges, ventricles, or the parenchyma of the brain where it becomes encysted and may calcify. In its racemose form it occupies frequently the basal meninges around the optic chiasm and brain stem. As the parasite undergoes disintegration, it sets up a granulomatous inflammatory reaction that may lead to communicating hydrocephalus.

*Case:* A 31-year-old Mexican woman was admitted to a mental hospital because of marked changes in personality in the previous nine months. She had become untidy, forgetful, and experienced visual hallucinations. She complained of headaches, impaired vision, deafness and tinnitus in the right ear, and poor balance. On admission she was distractible, emotionally labile, and showed defects in recent memory, decreased hearing on the right, anosmia, bitemporal hemianopsia, papilledema, impairment of fine movements, ataxia of gait, a positive Romberg sign, and spasticity of the right leg with ankle clonus. X-rays showed destruction of the base of the middle fossa and dorsum sellae. A ventriculogram showed generalized dilatation of all ventricles. On repeated examinations, the cerebrospinal fluid contained 11 to 66 cells/cmm, predominantly lymphocytes; total protein of 69 to 169 mg per 100 cc; and sugar of 37 mg per 100 cc. Craniotomy led to removal of a parasitic cyst from the region of the optic chiasm, but signs of increasing intracranial pressure supervened. She died approximately one and a half years following the onset of symptoms.

The brain contained numerous cysts in the ventricles and meninges. A section through the right frontal lobe showed a cyst containing a calcified cysticercus within the meninges of the mesial surface and operative trauma at the base of the right temporal lobe (Fig. 39a).

Microscopically, the segmented, partly necrotic larvum within the basal meninges (A) was surrounded by an inflammatory tissue (B) consisting of lymphocytes, eosinophils, epithelioid and foreign body giant cells, and fibroblasts (Fig. 39b).

In an old calcified intracortical cyst of another case, the scolex of the organism is shown (Fig. 39c).

*Reference*

Trelles, J. O. Cerebral Cysticercosis. World Neurology. 2: 488, 1961.

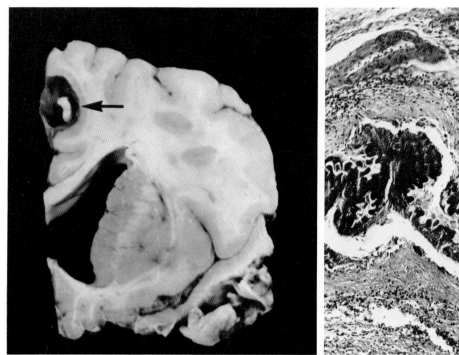

Fig. 39a. Cysticercosis

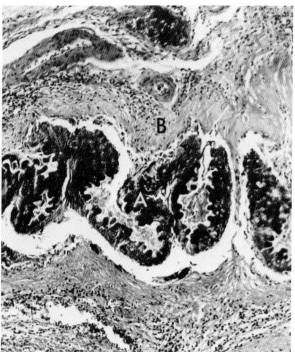

Fig. 39b. HE × 100

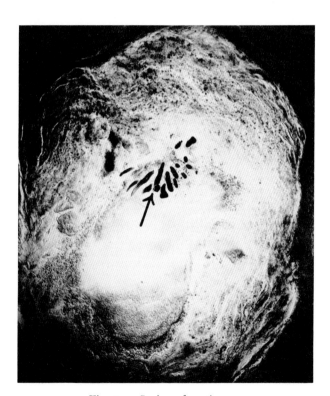

Fig. 39c. Scolex of cysticercus

Toxoplasmosis is an infection caused by the protozoan organism *Toxoplasma gondii*. It is found in all mammals and is transmitted to man by ingestion of uncooked meat. The portal of entry is the mouth inducing a regional lymphadenopathy. The acute generalized infection is caused by hematogenous dissemination producing symptoms of fever, rash, pneumonia, hepatitis, myocarditis, encephalitis and chorioretinitis.

The organism possesses a round or crescentic acidophil cell body with polar chromatin and is about $1-3\,\mu$ in diameter; it is found either extra- or intracellularly. Most frequently it occurs in the form of pseudocysts measuring about $15-30\,\mu$ in diameter. The diagnosis is based on a positive Sabin-Feldman antibody dye test.

The disorder occurs in two forms: acquired and congenital.

The *acquired* form is rare and tends to occur in individuals whose immunologic competence has been compromised such as in cases of malignant lymphoma or with the use of immunosuppressive drugs.

Pathologically, the lesions are more apt to be miliary glial nodules than large granulomas.

*Case:* A 46-year-old woman was admitted to a hospital with a seven weeks' history of severe upper respiratory infection and heavy menses. On admission pancytopenia was discovered. She was treated with Penicillin, Testosterone, Prednisone, Keflin, and several blood transfusions. Later scattered petechiae on the skin and jaundice developed. There were bilateral rales and liver and spleen were palpable 4–5 cm below the costal margin. EKG became abnormal; a mural biopsy revealed inflammatory reaction by lymphocytes and plasma cells. On the fourth hospital day, the patient exhibited choreiform movements; later developed seizures, became comatose and expired approximately a week following admission.

General autopsy revealed disseminated toxoplasmosis of lymph nodes, bone marrow, liver, and spleen. The brain showed no evidence of gross lesions. Microscopically, there were countless miliary glial nodules (Fig. 40a) consisting of pleomorphic microglial cells in the midst of which were scattered pseudocysts of toxoplasma organisms (Fig. 40b).

The *congenital* form is by far the more common. It is transmitted transplacentally from mothers who have a subclinical infection, generally during the second trimester of pregnancy. As a result there is no gross malformation of the brain (by contrast with the condition of cytomegalic inclusion encephalitis).

Pathologically, the gross appearance is one of focal discrete, yellowish and soft granulomas of variable size that are widely disseminated throughout the brain, most commonly in the vicinity of the meninges and ventricles (Fig. 40c).

Microscopically, the granulomas containing the pseudocysts consist of necrotic centers surrounded by epithelioid cells, lymphocytes, plasma cells, and occasional eosinophils but without giant cells; early calcification is a feature (Fig. 40d); the pseudocysts are scattered throughout the inflammatory zones (Fig. 40e).

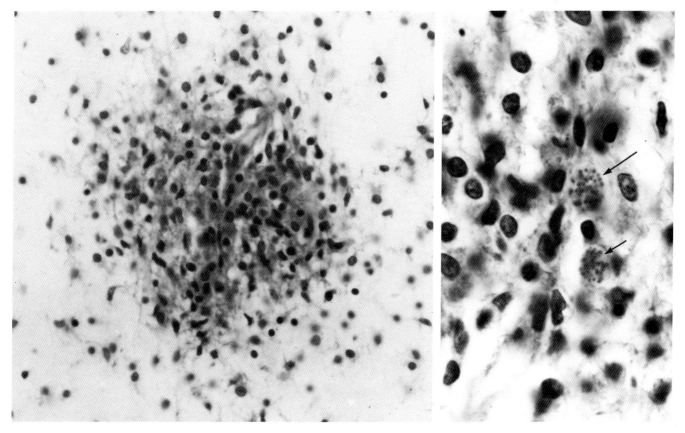

Fig. 40a. HE × 560                    Fig. 40b. HE × 900

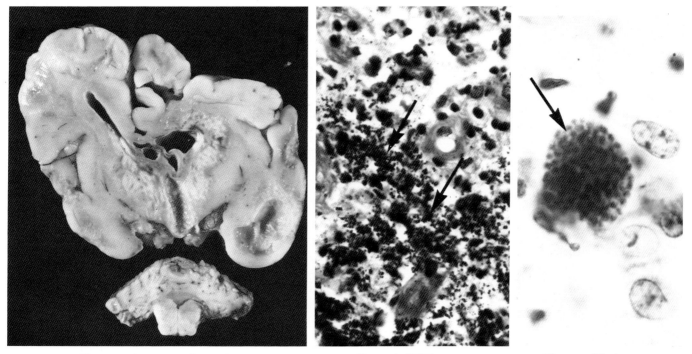

Fig. 40c. Acute toxoplasmosis        Fig. 40d. HVG × 300        Fig. 40e. Nissl × 1400

Toxoplasmosis may persist in a chronic progressive form. Therapy with sulfonamides or other drugs may reverse the changes in the cerebrospinal fluid but the neurologic sequelae of hydrocephalus, microcephaly, visual impairment, psychomotor retardation and intracranial calcification remain.

*Case:* A female infant had a normal birth and early development. At the age of eight weeks she developed fever, edema of the retina and optic disk, right facial palsy, ptosis of the left eyelid, and later acute chorioretinitis. The fever subsided under treatment with sulfonamides and streptomycin. At the age of four months she suffered a relapse. At this time white patches associated with black pigment were noted in the macular region. The spinal fluid contained 20–80 white cells/cmm, at first polymorphonuclear leucocytes, later lymphocytes; the total protein was 113 mg per 100 cc. With continued sulfonamide treatment the spinal fluid became normal at the age of 10 months. At this time intracerebral calcification was demonstrated by X-rays. Complement fixation studies on the blood serum were positive for toxoplasma in both the patient and her mother. The child's further course was one of progressive deterioration, and was characterized by blindness, idiocy, convulsions, spasticity of legs, left facial paresis, and microcephaly. The antibody dye test titer to toxoplasmosis continued to be elevated on repeated testing. The condition terminated at the age of seven years in marked disturbances of temperature regulation, the temperature before death dropping to 92° F.

The brain weighed 780 grams. It was small but well developed and showed focal areas of necrosis (A), granular opacity of the leptomeninges (B) and ependyma (C), atrophy of the optic nerves (D), corpus callosum (E), and cerebellum (F), and hydrocephalus ex vacuo (G) (Fig. 41a).

On section, focal areas of cortical atrophy were found, particularly in troughs of sulci (A); there were cysts in the lenticular area (B) and substantia nigra (C) (Fig. 41b).

Microscopically, the lesions were characterized by replacement of the parenchyma by either gliosis or cyst formation in which large amounts of calcium were deposited (Fig. 41c). The calcium appeared to be encrusted on colonies of toxoplasma organisms in addition to being deposited on surviving neurons and reactive macrophages. Scattered lymphocytes in the meninges and glial nodules in the nervous tissue suggested a still smouldering infection.

*Reference*

Wolf, A. and D. Cowen. Granulomatous Encephalomyelitis Due to Encephalitozoon. Bull. New York Neurol. Inst. 6: 306, 1937.
Nelson, T. L. Active Infantile Toxoplasmosis. J. Pediatrics, 35: 378–380 (Sept.) 1949.

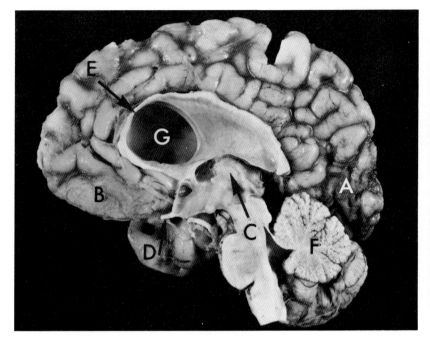

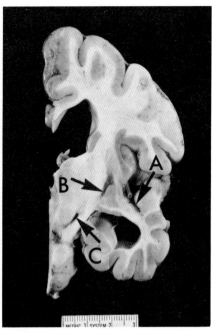

Fig. 41a. Chronic toxoplasmosis

Fig. 41b. Chronic toxoplasmosis

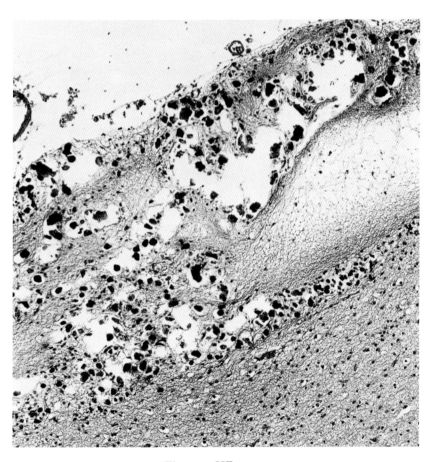

Fig. 41c. HE × 200

Infections of the nervous system caused by filterable viruses comprise a great variety of disorders caused by different infective agents that determine their epidemiologic and cultural characteristics and to a lesser degree their neurotropic, clinical, and pathologic manifestations.

They may be classified into a) those caused by RNA viruses, viz., enterovirus, arbovirus, rabies virus, and myxovirus; and b) those caused by DNA viruses, viz., herpes virus, cytomegalovirus and papova viruses. The diagnosis depends on serologic methods of demonstrating rising titers of specific immune antibodies and on isolation of the virus by animal inoculation or tissue culture.

Clinically, a variety of syndromes occurs, differing with the anatomic distribution of the lesions, particularly in their sequelae. The changes in the cerebrospinal fluid are usually characterized by moderate pleocytosis and elevated protein but normal sugars and chlorides.

Pathologically, the most common characteristics are predominance of inflammation in gray matter (although in some the white matter may also be involved), perivascular cuffing and meningeal infiltrates predominantly with lymphocytes, proliferation of microglia especially in the form of glial nodules and in some, intranuclear or intracytoplasmic inclusion bodies, regarded as virus particles.

### ENTEROVIRUS INFECTIONS

The virus of *poliomyelitis* is the most important of the enteroviruses, whose port of entry is by way of the upper alimentary tract whence it usually spreads along peripheral nerve fibers to invade the central nervous system.

Pathologically, the initial changes take place in nerve cells, largely the motor neurons, that show nonspecific degeneration and type B intranuclear inclusions. These are followed by inflammatory reaction, at the beginning by polys and later by microglia that surround the necrotic neurons (neuronophagia), accompanied by perivascular cuffing of lymphocytes. The distribution of the lesions is fairly constant, primarily in the anterior horns of the spinal cord, the tegmentum of the brain stem, the hypothalamus, and the motor cortex.

> *Case:* A 6-year-old boy developed, five days before admission to a hospital, headaches, malaise, a change in voice, vomiting, difficulty in swallowing, and pains in his legs and neck. On admission he had a slightly elevated temperature. He had a weak cough and a nasal twang to his voice. Gag reflex was diminished. Although there was no muscle weakness, the deep reflexes were hypoactive to absent. The spinal fluid was under a pressure of 90 mm $H_2O$ and contained 132 white cells/cmm, of which 72% were polymorphonuclear leucocytes and 28% lymphocytes. He followed a downhill course with increasing fever, inability to swallow and cough, and development of a right facial weakness. He died seven days after the onset of his symptoms The clinical diagnosis was bulbar poliomyelitis.

The spinal cord, at various levels, showed inflammatory and degenerative changes that were most intense in the anterior horns (Fig. 42a), manifested by neuronophagia (A), perivascular cuffing (B) and diffuse microglial proliferation (Fig. 42b). Similar changes were observed in the tegmentum of the medulla, particularly in the motor nuclei of cranial nerves and reticular formation (Fig. 42c), the tegmentum of the pons, the region of the oculomotor nuclei and substantia nigra of the midbrain, the dentate nucleus of the cerebellum, the hypothalamus, globus pallidus, and the Betz cell layer of the motor cortex (Fig. 42d).

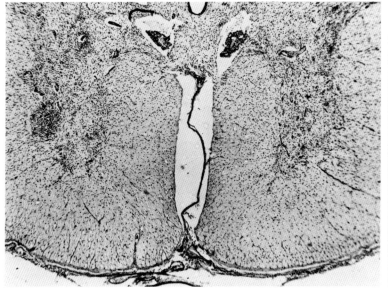

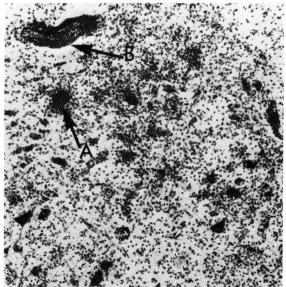

Fig. 42a. Nissl × 32

Fig. 42b. Nissl × 100

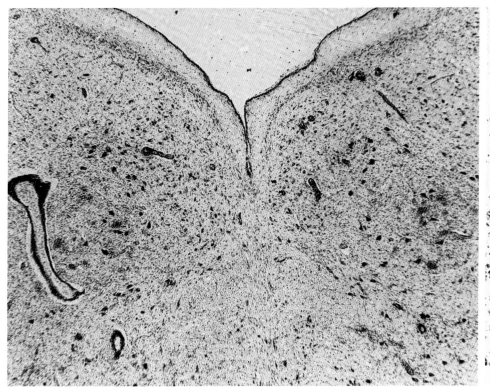

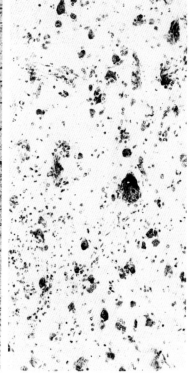

Fig. 42c. Nissl × 45

Fig. 42d. Nissl × 200

Arthropod-borne viruses occur throughout the world in a great variety of forms that have in common transmission by mosquitoes or tics, an intermediate vector such as mammals and birds, seasonal occurrence, similarity in appearance, though differing antigenically, and antibody production during convalescence.

The most common forms of encephalitis caused by arboviruses are St. Louis, Japanese B, and Eastern and Western equine encephalitis.

## St. Louis Encephalitis

Following the epidemics in the 1930s, St. Louis Encephalitis has been sporadic; it is endemic in the Central Valley of California and Texas. It is transmitted by mosquitoes; nestling birds form the reservoir. It occurs at all ages, has a low mortality rate and rare sequelae.

Pathologically, the lesions show the characteristic histologic features of viral infection, with predilection for the tegmentum of the pons and medulla (Fig. 43a), the substantia nigra of the midbrain (Fig. 43b), the basal ganglia, hypothalamus, and the cerebellum (Fig. 43c).

## Japanese (B) Encephalitis

Epidemics of Japanese encephalitis have occurred periodically in Japan and throughout Asia. It is transmitted by mosquitoes and the infection is carried by birds. It occurs at all ages, the mortality is high and the sequelae are common, consisting of mental changes, seizures and motor impairment.

Pathologically, the acute lesions show variations from nodules of hematogenous mononuclear and microglial cells, neuronophagias and perivascular cuffing to foci of rarefaction necrosis with or without vascular relationship. In chronic stages, cysts and focal calcification have been reported.

*Case:* A 22-year-old soldier was admitted to a hospital in Vietnam on October 10, 1971 because he developed fever, stiff neck, and headaches on the previous day. The cerebrospinal fluid contained 1,000 polymorphonuclear leucocytes per cmm, a total protein of 110 mg % and sugar of 80 mg %, but smears and cultures were negative for bacteria. He was treated with various antibiotics. Over the next two weeks his temperature remained at 104–105° F. He showed increasing mental confusion and inappropriate behavior. Repeated lumbar punctures revealed decreasing leucocytes but increasing pressures to 400 mm. of water. Titers of 1:5120 for Japanese B encephalitis were determined. He later developed anisocoria, paresis of the right arm, semicoma and bilateral ankle clonus. He expired of bronchopneumonia six weeks following the onset of symptoms.

Grossly, the brain was edematous and showed scattered petechial hemorrhages.

Microscopically, the cerebral white matter contained large microglial nodules (Fig. 43d). Some lesions were perivascular foci of necrosis containing macrophages, surrounded by rarefaction (Fig. 43e) while others were perivascular hemorrhages. In the gray matter, the changes were milder, more diffuse and consisted of scattered perivascular lymphocytes, dropout of neurons, and diffuse proliferation of microglia.

*Reference*

Zimmerman, H. M. The Pathology of Japanese B Encephalitis. Am. J. Path. 22: 965, 1946.

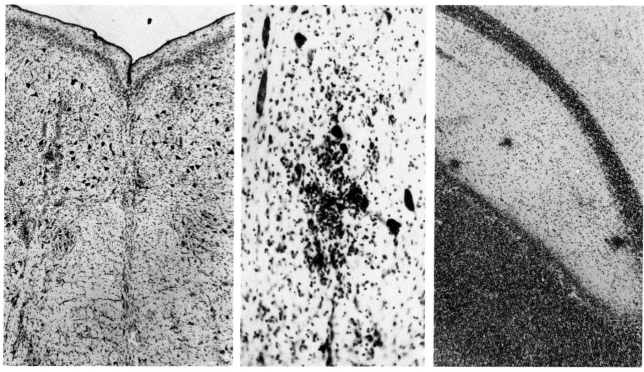

Fig. 43a. Nissl × 35          Fig. 43b. Nissl × 125          Fig. 43c. Nissl × 32

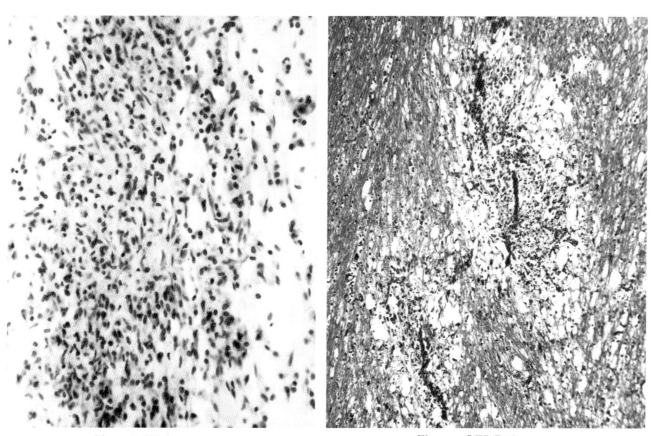

Fig. 43d. Nissl × 250          Fig. 43e. LFB-PAS × 100

## Equine Encephalitis

There are two forms of equine encephalitis, Eastern and Western, both being transmitted to horses and humans by mosquitoes with wild birds serving as the primary reservoir hosts. Both have occurred in epidemic form, the Eastern variety being much the more severe with a greater mortality rate.

The Western form is endemic in the Central Valley of California. It has a predilection for infants and although the mortality rate is relatively low, it often leaves severe residua of cerebral palsy and mental retardation.

The pathology in the acute phase resembles that of Japanese B encephalitis, the lesions varying from foci of rarefaction necrosis to perivascular cuffing with lymphocytes and glial nodules, distributed in basal ganglia, cortex, brain stem, and cerebellum. The white matter is least involved and vascular changes are usually absent, however some have reported extensive damage to white matter with prominent vascular lesions, such findings being especially pronounced in chronic stages.

*Case:* A 5-year-old boy had a normal birth and early development until the onset at the age of one month of an acute illness at a time when an epidemic of Western equine encephalitis was occurring in the Central Valley of California, where he was born. The symptoms were characterized by irritability, fever, and episodes of decerebrate rigidity. When admitted to a hospital, he was semicomatose. The cerebrospinal fluid contained 270 white blood cells with 46% polys and 54% lymphocytes per cmm; the total protein was 150 mg %, but there was no growth on culture. Serologic studies against the virus of Western equine encephalitis were positive with the complement fixation test showing a rise in titer from 400 $LD_{50}$ to 5,000 $LD_{50}$ in the course of about a month. As the acute phase subsided, the patient began showing signs of arrested mental and motor development. His I.Q. was estimated at 40. Neurologically, he showed a scissor-like gait, poor coordination, hyperactive reflexes, failure of speech development and occasional seizures. He was admitted to a State hospital for the retarded where he died at the age of five years.

The brain weighed 815 grams and showed on section scattered areas of cortical atrophy and cysts (Fig. 44a).

Microscopically, the most severe lesions were characterized by demyelination (Fig. 44b) and gliosis (Fig. 44c) with cyst formation, that had their predilection in the cortex about the troughs of sulci and in the underlying white matter. Similar foci were encountered in subcortical regions such as the thalamus and substantia nigra. Many of the lesions contained large amounts of calcium salts (Fig. 44d), as well as disseminated perivascular cuffing and glial nodules (Fig. 44e) indicative of persistent viral activity. In addition there were mild diffuse changes of neuronal dropout and microglial and astroglial proliferation.

*References*

Finley, K. H. and A. C. Hollister. Western Equine and St. Louis Encephalomyelitis: the Distribution and Histological Nature of CNS Lesions. Calif. Med. 74: 225, 1951.
Herzon, H., J. T. Shelton, and H. B. Bruyn. Sequelae of Western Equine and Other Arthropod-borne Encephalitides. Neurology. 7: 535, 1957.
Noran, H. H. and A. B. Baker. Western Equine Encephalitis. J. Neuropath. and Expt. Neurol. 4: 269, 1945.

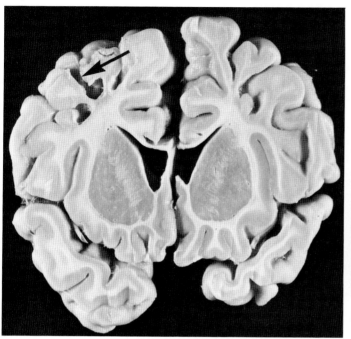

Fig. 44a. Chronic Western equine encephalitis

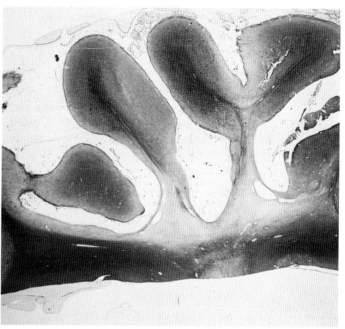

Fig. 44b. Weil stain

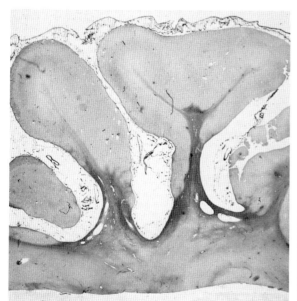

Fig. 44c. Holzer stain

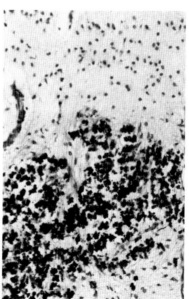

Fig. 44d. Nissl × 125

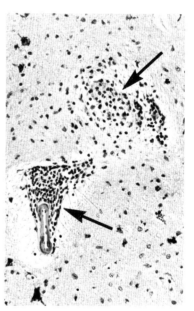

Fig. 44e. Nissl × 170

## Lethargic Encephalitis (of von Economo)

Lethargic encephalitis was first reported by von Economo in the period around World War I when it occurred in association with epidemics of influenza. Since then sporadic cases in decreasing incidence have been observed. A virus etiology has been assumed from its pathologic findings but has never been proven.

Clinically, the disorder is especially noteworthy for its tendency to occur in a chronic form, usually after a free interval following the acute illness, giving rise to a great variety of psychiatric and neurologic syndromes especially of behavior disorder, inversion of sleep rhythm, oculogyric crises, and Parkinsonism.

Pathologically, the acute stages resemble those of St. Louis encephalitis with disseminated perivascular cuffing and glial nodules and predilection for the brain stem, especially the substantia nigra, and basal ganglia, however, with virtually no involvement of the cortex and the cerebellum. In its chronic stage, the disease is restricted to the midbrain, involving exclusively the substantia nigra and the periaqueductal region. Here the neurons are greatly diminished and replaced by gliosis, at times accompanied by low grade inflammatory reaction. A feature of the chronic stage is the consistent finding of neurofibrillary tangles of Alzheimer in the affected areas.

*Case:* A 42-year-old man developed in 1915, at the age of three years an attack of influenza, a few years following which, increasing disturbance in behavior became apparent. He began running away from school and home; slept a lot and was finally committed to a State school because of delinquent behavior. Later he complained that people were talking about him, saying "his eyes were going up and down." At age twenty-two, he was admitted to a State hospital because he was thought to show symptoms of schizophrenia; however, neurologic examination revealed dysarthria, anisocoria, with the right pupil being larger than the left, and poor reaction of both pupils. At the age of thirty-six, it was noted that he was dragging his right leg and walking stiff-legged, spoke indistinctly, tended to fix his eyes on something above his head for long periods of time, and slept all day and was awake during the night. Tremor of hands, lips, and eyelids, masked facies and drooling then developed. At this time, a diagnosis of postencephalitic Parkinsonism was made, and he was started on Artane with some improvement. During the following four years he had an occasional seizure, during one of which he died.

Grossly, the brain appeared normal with the exception of distinct bilateral depigmentation of the substantia nigra (Fig. 45a) as compared with the normal appearance of this region (Fig. 45b).

Microscopically, bilateral dense gliosis replaced the degenerated substantia nigra and the periaqueductal region, including the area of the oculomotor nuclei (Fig. 45c). The compact layer of the substantia nigra showed a marked reduction of the melanin-bearing nerve cells accompanied by proliferation of glial nuclei but without distinct inflammatory reaction (Fig. 45d). Scattered argentophilic neurofibrillary tangles were seen in both the nigral and oculomotor regions (Fig. 45e).

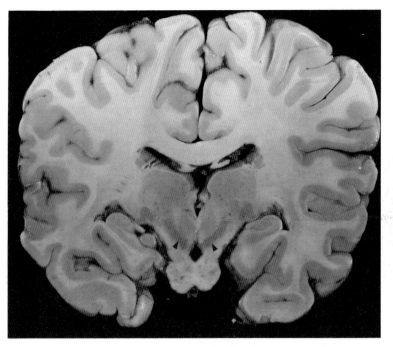

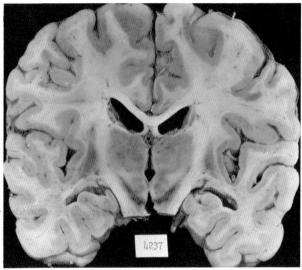

Fig. 45b. Normal substantia nigra

Fig. 45a. Chronic lethargic encephalitis (depigmentation of substantia nigra)

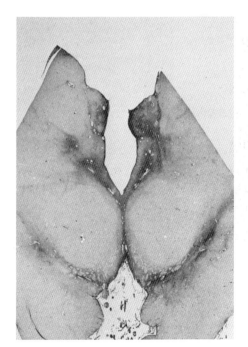

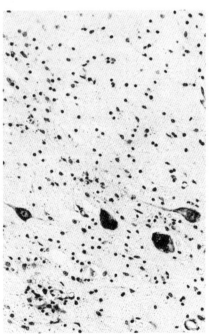

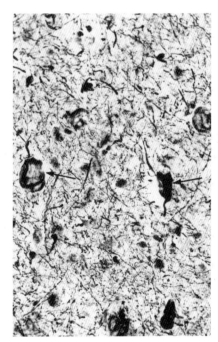

Fig. 45c. Holzer stain

Fig. 45d. Nissl × 130

Fig. 45e. von Braunmühl × 280

## Herpes Simplex Encephalitis

Infection by herpes simplex virus is transmitted by direct or indirect contact with secretions from conjunctiva, saliva, skin and genital mucosa. In the majority of humans, infection occurs in early life, followed by a latent state in which circulating antibodies are found, when it may become overt by a variety of precipitating factors. Herpes simplex encephalitis however is regarded as a primary infection. It occurs at all ages. Until recently it has been considered to be invariably fatal, however, increasingly cases showing recovery, with or without sequelae, have been reported.

Clinically, the onset is acute, characterized by fever, meningeal signs, anosmia, seizures, prominent mental signs and alterations in consciousness. The cerebrospinal fluid shows pleocytosis and raised total protein. Diagnosis is based on fourfold rise in serum antibodies, fluorescent antibody staining of specific antigen, demonstration of intranuclear inclusions by biopsy and, above all, by isolation of the virus from the brain.

Pathologically, the pathognomonic findings are a) an acute necrotizing hemorrhagic encephalitis, located predominantly in limbic structures of the temporal lobes and orbito-frontal regions with limited extension into adjacent structures; it is usually bilateral but at times unilateral when it gives rise to symptoms of a space-occupying lesion; and b) intranuclear inclusions of Cowdry's type A in nerve cells and in oligodendroglia. In some cases of necrotizing encephalitis, inclusions have not been found and their classification with herpes simplex encephalitis has remained controversial.

*Case:* A 25-year-old woman developed an acute illness, characterized by headaches, a temperature of 104.6° F., nausea, vomiting, and mental confusion. She was admitted to a hospital where examination of the cerebrospinal fluid showed a cell count of 686 with 96% mononuclears per cmm, a total protein, varying from 60 to 155 mg%; sugar of 45 mg%; and chlorides of 118 mEq. There were no organisms demonstrated on smears, and cultures were negative. The single serum herpes titer was 1:16, interpreted as inconclusive. The patient expired ten days after the onset of the illness. At autopsy, herpes simplex virus was isolated from the brain and by fluorescent antibody techniques.

The brain showed acute necrosis of both temporal lobes and adjacent insula, in which there were scattered petechial hemorrhages that became diffuse in the adjacent subarachnoid spaces, especially of the Sylvian fissure (Fig. 46a).

Microscopically, the leptomeninges and perivascular spaces within the cortex were infiltrated with lymphocytes and plasma cells while the cytoarchitecture of the cortex was completely destroyed and replaced by countless macrophages and sparse astrocytes (Fig. 46b). In the vicinity of the necrotic areas were scattered neurons and oligodendroglia with granular to homogeneous intranuclear eosinophilic inclusions, surrounded by halos and marginated chromatin near the nuclear membrane (Fig. 46c). Electron microscopic study revealed intranuclear particles, approximately 900–1000 Å wide, containing either empty or dense cores, the latter about 300–400 Å in diameter; there was evagination and duplication of the nuclear membrane (Fig. 46d).

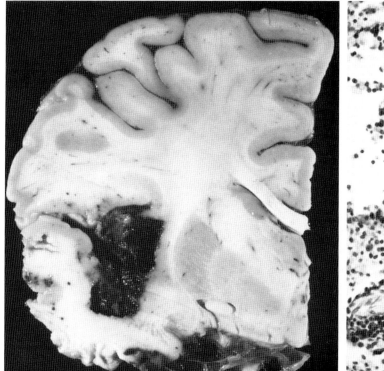

Fig. 46a. Acute herpes simplex encephalitis

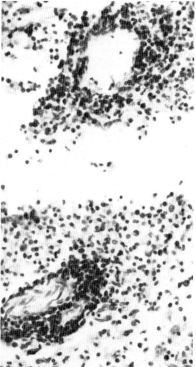

Fig. 46b. Nissl × 175

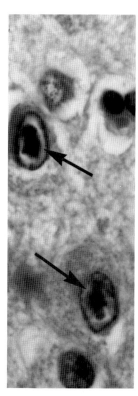

Fig. 46c. Lendrum
× 560

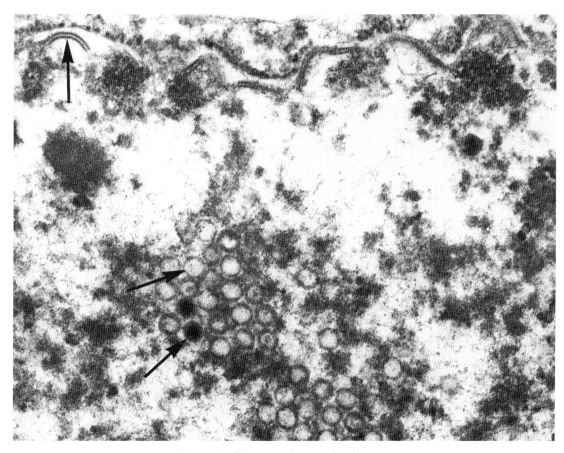

Fig. 46d. Electron micrograph × 60,000

## Herpes Simplex Encephalitis (continued)

The pathology of the chronic stage in herpes simplex encephalitis has seldom been reported. The following case is of special interest because of the clinical picture suggestive of a Klüver-Bucy syndrome, produced by the characteristic location of the lesions in limbic structures of the temporal lobe.

*Case:* A 60-year-old male school teacher developed vertigo, headaches, and nausea, and when admitted to a hospital four days later, was noted to have a temperature of 108° F., disorientation, dysphasia, nystagmus, and twitching facial movements. A lumbar puncture revealed an elevated pressure, 200 cells per cmm, mostly lymphocytes, a total protein of 200 mg %, normal sugar and chlorides, and negative cultures of bacteria and fungi. Patient remained febrile and stuporous during the next two weeks, receiving Penicillin and Dilantin empirically. Repeated lumbar punctures continued to show pleocytosis and elevated protein. Complement fixation titers for herpes simplex were reported to have risen from 1:16 on acute phase serum to 1:128 after two weeks. He gradually became afebrile but remained markedly confused and dysphasic. He was committed to a State mental hospital where he was reported to be combative and exhibited "oral tendencies," eating anything "which he could get his hands on" so that he developed repeated attacks of gastritis. He expired of bronchopneumonia approximately two years after the onset of his symptoms.

The brain showed bilaterally symmetrical cystic necrosis of the temporal lobes with the exception of the superior temporal gyri (Fig. 47a).

Microscopically, the lesions showed necrosis in a chronic stage with subpial astrogliosis and cystic transformation of the remaining gray matter in which sparse glial and collagenous fibers were interspersed with macrophages, astrocytes and lymphocytes (Fig. 47b). In adjacent areas, rare intranuclear inclusion bodies within degenerating nerve cells (Fig. 47c) attested to persistence of the specific infection.

*References*

Baringer, J. R., and J. F. Griffith. Experimental Herpes Simplex Encephalitis: Early Neuropathologic Changes. J. Neuropath. and Expt. Neurol. 29: 89, 1968.

Chou, S. M., and J. D. Cherry. Ultrastructure of Cowdry Type A Inclusions. I. In Human Herpes Simplex Encephalitis. Neurology 17: 575, 1967.

Drachman, D. A., and R. D. Adams. Herpes Simplex Encephalitis and Acute Inclusion Body Encephalitis. Arch. Neurol. Psychiat. 7: 45, 1962.

Haymaker, W. Herpes Simplex Encephalitis in Man. J. Neuropath. and Expt. Neurol. 8: 132, 1949.

Itabashi, H. H., D. M. Bass, and J. R. McCulloch. Inclusion Body of Acute Inclusion Encephalitis. Arch. Neurol. 14: 493, 1966.

Leestma, J. E., M. B. Bornstein, R. D. Sheppard, and L. A. Feldman. Ultrastructural Aspects of Herpes Simplex Virus Infection in Organized Cultures of Mammalian Nervous Tissue. Lab. Invest. 20: 70, 1969.

Morecki, R., and N. H. Becker. Human Herpes Virus Infection. Its Fine Structure Identification in Paraffin-embedded Tissue. Arch. Path. 86: 292, 1968.

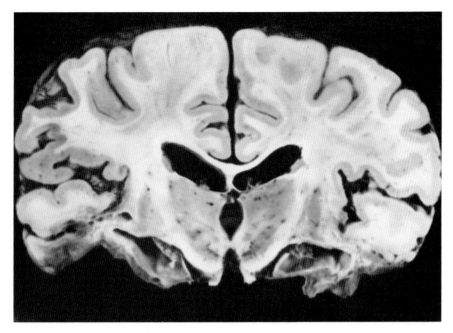

Fig. 47a. Chronic herpes simplex encephalitis

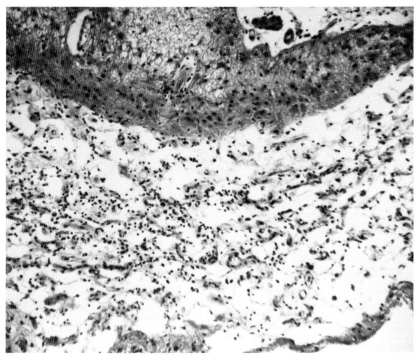

Fig. 47b. HE × 100

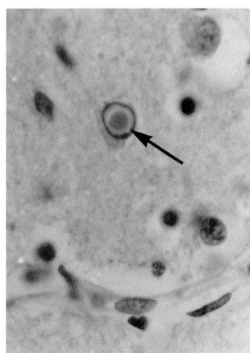

Fig. 47c. HE × 800

## Cytomegalic Inclusion Disease (CID)

CID, a disease caused by cytomegalo- or salivary gland virus, is primarily a disease of the newborn that is acquired in utero. It has also been found on occasion in patients suffering from debilitating diseases and in the presence of immunosuppression.

In the fetus, it is transmitted through the placenta and causes generalized visceral infection, with the central nervous system being involved in about 10% of the cases.

The clinical manifestations are jaundice, hepatosplenomegaly, purpura of skin due to erythroblastemia and thrombocytopenia, chorioretinitis and evidence of cerebral involvement manifested by seizures, hydrocephalus, microcephaly and intracranial calcification. As such it bears a resemblance to congenital toxoplasmosis. Diagnosis is based on demonstration of cytomegaly in desquamated epithelial cells of renal tubules in the urine, the presence of specific antibodies in the blood of infant and mother and recovery of virus.

The pathologic changes in the central nervous system are a complex combination of malformations and of active and healed inflammation. It is assumed from the nature of the anomalies that the infection attacks the fetus during the third or fourth month of pregnancy (thus distinguishing it from toxoplasmosis). As such it is one of the most significant examples of a teratogenic agent acting on the nervous system.

Histologically, it is characterized by disseminated calcifying encephalitis with predilection for periventricular tissues, with variations from granulomas to microglial nodules and perivascular cuffing with lymphocytes. The pathognomonic feature is the presence of cytomegaly with intranuclear and intracytoplasmic inclusions of type A, in various glial, neuronal, endothelial and meningeal cells.

> *Case 1:* A 6-week-old, white male was admitted to a hospital with a history that he was the product of a full-term, normal pregnancy and was one of fraternal non-identical twins (twin was normal). It was a breech presentation and he weighed 3 lb and 3 oz. The head measured 26 cm in circumference. Oxygen administration was required at birth and soon after he was noted to be twitching, to be irritable, difficult to feed, and having respiratory difficulties. On admission, he weighed 5 lb. Head circumference was 28 cm; anterior fontanelle was small and the sutures appeared "rigid." Liver and spleen were enlarged. Neurologically, he was restless, with a high pitched, weak cry, and with hyperactive deep tendon reflexes. The blood contained 4,060,000 R.B.C., a hemoglobin of 11.8 and 17,450 W.B.C. The clinical course was progressively downhill, leading to his ultimate demise.

Grossly, the brain was abnormally small, weighing 70 gms. and showed widespread anomalies in the form of micropolygyria, arhinencephaly, granular ependymitis and periventricular calcification.

Microscopically, widespread active inflammation in the form of infiltrations of meninges and perivascular spaces with lymphocytes was associated with anomalous development of the cerebral cortex showing a pattern of micropolygyria (Fig. 48a). The cerebral white matter and especially the subependymal tissue were inundated with lymphocytes, plasma cells, macrophages, and large amounts of calcific deposits (Fig. 48b). There were numerous large cells with intranuclear inclusions that stained with hematoxylin-eosin and Feulgen methods and fewer intracytoplasmic granular inclusions that did not stain with the Feulgen method (Fig. 48c).

Similar inclusions were found in kidneys, lungs, and pancreas.

Electron microscopic study of a nuclear inclusion body showed virions, approximately 1400 Å wide, some with empty or dense cores and others with inner circles (Fig. 48d).

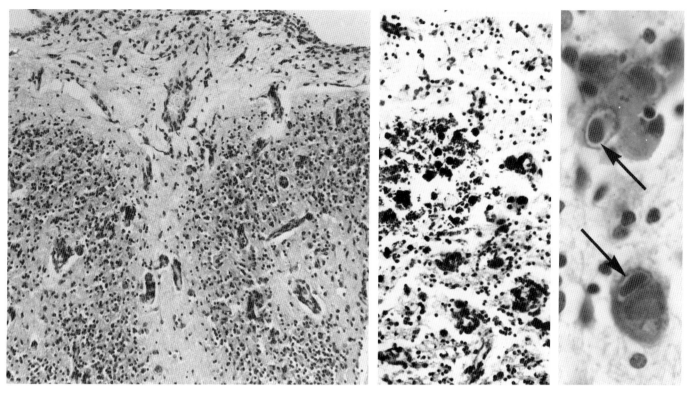

Fig. 48a. Nissl × 130          Fig. 48b. Nissl × 225          Fig. 48c. HE × 720

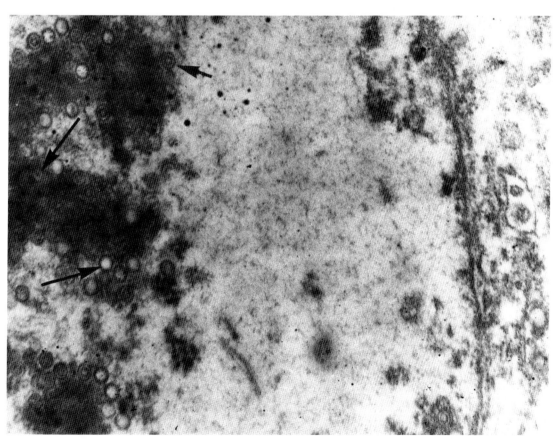

Fig. 48d. Electron micrograph × 30,000

## Cytomegalic Inclusion Disease (CID) (continued)

In the majority of cases, CID proves fatal, however, in those that survive, characteristic pathologic residua are observed in the form of gross malformations and calcification of the brain, as illustrated in the following:

*Case 2:* A white male child was a 4-pound product of a thirty-six-week gestation complicated by an attack of severe "flu" during the fourth month of pregnancy and intermittent vaginal bleeding through the seventh month. Delivery was precipitous. A purpuric rash and jaundice were noted in the first day of life. There was hepatosplenomegaly and thrombocytopenia. The head was small and showed intracranial calcifications. The cerebrospinal fluid contained 9 cells/cmm and 180 mg% of total protein. A diagnosis of cytomegalic inclusion disease was confirmed by finding the characteristic cytomegaly in the urinary sediment. Reexamination at seven weeks of age revealed microcephaly with head circumference of 27.7 cm; lesions of chorioretinitis, jaundice, and hepatosplenomegaly; a bilirubin of 2.2 mg%; a PCV of 32% and W.B.C. of 24,000; urine contained W.B.C. Readmitted to a hospital at the age of two years, he showed deafness, bilateral optic atrophy, and spastic quadriplegia. Liver and spleen at this time were only slightly enlarged. EEG disclosed a left temporo-occipital focus of slow spiking waves. He was subject to fever and respiratory distress. Towards the end he had a grand mal convulsion and expired at the age of two years and eight months.

The brain was extremely small, weighing 320 gms, and showed diffuse micropolygyria, large ventricles, absence of septum pellucidum, minute subependymal heterotopia and calcific deposits, and hypoplasia of left cerebellar hemisphere, of right inferior olivary nucleus and of both medullary pyramids (Fig. 49a).

Microscopically, a typical pattern of micropolygyria with rudimentary sulci and two to three layered cortex, was noted (Fig. 49b). There were deposits of calcium associated with gliosis at the site of the cerebellar hypoplasia (Fig. 49c) and in the walls of the lateral ventricles (Fig. 49d).

*References*

Diezel, P. B. Mikrogyrie infolge cerebraler Speicheldrüsen Virusinfektion im Rahmen generalisierter Cytomegalie be einem Säugling. Virchow's Archiv. 325: 109, 1954.

Haymaker, W., B. R. Girdany, J. Stephans, and R. D. Lillie. Cerebral Involvement with Advanced Periventricular Calcification in Generalized Cytomegalic Inclusion Disease in the Newborn. J. Neuropath. and Expt. Neurol. 13: 562, 1954.

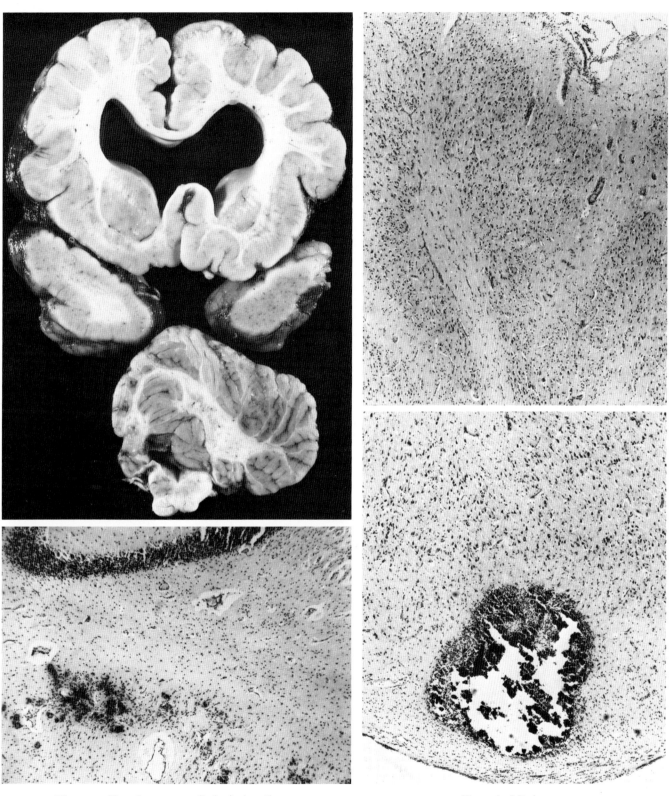

Fig. 49a. Chronic cytomegalic inclusion disease
Fig. 49c. Nissl × 50

Fig. 49b. Nissl × 10
Fig. 49d. Nissl × 50

### Subacute Sclerosing Panencephalitis (SSPE)

SSPE is a disorder that was previously described as inclusion encephalitis by Dawson, as subacute sclerosing leukoencephalitis by Van Bogaert, and, probably, also, as panencephalitis by Pette and Döring.

The disease involves primarily children and adolescents, rarely adults. It has an insidious onset and a subacute to chronic clinical course, varying from several months to many years. The symptoms are progressive, consisting of prominent mental changes, seizures, myoclonus, dyskinesias, spasticity, retinitis, optic atrophy and macular degeneration. The cerebrospinal fluid contains increased gamma globulins in the absence of pleocytosis. The EEG shows a characteristic pattern of episodic rhythmic paroxysmal slow-wave discharges. Diagnosis can be made by demonstration of intranuclear inclusions in a cortical biopsy. Although a specific virus has not been isolated, recent investigations have incriminated measles virus as the probable etiologic agent by the demonstration of elevated levels of measles antibodies in the blood stream and cerebrospinal fluid and by immunofluorescence of the antigen in neurons and glia.

Pathologically, subacute to chronic diffuse inflammatory changes occur in the form of perivascular cuffing with lymphocytes and plasma cells and of microglia, as rod cells and glial nodules. These are equally present in cerebral gray and white matter with varying intensity, resulting in either degeneration of gray matter and/or demyelination and gliosis of white matter. There are less marked changes in subcortical areas, the condition decreasing rostro-caudally. The specific feature is the presence of intranuclear eosinophilic inclusions of type A in nerve cells and oligodendroglia, with less common intracytoplasmic inclusions.

> *Case:* A 10-year-old white girl was in good health until the age of seventeen months when she had a convulsion affecting her left side. Since then she continued to have convulsions for which she received anticonvulsant medication. At the age of three years a cortical biopsy was performed which was diagnostic of inclusion encephalitis. (There was no record of a cerebrospinal fluid examination.) Her further course was one of progressive deterioration, both mentally and neurologically. At the age of seven years she was committed to a State hospital where examination revealed virtually complete unresponsiveness, sluggish pupillary reaction to light, constant roving movements of the eyes, nystagmus on right lateral gaze, and spastic quadriplegia with bilateral ankle clonus and Babinski signs. She expired there of bronchopneumonia at the age of ten years.

The cortical biopsy showed signs of an active and diffuse inflammatory process, characterized by proliferation of countless microglia in the form of rod cells, moderate numbers of hypertrophied astrocytes, perivascular cuffing with lymphocytes and plasma cells, and degeneration and depletion of neurons (Fig. 50a). Numerous intranuclear eosinophilic inclusions of variable size, with or without halos, were found in surviving neurons (Fig. 50b) and oligodendroglia (Fig. 50c).

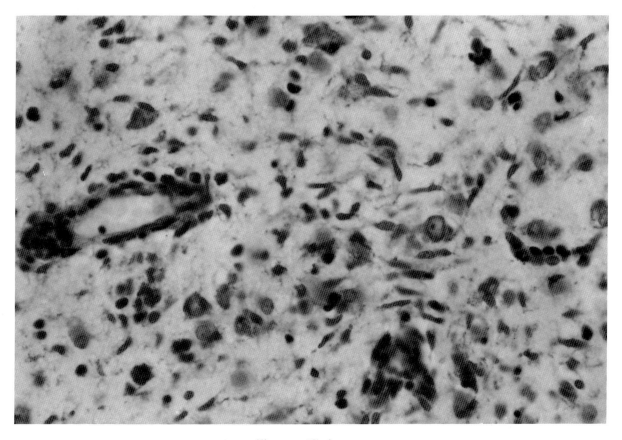

Fig. 50a. Nissl × 300

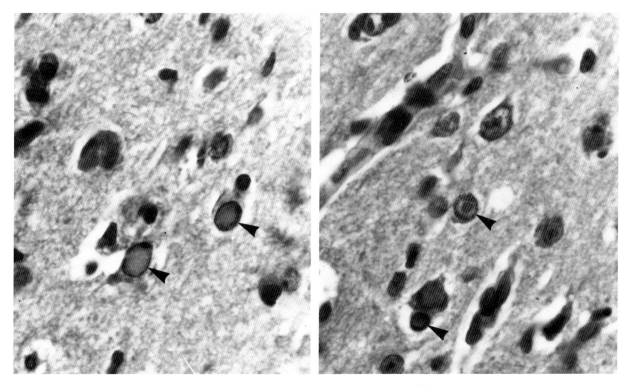

Fig. 50b. HE × 720

Fig. 50c. HE × 900

## Subacute Sclerosing Panencephalitis (SSPE) (continued)

The brain at autopsy was severely atrophied, weighing 750 gms. In coronal sections, there was diffuse atrophy of the gray and white matter, the latter showing demyelination, both in the cerebrum and cerebellum, associated with corresponding dilatation of the sub-arachnoid spaces and ventricles (Fig. 51a).

Microscopically, diffuse loss of neurons without any trace of inflammation indicated a burnt out pathologic process (Fig. 51b). There were neurofibrillary tangles of Alzheimer in surviving neurons (Fig. 51c). The white matter was the site of extensive and diffuse demyelination in which fat-containing lipids were still present (Fig. 51d) but in which a dense gliosis prevailed (Fig. 51e).

*References*

### General Neuropathology

Dawson, J. R. Cellular Inclusions in Cerebral Lesions of Lethargic Encephalitis. Am. J. Path. 9: 7, 1933.
Katz, S. L. and J. F. Griffith. Slow Virus Infections. Hospital Practice. 6: 64, 1971.
Malamud, N., W. Haymaker, and H. Pinkerton. Inclusion Encephalitis. Am. J. Path. 26: 133, 1950.
Van Bogaert, L. Une leuco-encéphalite sclérosante subaigue. J. Neurol. Neurosurg. Psychiat. 8: 101, 1945.

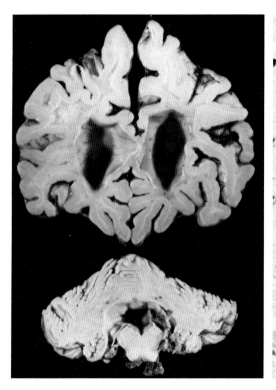

Fig. 51a. Chronic subacute
sclerosing panencephalitis

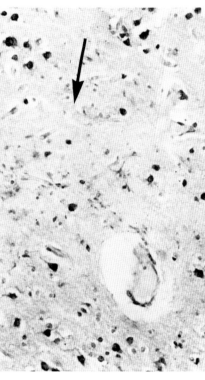

Fig. 51b. Nissl × 125

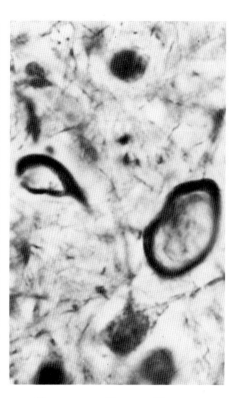

Fig. 51c. von Braunmühl × 400

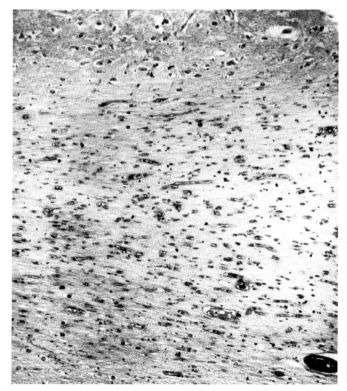

Fig. 51d. LFB-PAS × 100

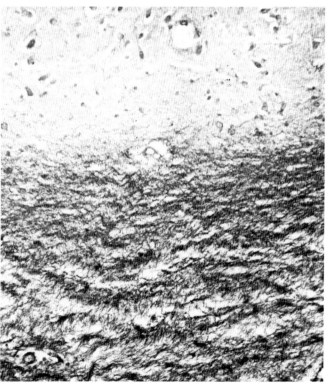

Fig. 51e. Holzer × 125

## Subacute Sclerosing Panencephalitis (SSPE) in Electron Microscopy

In the electron microscope, large intranuclear aggregates of tubules, approximately 150 Å in diameter, are seen in neurons and oligodendroglia (Fig. 52a). In addition, the cytoplasm sometimes contains aggregates of "granular filaments," about 240 Å in diameter. These structures are indistinguishable from measles virus. However, Oyanagi, et al., have demonstrated that despite their morphological identity, SSPE particles and measles particles behave differently when inoculated into cells in culture.

Astrocytic changes are especially pronounced in SSPE. They contain "nuclear bodies" from 2–3$\mu$ in diameter which usually consist of central cores of dense granules, 100–300 Å in diameter, surrounded by a circular network of fine filaments (Fig. 52b). These structures are probably not unique to SSPE, since, apparently, identical structures have been seen in astrocytic nuclei in a variety of conditions, especially viral infections and neoplasms (Popoff and Steward, 1968). In SSPE, however, they are especially widespread and, unlike the tubular inclusions of neurons and oligodendroglia, they are seen in virtually every case reported. The astrocytic cytoplasm also displays the usual reactive changes including pronounced increase of glial filaments and the appearance of dense-cored, membrane-bounded particles, approximately 500–800 Å in diameter (Gonatas, 1966; Gonatas, et al., 1967; Tellez-Nagel and Harter, 1966).

In addition, some affected cells in SSPE may contain filamentous or lattice-like structures in their nuclei. These structures are also nonspecific and have been observed in nuclei in other conditions.

*References*

### Electron Microscopy

Bouteille, M., C. Fontaine, C. Vedrenne, and J. Delarue. Sur un cas d'encephalite Subaigue a Inclusions. Etude Anatomoclinique et Ultrastructurale. Rev. Neurol. 113: 454, 1965.

Gonatas, N. K. Subacute Sclerosing Leucoencephalitis: Electron Microscopic and Cytochemical Observations on a Cerebral Biopsy. J. Neuropath. and Expt. Neurol. 25: 177, 1966.

Gonatas, N. K., J. Martin, and I. Evangelista. The Osmiophilic Particles of Astrocytes. Virus, Lipid Droplets or Products of Secretion? J. Neuropath. and Expt. Neurol. 26: 369, 1967.

Herndon, R. M., and L. J. Rubinstein. Light and Electron Microscopy Observations on the Development of Viral Particles in the Inclusions of Dawson's Encephalitis (Subacute Sclerosing Panencephalitis). Neurology. 18: 8, 1968.

Masurovsky, E. B., H. H. Bentiez, S. U. Kim, and M. R. Murray. Origin, Development, and Nature of Intranuclear Rodlets and Associated Bodies in Chicken Sympathetic Neurons. J. Cell Biol. 44: 172, 1970.

Oyanagi, S., L. Be. Rorke, M. Katz, and H. Koprowski. Histopathology and Electron Microscopy of Three Cases of Subacute Sclerosing Panencephalitis (SSPE). Acta Neuropath. 18: 58, 1971.

Oyanagi, S., V. ter Meulen, M. Katz, and H. Koprowski. Comparison of Subacute Sclerosing Panencephalitis and Measles Viruses: An Electron Microscope Study. J. Virol. 7: 176, 1971.

Popoff, N., and S. Stewart. The Fine Structure of Nuclear Inclusions in the Brain of Experimental Golden Hamsters. J. Ultrastruct. Res. 23: 374, 1968.

Server, J. L., and W. Zeman (ed.). Measles, Virus and Subacute Sclerosing Panencephalitis. Neurol. 18: 1, Part 2, 1968.

Tellez-Nagel, I., and D. H. Harter. Subacute Sclerosing Leukoencephalitis. I. Clinico-pathological, Electron Microscopic and Virological Observations. J. Neuropath and Expt. Neurol. 25: 560, 1966.

ZuRhein, G. M., and S. M. Chou. Subacute Sclerosing Panencephalitis. Ultrastructural Study of a Brain Biopsy. Neurology. 18: 146, 1968.

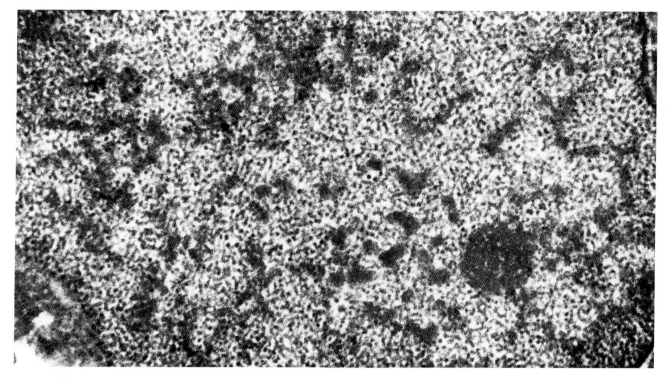

Fig. 52a. An electron micrograph of an intranuclear aggregate of tubules in an affected cell in the brain of a case of subacute sclerosing panencephalitis. This micrograph was prepared from paraffin-embedded, formalin-fixed autopsy material. × 40,000.

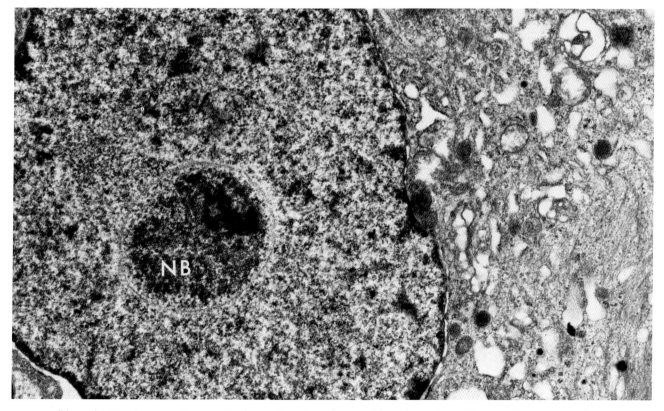

Fig. 52b. An electron micrograph of a nuclear body (NB) within the nucleus of a reactive astrocyte from a biopsy specimen of a case of subacute sclerosing panencephalitis. × 20,000.

# III

## *Demyelinating Disorders*

Demyelinating disorders of the central nervous system may be grouped together on the basis that the fundamental pathologic process is a primary degeneration of myelin, even though their nosologic relationship remains unclear and their clinical and pathologic manifestations differ widely.

They may be classified into: a) acute disseminated or perivenous encephalomyelitis, b) acute hemorrhagic leukoencephalitis, c) neuromyelitis optica, d) multiple sclerosis, and e) diffuse sclerosis (Schilder's disease).

Acute infectious polyneuritis, which is essentially a demyelinative disorder of the peripheral nervous system may be considered as a related disorder.

### Acute Disseminated Encephalomyelitis

Known also as perivenous, post- or parainfectious encephalomyelitis, it is characterized by a remarkably similar pathologic reaction that is evoked by a great variety of precipitating conditions, viz., vaccination (cowpox, antirabies, and typhoid vaccines), exanthematous diseases (rubeola, rubella, variola, varicella), mumps, and influenza.

Clinically, the manifestations are similar to those of encephalitis, however, characteristically they develop during convalescence from the precipitating condition.

Pathologically, the essential features are perivascular (most often perivenous) demyelination (Figs. 53a and b) with relative preservation of axons (Fig. 53c). Reaction occurs by microglia and hematogenous reticuloendothelial cells during the initial phase that progresses in the next stage to formation of sudanophilic macrophages and that regresses ultimately to an end stage of astrogliosis. It is thus at any given time a monophasic disorder. Inflammatory reaction is either minimal or lacking. The white matter and the subendymal and subpial zones are primarily involved, corresponding to venous distribution, with limited extension into adjacent gray matter.

The pathogenesis of acute disseminated encephalomyelitis has been variously interpreted. The most acceptable theory has been that the lesion represents an antigen-antibody reaction, somewhat similar to that of experimental allergic encephalomyelitis. Some, however, have argued for a direct invasion of the central nervous system by the virus of the antecedent infection although the virus has not been recovered from the nervous tissue.

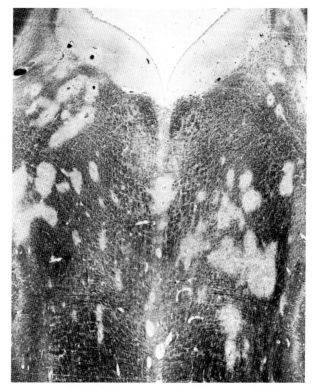

Fig. 53a. Weil × 8

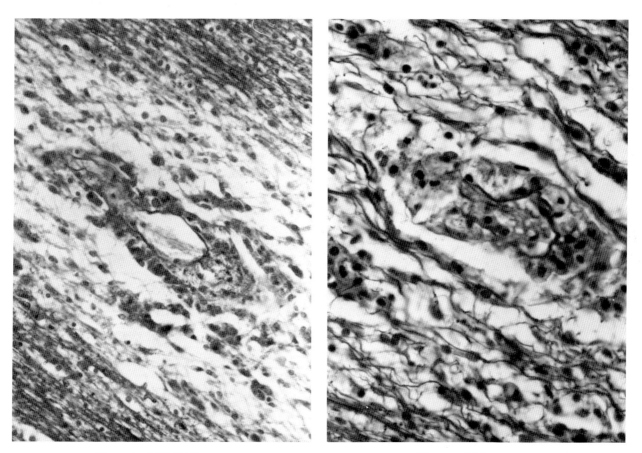

Fig. 53b. LFB-PAS × 100

Fig. 53c. Holmes × 450

Measles is probably the most common disorder to evoke the demyelinating reaction.

*Case 1:* An 8-year-old girl developed measles. Five days after the onset, as she was beginning to convalesce, her temperature climbed to 104° F., and she complained of headaches, became lethargic and developed muscle twitchings. The next day she was admitted to a hospital in a state of semicoma. Her temperature was 101° F.; there was a fading rubeola rash, and residual Koplik's lesions were seen in the mouth. There was resistance to flexion of the neck and deep reflexes were hypoactive. The cerebrospinal fluid contained 864 W.B.C. per cmm with 90% "polys"; the total protein was 54 mg %; sugar 75 mg %; chloride 128 mEq, and cultures were negative. Her further course was characterized by increasing depth of coma, despite treatment with intravenous hydrocortisone and ACTH. Temperatures then began to drop to subnormal levels, and following a convulsion on the eleventh day of her neurologic symptoms, she expired.

Grossly, the brain weighed 1,380 grams, was edematous but not otherwise remarkable. Microscopically, discrete foci of demyelination surrounded the venules of the white matter of the cerebrum (Fig. 54a), at times tending to coalesce and transgress into the adjacent gray matter. The demyelinating foci showed a cellular reaction (Fig. 54b), that consisted of lipid-containing macrophages around distended and congested blood vessels replacing the disintegrated myelin.

Measles encephalomyelitis is particularly prone to develop sequelae in the form of mental retardation and cerebral palsy.

*Case 2:* A 13-year-old boy had an attack of measles, after which he developed symptoms of coma and convulsions for a period of one month. As the coma passed he presented clinical signs of mental deterioration, aggressive-impulsive behavior, purposeless movements, and a stumbling, wide-based gait. He functioned at an imbecile level, and died in status epilepticus four years after the onset of the illness.

In myelin stains, the central white matter showed diffuse and patchy areas of demyelination, associated with enlargement of the ventricles, while the cortex appeared intact (Fig. 54c). Microscopically, perivenous foci of a cellular gliosis were disseminated throughout the white matter (Fig. 54d).

*References*

Malamud, N. a) Encephalomyelitis Complicating Measles. Arch. Neurol. and Psychiat. 38: 1025, 1937.
   b) Sequelae of Postmeasles Encephalomyelitis. Arch. Neurol. and Psychiat. 41: 943, 1939.

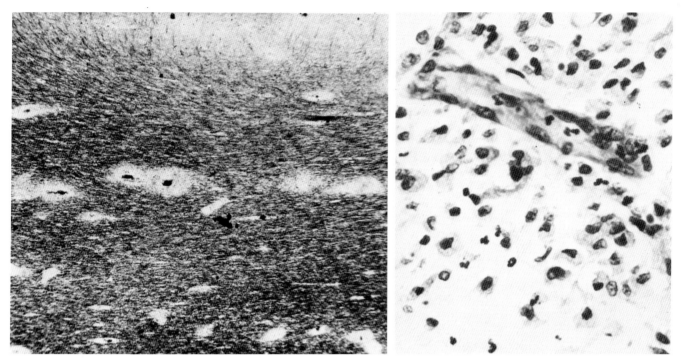

Fig. 54a. Weigert-Kulschitzky × 42

Fig. 54b. Nissl × 475

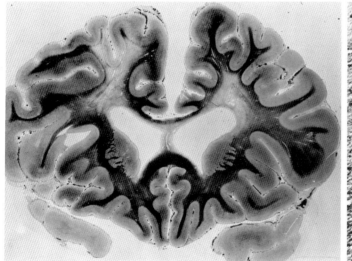

Fig. 54c. Weigert-Kulschitsky

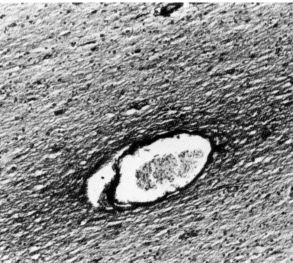

Fig. 54d. Holzer × 145

Encephalomyelitis complicating vaccination for smallpox has been almost as common as following measles infection.

> *Case:* A 21-year-old man had been vaccinated twice with cowpox vaccine. A week later he had a severe local ulcerative reaction, followed by coma, nuchal rigidity, opisthotonus, and hyperactive reflexes with ankle clonus. The spinal fluid contained 204 lymphocytes and 24 polymorphonuclear leucocytes per cu. mm., but virus culture was negative. Death occurred three weeks following the first vaccination.

Disseminated perivenous demyelinating lesions were scattered throughout the white matter as shown by a reaction with lymphocytes and macrophages in the perivascular spaces, surrounded by zones of proliferating microglia (Fig. 55a).

### POSTMUMPS ENCEPHALOMYELITIS

Mumps may be complicated by meningitis or encephalitis in the acute phase or by an encephalomyelitis during convalescence.

> *Case:* A 22-year-old man developed, twelve days after the onset of parotitis, nausea, vomiting, lethargy, nystagmus, dysarthria, ophthalmoplegia, a right facial paralysis, bilateral ankle clonus, and a Kernig sign. Death occurred on the fifth day of the neurologic disorder.

Perivenous demyelinating lesions were manifested by infiltrations with lymphocytes in perivascular spaces and by surrounding zones of proliferating microglia, as in the white matter near the inferior olivary nucleus (Fig. 55b).

### POSTCHICKENPOX ENCEPHALOMYELITIS

In some cases of perivenous encephalomyelitis, the brunt of the reaction is borne by the spinal cord where it induces a peripheral myelitis.

> In a case of encephalomyelitis that followed chickenpox infection, besides scattered demyelinating foci in the cerebral white matter (Fig. 55c) there was severe involvement of the spinal cord. Alternating bands of demyelinization surrounded the veins as they coursed through the columns of white matter to drain into the venous plexuses on the periphery of the cord (Fig. 55d).

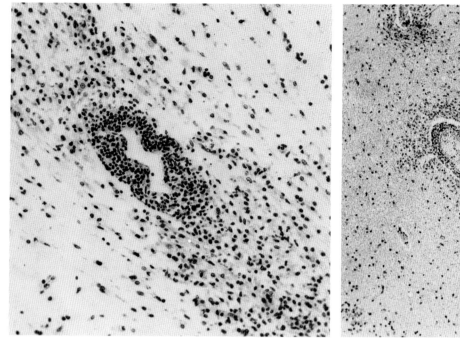

Fig. 55a.  Nissl × 200

Fig. 55b.  Nissl × 100

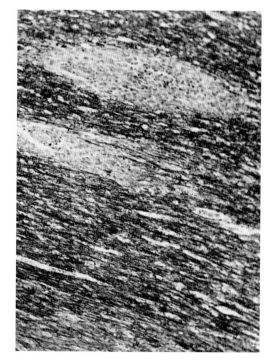

Fig. 55c.  Weil × 100

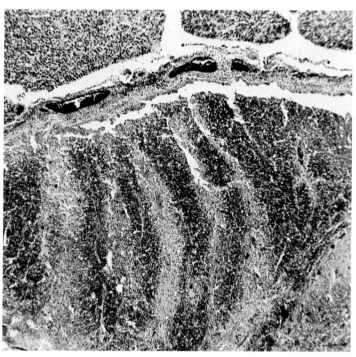

Fig. 55d.  Weil × 50

Influenza, upper respiratory infections, and pneumonia may be complicated by the condition of perivenous encephalomyelitis.

*Case:* A 39-year-old man, as he was convalescing from a "cold," suddenly developed headaches, nausea, vomiting, and diplopia. When admitted to a hospital he showed signs of pneumonia, and was in coma. The deep reflexes were absent, as were the superficial abdominals on the right, and there was a Babinski sign on the left side. The cerebrospinal fluid contained 210 cells/cmm, mostly polymorphonuclear leucocytes. He died ten days after the onset of his symptoms.

The cerebral white matter contained numerous foci of demyelination surrounding congested veins (Fig. 56a). Under higher magnification, a complete loss of myelin in the vicinity of the veins was replaced by a cellular reaction of macrophages (Fig. 56b).

## ACUTE HEMORRHAGIC LEUKOENCEPHALITIS

First described by Hurst in 1941, the disorder appears to be a variant, although a more fulminant form, of acute disseminated encephalomyelitis since transitions occur with the latter condition. It commonly develops after influenza or upper respiratory infections, ushered in by an abrupt onset of coma and seizures that rapidly progresses to a fatal termination.

The most striking pathology is one of disseminated perivascular and ring hemorrhages, attributed to fibrinoid necrosis of vessel walls, that are often intermingled with perivenous nonhemorrhagic foci of demyelination.

*Case:* A 53-year-old woman became acutely ill with symptoms of chills, malaise, and fever, the temperature rising to 103° F. During the next few days there was intermittent fever and she developed chest rales. Three days after the onset she suddenly became mentally confused, later semicomatose, and was admitted to a hospital. On admission her temperature was 104° F. Chest x-rays revealed evidence of pneumonia and pneumococci were cultured from blood and sputum. She was treated with penicillin without improvement. About a week following the onset she went into cardiac collapse, showed signs of renal shutdown, became more deeply comatose, and expired.

Grossly, the brain showed countless petechial hemorrhages confined to the cerebral white matter, including the corpus callosum and internal capsules (Fig. 56c).

Microscopically, ring hemorrhages surrounded the venules in the white matter, along with perivascular foci of demyelination (Fig. 56d). The walls of some venules showed signs of fibrinoid necrosis.

*Reference*

Hurst, E. W. Acute Hemorrhagic Leukoencephalitis. Med. J. Australia, 2: 1, 1941.

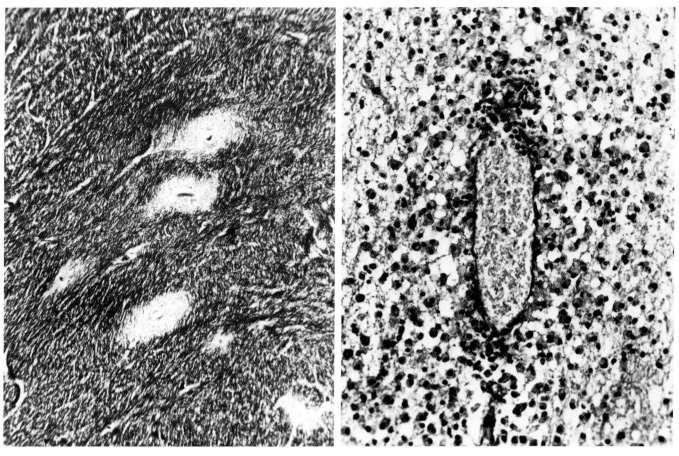

Fig. 56a. Weil × 32

Fig. 56b. Weil × 200

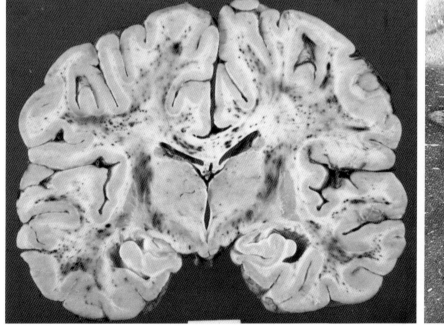

Fig. 56c. Acute hemorrhagic leukoencephalitis

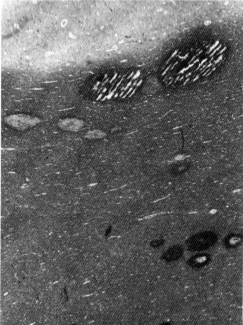

Fig. 56d. Weil × 20

EAE is considered to be a good experimental model of human autoimmune demyelinating encephalomyelitis. It is produced in animals by injecting a mixture of myelin and Freund's adjuvant. Demyelination begins within about three weeks. The demyelination is preceded by the appearance of sensitized mononuclear cells which penetrate the venules of the central nervous system (Figs. 57a and b) and may be found in large numbers in both the perivascular space and nearby involved parenchyma. Hematogenous edema fluid accompanies the cells and constitutes an essential feature of the lesion.

Electron microscopy has been used to examine the details of the demyelinating process. Among the first stages of demyelination is a regular separation of the myelin lamellae at the intraperiod line. This is followed by a so-called "vesicular" disintegration and further destruction. These processes are highly characteristic of EAE but are not unique to this condition. The precise role of mononuclear cells in this process is not entirely clear. Interestingly, cell processes have often been observed penetrating between adjacent myelin lamellae and apparently stripping the myelin from the axon.

In some advanced stages, macrophages containing the remains of myelin sheaths are found. In addition, reactive glial cells are seen as well as alterations of the axoplasm. Finally, remyelination seems to occur although this process is slow and incomplete.

In addition to ordinary EAE, a hyperacute form can be induced by adding pertussis vaccine to the myelin. In this case, the hematogenous elements include polymorphonuclear cells and erythrocytes associated with fibrin in addition to the mononuclear cells and plasma. Hyperacute EAE has a short incubation period and the animal dies in a short time. It has been compared to acute hemorrhagic leukoencephalitis of Hurst.

*References*

Hirano, A., H. M. Dembitzer, N. H. Becker, S. Levine, and H. M. Zimmerman. Fine Structural Alterations of the Blood-brain Barrier in Experimental Allergic Encephalomyelitis. J. Neuropath. and Expt. Neurol. 29: 432, 1970.

Lampert, P. Electron Microscopic Studies on Ordinary and Hyperacute Experimental Allergic Encephalomyelitis. Acta Neuropathologica. 9: 99, 1967.

Levine, S., A. Hirano, and H. M. Zimmerman. Hyperacute Allergic Encephalomyelitis. Electron Microscopic Observations. Amer. J. Path. 47: 209, 1965.

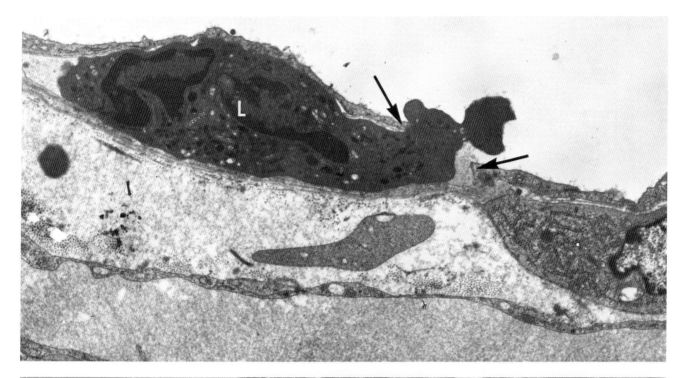

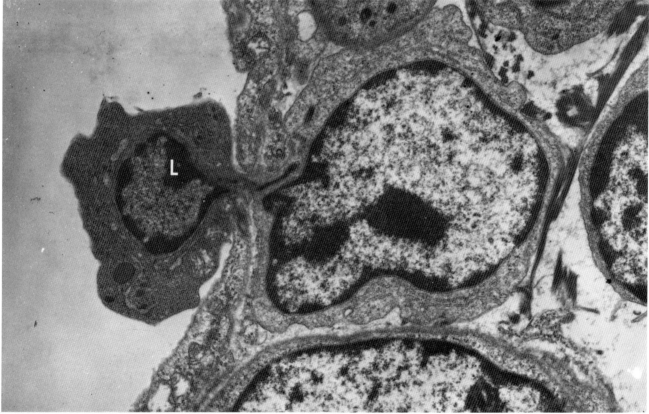

Fig. 57a. An electron micrograph of a blood vessel in a case of hyperacute experimental allergic encephalo-myelitis. A polymorphonuclear leukocyte (L) is seen penetrating between endothelial cells (arrows). × 10,000 (Levine et al., Am. J. Pathol. 47: 209, 1965)

Fig. 57b. An electron micrograph similar to Figure 57a showing a leukocyte (L) penetrating the endothelial cell. × 15,000 (Levine et al., Am. J. Pathol. 47: 209, 1965)

# ACUTE INFECTIOUS POLYNEURITIS

## (LANDRY-GUILLAIN-BARRÉ SYNDROME)

Acute infectious polyneuritis is characterized clinically by a sensorimotor polyneuropathy, with manifestations of Landry's ascending paralysis and Guillain-Barré syndrome, characterized by dissociation between an elevated protein and few or no cells in the cerebrospinal fluid. It often follows flulike and exanthematous illnesses or antirabies vaccination, and thus bears resemblance to acute disseminated encephalomyelitis. Like the latter, no specific virus has been recovered, and, by analogy with experimental allergic neuritis, may represent a delayed hypersensitivity reaction.

Pathologically, it is essentially a demyelinative neuropathy, showing segmental demyelination, with loss of myelin and relative preservation of axons. There have been some differences of opinion as to whether or not an inflammatory reaction by lymphocytes is an essential feature.

*Case:* A 38-year-old woman was admitted to the hospital because of complete paralysis and inability to breathe. One week prior to admission, she had suffered an upper respiratory infection and on the day prior to admission, she suddenly experienced muscular aches and weakness progressing from the legs to thighs and back. Examination revealed complete motor paralysis, except for ability to wiggle toes and fingers, and involvement of cranial nerves VII, X, XI, and XII. She complained of deep pain, tinnitus and diplopia, and subsequently developed paresthesias. By the fifth hospital day, there was complete paralysis of the left lateral rectus muscle with weak, disconjugate eye movements and absent pupillary reflexes. Cerebrospinal fluid showed an opening pressure of 430 mm. of water and contained 124 mg % protein and 1 lymphocyte per cmm. Treatment consisted of hydrocortisone, tracheostomy, fluids and potassium. She later developed absent bowel sounds, blood pressure of 220/130, pulse rate of 148, and changes in the electrocardiogram. On the twelfth hospital day, cardiac arrest occurred and she expired.

The peripheral nervous system showed evidence of generalized polyneuropathy, including the dorsal and ventral nerve roots, characterized by disruption and loss of myelin sheaths with reaction by mononuclear cells containing granular, PAS positive, lipid material in the absence of any inflammatory cells (Figs. 58a and b).

Axonal reaction changes with central chromatolysis, accompanied by proliferation of micro- and astroglia, were observed in the remaining motor cells of the anterior horns and of the facial nucleus (Figs. 58c and d), as well as in some other motor cranial nuclei.

*References*

Asbury, A. K., B. G. Arnason, and R. D. Adams. The Inflammatory Lesion in Idiopathic Polyneuritis; Its Role in Pathogenesis. Med. 48: 173, 1969.
Haymaker, W., and J. Kernohan. The Landry-Guillain-Barré Syndrome. Med. 28: 59, 1949.

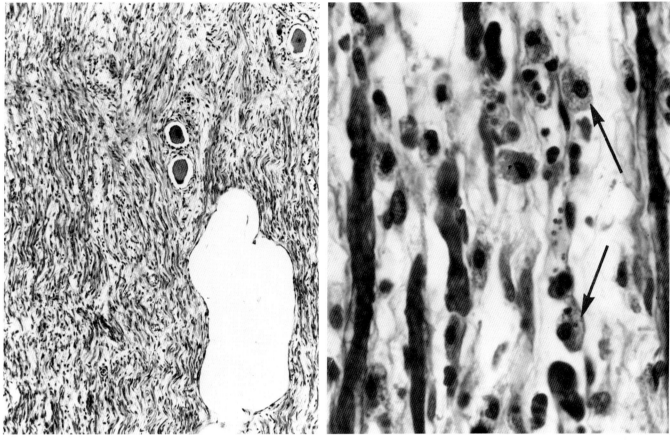

Fig. 58a. LFB-PAS × 90

Fig. 58b. LFB-PAS × 560

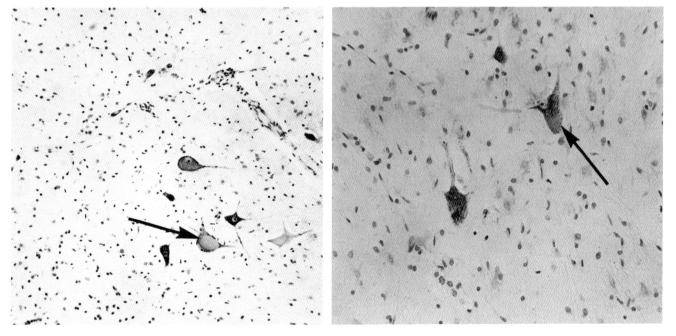

Fig. 58c. Nissl × 100

Fig. 58d. Nissl × 200

Electron microscopic studies of GBS have included examination of postmortem tissue of patients with GBS and of cultures of myelinated dorsal root ganglia treated with serum from patients with GBS (Figs. 59a and b). In addition, fine structural studies have been performed on what is considered an experimental model of GBS, namely, experimental allergic neuritis (EAN). This condition is induced by the administration of peripheral myelin and Freund's adjuvant.

In all cases, demyelination is found in the peripheral nervous system with apparent sparing of the axons. In postmortem human material and in EAN, hematogenous mononuclear cells are found in the demyelinating areas as is abundant edema fluid.

The exact means by which the mononuclear cells find their way out of the blood stream has been studied in EAN. Apparently, these cells penetrate the vascular wall at the level of the venules. Whether they pass between adjacent endothelial cells or somehow penetrate directly through the endothelial cells, or both, is presently controversial.

Likewise, the precise role of the mononuclear cell in the demyelinating process itself is not entirely clear. Some consider that the immediate presence of mononuclear cells is an absolute requirement for demyelination. Indeed, micrographs illustrating cell processes separating adjacent myelin lamellae have been published. Such illustrations also demonstrated destructive alterations of the myelin in areas immediately abutting such invading processes. Other studies, however, suggest that demyelination may occur without the immediate presence of mononuclear cells. It has also been pointed out by Lampert that it is apparently the myelin lamellae themselves which are attacked and not the Schwann cell proper.

Phagocytic activity follows demyelination. Finally, active and rapid remyelination occurs.

*References*

Aström, K. E., H. deF. Webster, and B. G. Arnason. The Initial Lesion in Experimental Allergic Neuritis. A Phase and Electron Microscopic Study. J. Exper. Med. 128: 469, 1968.

Carpenter, S. An Ultrastructural Study of an Acute Fatal Case of the Guillain-Barré Syndrome. J. Neurol. Sci. 15: 125, 1972.

Hirano, A., S. D. Cook, J. N. Whitaker, P. C. Dowling, and M. R. Murray. Fine Structural Aspects of Demyelination in Vitro. The Effects of Guillain-Barré Serum. J. Neuropath. and Expt. Neurol. 30: 249, 1971.

Lampert, P. W. Mechanism of Demyelination in Experimental Allergic Neuritis. Electron Microscopic Studies. Lab. Invest. 20: 127, 1969.

Lampert, P. W., and R. S. Garrett. Mechanism of Demyelination in Tellurium Neuropathy. Electron Microscopic Observations. Lab. Invest. 25: 380, 1971.

Raine, C. S., H. Wisniewski, and J. Prineas. An Ultrastructural Study of Experimental Demyelination and Remyelination. II. Chronic Experimental Allergic Encephalomyelitis in the Peripheral Nervous System. Lab. Invest. 21: 316, 1969.

Wisniewski, H., J. Prineas, and C. S. Raine. An Ultrastructural Study of Experimental Demyelination and Remyelination. I. Acute Experimental Allergic Encephalomyelitis in the Peripheral Nervous System. Lab. Invest. 21: 105, 1969.

Wisniewski, H., R. D. Terry, J. N. Whitaker, S. D. Cook, and P. C. Dowling. Landry-Guillain-Barré Syndrome. A Primary Demyelinating Disease. Arch. Neurol. 21: 269, 1969.

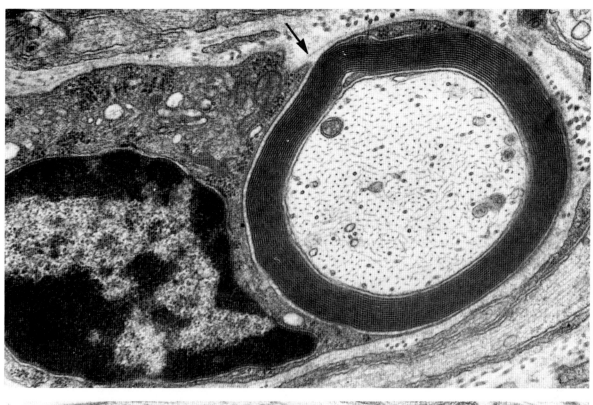

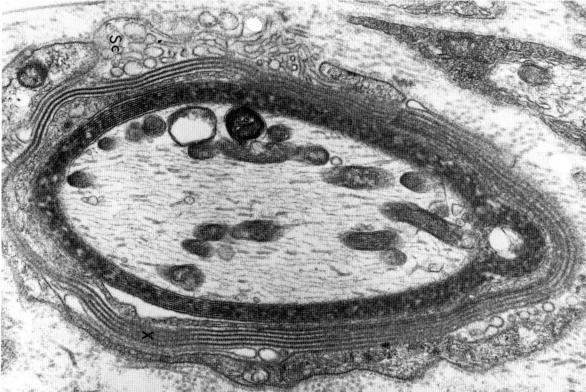

Fig. 59a. An electron micrograph of a culture of dorsal root ganglion treated with serum prepared from a patient with Guillain-Barré syndrome. The external mesaxon shows a distinct separation (arrow) which extends almost completely around the sheath. × 32,000 (Hirano et al., J. Neuropathol. Exper. Neurol. 30: 249, 1971)

Fig. 59b. An electron micrograph similar to that of Figure 59a showing loosened (X) and degenerated myelin lamellae as well as vesiculated Schwann cell cytoplasm (SC). The axon appears relatively intact. × 30,000 (Hirano et al., J. Neuropathol. Exper. Neurol. 30: 249, 1971)

# Neuromyelitis Optica

First described by Devic in 1894, the condition is characterized by an abrupt onset of blindness, followed after an interval of time by development of a paraplegia with a sensory level and cerebrospinal fluid findings of pleocytosis and elevated protein.

It has become increasingly evident that neuromyelitis optica is a syndrome, represented by at least three different pathologic conditions, viz., an optic neuritis in association with a) necrotic myelitis, b) acute disseminated and/or hemorrhagic encephalomyelitis, and c) multiple sclerosis.

## NEUROMYELITIS OPTICA WITH NECROTIC MYELITIS

*Case:* A 32-year-old woman, while convalescing from the "flu," developed progressive weakness and paralysis of her legs, a complete anesthesia up to the level of the nipple line, clonic flexion spasms, and radiating pains in the extremities and back, followed later by numbness in the ulnar nerve distribution. Four years earlier she had had a sudden episode of complete blindness, followed by some recovery of vision in the left eye but permanent visual impairment of the right eye. Her symptoms underwent remissions and exacerbations, and she died one year following the onset of her illness.

Sections through the upper dorsal and lower cervical levels revealed complete demyelinization and necrosis of the spinal cord that equally affected the gray and white matter so that the normal landmarks were no longer distinguished (Fig. 60a). On higher magnification, the cord was replaced by diffuse and focal fat-laden macrophages (arrows) lying freely in the tissue and in perivascular spaces, among which fibrous astrocytes formed a sparse framework (Fig. 60b). There was no sign of inflammation or of vascular disease. Above and below the necrotic segments there was ascending and descending Wallerian degeneration similar to the effects of a cord transection. The optic chiasm was demyelinated and replaced by gliosis (Fig. 60c). The pathologic process in the optic pathways was obviously chronic, in contrast to the subacute lesions in the cord.

This form of neuromyelitis optica with its massive necrosis of gray and white matter, differs essentially from the acute demyelinating disorders although, presumably, it has a similar precipitating influenzal illness.

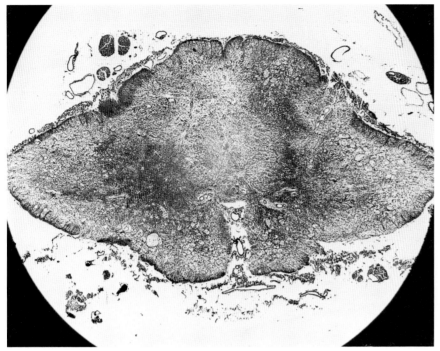

Fig. 60a. HE of cord × 7

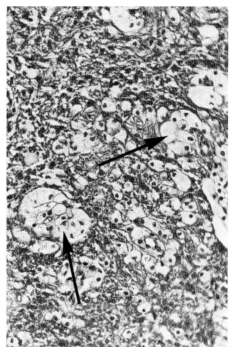

Fig. 60b. HE × 200

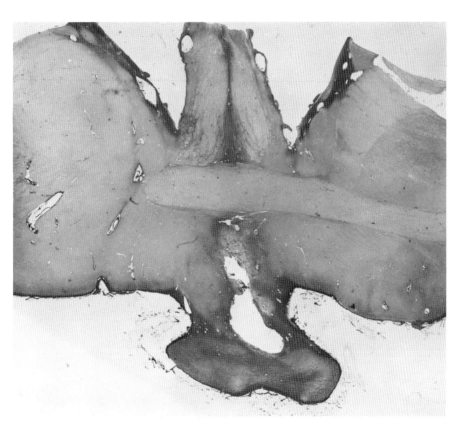

Fig. 60c. Holzer × 5

*Case:* A 53-year-old man had an influenzal type illness over a period of five days followed by recovery except for a mild residual weakness. Four months later he developed rapidly a decrease in visual acuity, first of the left and then of the right eye, becoming totally blind. A month later he suddenly developed fever, numbness and weakness of the extremities, started vomiting and lapsed into semicoma. On admission to the hospital he showed bilateral optic atrophy, a left facial palsy, gross weakness of trunk and legs, a vague sensory level at $T_2$ and urinary retention. The cerebrospinal fluid contained 108 lymphocytes per cmm and a total protein of 123 mg %. His condition progressively deteriorated and he expired about ten days following the acute febrile episode.

The brain showed grossly two discrete areas of acute hemorrhagic necrosis: in the splenium of the corpus callosum and adjacent right cingulate region, and in the white matter of the left cerebellar hemisphere (Fig. 61a).

Microscopically, the optic nerves were largely demyelinated (Fig. 61b) and replaced by diffuse astrogliosis.

The lesions in the corpus callosum and in the cerebellum (Fig. 61c) were characterized by perivascular and coalescing hemorrhages (A) and perivenous foci of demyelination (B). The latter change was equally seen in the medulla, bilaterally, although more on the left side. The spinal cord showed no significant changes and the vague syndrome of transverse myelitis was more likely owing to the lesions in the medulla.

In this case, the syndrome of neuromyelitis optica developed as a postinfluenzal demyelinating disorder showing features of both perivenous and hemorrhagic encephalomyelitis.

Cases of multiple sclerosis with episodes of acute retrobulbar neuritis followed by symptoms of spinal cord involvement are well known, their pathology being that of multiple sclerosis.

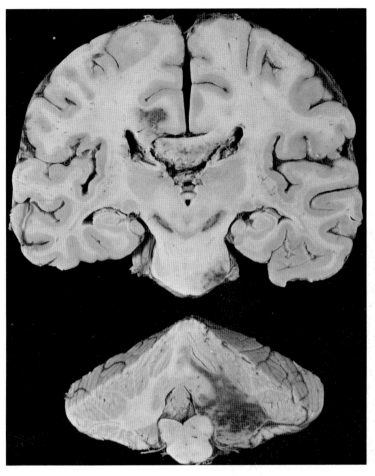

Fig. 61a. Disseminated hemorrhagic encephalomyelitis

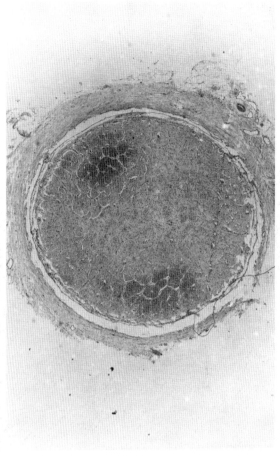

Fig. 61b. Weil × 16

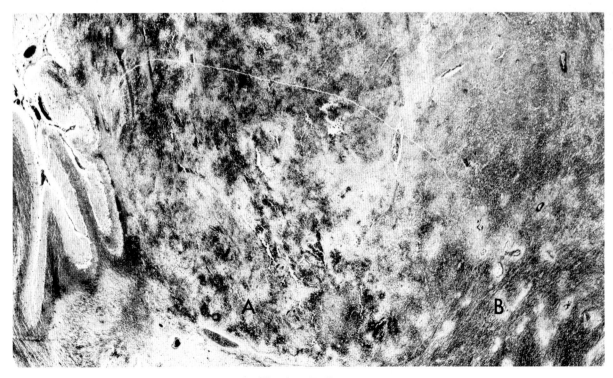

Fig. 61c. Weil × 10

Multiple or disseminated sclerosis is one of the most common neurologic disorders. Its clinical manifestations are noteworthy for their manifold manifestations, depending on the variable localization of recurrent and widespread lesions throughout the cerebrospinal structures, their tendency to remissions and exacerbations and the finding of raised gamma globulins in the cerebrospinal fluid.

Pathologically, the pathognomonic lesion is the formation of plaques of demyelination. These are circumscribed, grossly visible lesions of various sizes, shapes and colors that are distributed in an unsystematized and discontinuous manner (Fig. 62a). Their starting point may be a blood vessel, usually a vein, in the white matter or periventricular regions (Fig. 62b), whence they extend in a manner that does not correspond to the territory of vascular supply. In their development they undergo progressive reaction of phagocytosis and gliosis (Fig. 62c) in a centrifugal manner so that the margin of the plaque is more active, as indicated by its greater cellularity, than the center which is less cellular and sclerotic. At any given time the disease is characterized by polyphasic recent and old lesions. The primary site of the change in the myelin sheaths contrasts with the relative preservation of the neurons and axons (Figs. 62d and e). Because of the myeloaxonal dissociation, Wallerian degeneration of tracts is usually absent. The myelin byproducts stain with Sudan, the sudanophilic content representing an increase in cholesterol esters and neutral fats as the phospholipids are depleted. The oligodendroglia within the plaque disappear early but whether this is a primary or secondary phenomenon is unclear. Necrosis is not a feature of the lesions and inflammatory reaction is inconstant. While the principal changes occur in the white matter, the gray matter is often involved, largely in border zones with the white matter.

The etiology of multiple sclerosis remains undetermined. Its pathogenesis has given rise to a number of theories in which allergy and infection have received major attention. No infective agent however has yet been discovered. The concept of an autoimmune response has found some support in analogies with experimental allergic encephalomyelitis although there are distinct morphologic differences. The finding by Japanese investigators of lesions resembling acute multiple sclerosis following antirabies vaccination has afforded further evidence that sensitization may be an etiologic factor.

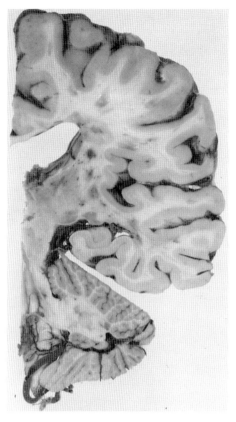

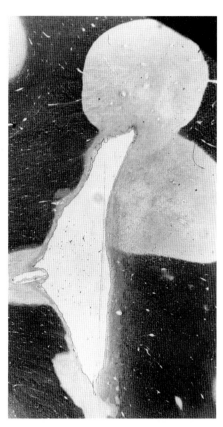

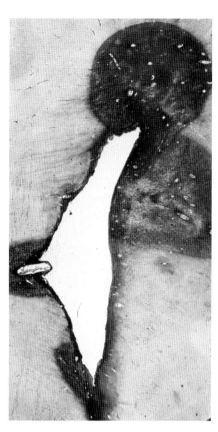

Fig. 62a. Multiple sclerosis

Fig. 62b. Weil method

Fig. 62c. Holzer method

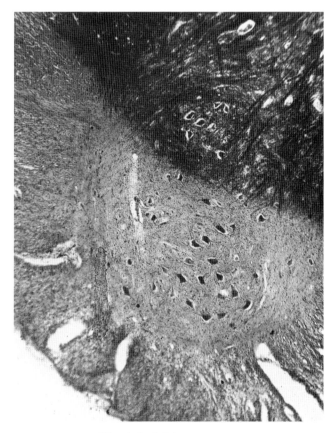

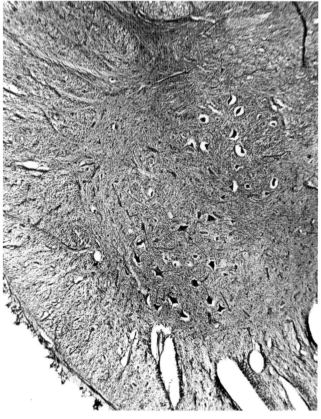

Fig. 62d. Spielmeyer × 32

Fig. 62e. von Braunmühl × 32

Acute multiple sclerosis is a rapidly developing form of the disease that on clinical grounds cannot be distinguished from acute encephalomyelitis, discussed previously. There is, however, reason to believe that on pathoanatomic grounds the acute does not differ fundamentally from the chronic forms of multiple sclerosis, and that it is merely the result of the more rapid tempo of the process. Moreover, the findings in the acute case can be assumed to form the basis for the acute exacerbations in the course of the chronic disease.

> *Case:* A 23-year-old woman had an acute onset of increasing mental confusion, somnolence, inability to walk, and urinary retention for four weeks before admission to the hospital. On examination, she was in semicoma and had diminished vision, horizontal and vertical nystagmus, ptosis on the right side, a central facial paralysis on the left side, incoordination in the upper extremities, and spastic paralysis of the lower extremities with bilateral pyramidal tract signs. She died approximately six weeks following admission. The clinical diagnosis was encephalitis.

Grossly, there were multiple discrete plaque-like lesions, of variable shape and size, and of a reddish-brown color.

Microscopically, the foci of demyelination were characterized in Nissl preparations by their intense staining, were frequently perivascular and were scattered throughout the white matter at border zones with gray matter (Fig. 63a). Some of the lesions were uniformly dark because of their compact cellular content, but others had pale centers and dark margins that under higher magnification (Fig. 63b) showed the pale centers to be composed predominantly of protoplasmic and fibrillary astrocytes (A) whereas the margins contained mostly macrophages (B); inflammatory reaction with perivascular lymphocytes was minimal. In fat stains, the same difference was reflected in the higher sudanophilic fat content on the periphery (A) than in the center of the plaques (B) (Fig. 63c).

Despite the predominance of acute densely cellular lesions (A) there were scattered rarefied pale plaques (B) that appeared to be more chronic, consisting primarily of astrocytes and sparse macrophages (Fig. 63d). Such coexistence of lesions of varying age demonstrates the essential similarity between the acute and the average chronic form of multiple sclerosis.

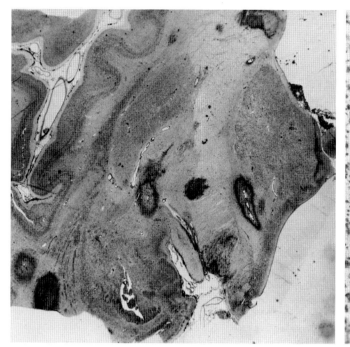

Fig. 63a. Nissl × 2

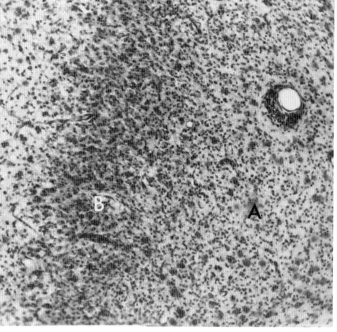

Fig. 63b. Nissl × 100

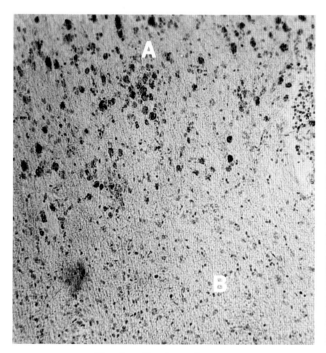

Fig. 63c. Scarlet red × 100

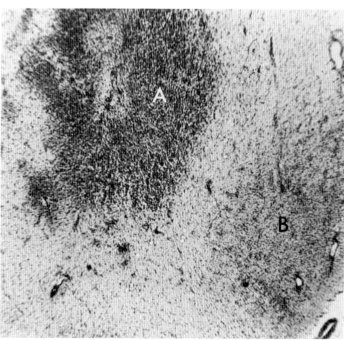

Fig. 63d. Nissl × 50

*Case:* A 32-year-old woman developed slowly progressive difficulty in walking, which was worse on the right side. Two years later there were additional symptoms of numbess of the left side of the face and leg and of blurring of vision. This was followed by a spontaneous remission lasting a year. Subsequently she suffered a relapse, with development of permanent spastic paralysis associated with pyramidal tract signs, muscular atrophy, incontinence of bladder and bowels, and euphoria. Examination of the cerebrospinal fluid showed a positive Pandy reaction, a total protein of 75 mg per 100 cc, and a midzone rise in the colloidal gold curve. She died in the eighth year of her illness of a ruptured duodenal ulcer, of which she had not complained.

The outward appearance of the brain was normal except for grayish-brown plaques of varying size scattered through the basal surface of the pons. On section, numerous lesions were found in the cerebral white matter and the brain stem with predilection for periventricular areas (Fig. 64a).

Microscopically, sharply circumscribed foci of demyelination were observed, especially in the periventricular regions of the lateral and third ventricles (Fig. 64b).

Similar plaque formation extended throughout the brain stem and cerebellum with predilection for the walls of the fourth ventricle and in the spinal cord where the lesions concentrated around the dorsal and ventral fissures, spreading bilaterally but asymmetrically into the gray and white matter.

The more active lesions were moderately cellular, consisting of hypertrophied fibrillary astrocytes intermingled with fat-laden macrophages, the latter being especially concentrated in perivascular spaces (Fig. 64c).

The older lesions contained few remaining oligodendroglia and sparse fibrous astrocytes, associated with abundant glial fibers forming an isomorphic gliosis, representing a sclerotic end-stage (Fig. 64d). On the edges of the plaques, the myelin sheaths usually showed variable degrees of fragmentation and beading. Some lesions showed only reduced staining without loss of myelin—so-called shadow plaques.

In some cases of multiple sclerosis, there may be a characteristic pattern of demyelination in which alternating bands of demyelination and of intact myelin occurs. When this pattern supervenes, the condition has been designated as concentric sclerosis or Balo's disease.

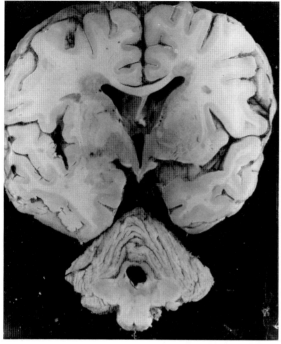

Fig. 64a. Multiple sclerosis

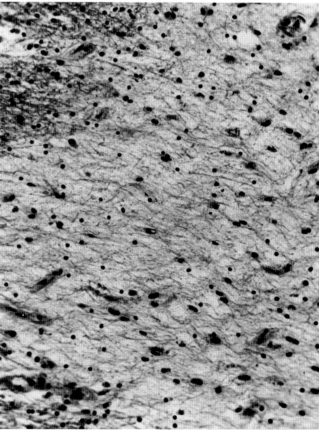

Fig. 64b. Weil × 2

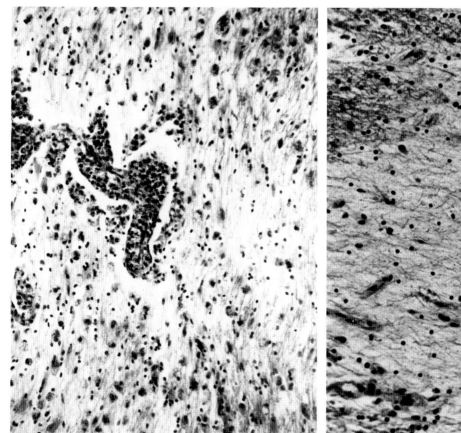

Fig. 64c. LFB-PAS × 150

Fig. 64d. HVG × 200

Diffuse sclerosis has been applied historically to a heterogeneous group of primary demyelinating disorders in which widespread demyelination and gliosis is the common feature, by contrast with the patchy lesions characteristic of multiple sclerosis. In recent years, a distinct separation has been introduced, between certain hereditary metabolic disorders known as leukodystrophies, and a disorder that is closely related to multiple sclerosis and to which the term Schilder's disease might best be applied. It is this latter condition that will be discussed in this chapter, while the leukodystrophies will be considered with the metabolic disorders (Chapter IX).

Clinically, Schilder's disease is considered to be sporadic, occurring at all ages, but predominantly in children and young adults. It is characterized by a variable course of weeks to many years with prominent mental signs, seizures, and signs of involvement of visual, auditory, and motor pathways. The cerebrospinal fluid often contains an increased amount of protein.

Pathologically, large hemispheral areas of demyelination occur in the white matter of any of the lobes, more commonly in the occipital regions, associated with variable involvement of the white matter of the brain stem and cerebellum. The lesions generally stop short of the gray matter and do not involve the U-fibers. At times plaques, typical of multiple sclerosis, may also be present to which the term transitional sclerosis has been applied. The histopathology and pathogenesis do not differ essentially from multiple sclerosis. The disintegrating myelin byproducts are likewise sudanophilic, the degree of axonal damage is somewhat more severe than in multiple sclerosis, and the reactive gliosis tends to be more anisomorphic.

The following two cases illustrate Schilder's disease, as it occurs respectively in childhood and in adults:

Case 1: A 9-year-old boy, whose family history was negative, began showing a loss of interest in his school work at the age of seven years. Examination revealed impaired hearing, and episodic mental confusion. Two months later he was almost totally deaf; pupils were dilated and equal, reacting sluggishly to light; speech was slurred; there was incoordination of arms and legs, the gait was ataxic; there was slight spasticity of both legs; knee and ankle jerks were hyperactive and there were bilateral Babinski signs. The cerebrospinal fluid contained 108 mg % of total protein. Contrast studies, and rectal, sural nerve and cortical biopsies were negative. Six months later he was committed to a State hospital for the retarded where he exhibited profound mental retardation, virtually no speech, marked visual impairment, frequent convulsions, and spastic quadriparesis. EEGs showed evidence of diffuse brain damage. His course in the hospital was progressively downhill and he expired of pneumonia, approximately two years after the onset.

The brain weighed 1,340 grams and was normal on external inspection. Sections revealed extensive areas of demyelination, showing a grayish and gelatinous transformation of the cerebral white matter of all lobes, though leaving parts of it intact, associated with plaque-like foci of demyelination in the cerebellar white matter (Fig. 65a).

Microscopically, diffuse demyelination extended up to the U-fibers which were largely spared (Fig. 65b), associated with corresponding gliosis (Fig. 65c). There was also severe destruction of axis cylinders. Sudanophilic fat was present in many areas (Fig. 65d).

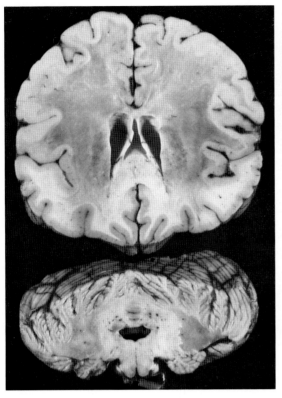

Fig. 65a. Schilder's disease

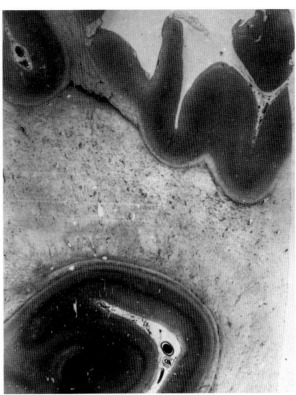

Fig. 65b. Weil method

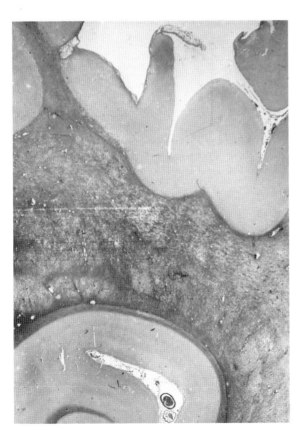

Fig. 65c. Holzer method

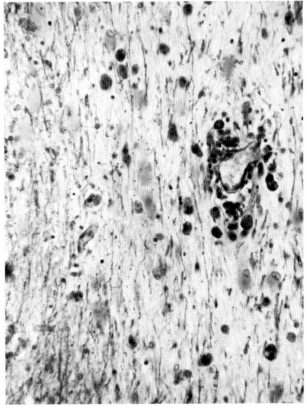

Fig. 65d. LFB-PAS × 200

*Case 2:* A 35-year-old man had an onset of mental symptoms, four years prior to death, characterized by loss of interest, impulsive and abusive behavior, and impotence. He was hospitalized two years later when a neurologic examination and various diagnostic tests, including angiography, were negative, with the exception of an "organic profile" in the mental status and diffuse slowing in the EEG. He was committed to a State hospital. While there, he showed increasing confusion, disorientation and hyperactivity. Several grand mal seizures occurred and later visual impairment became apparent. He was then transferred to a university hospital where repeat cerebrospinal fluid examination, angiography, brain scan and pneumoencephalography were again negative. A cortical biopsy failed to show any specific changes. His course was one of progressive deterioration to the point of mutism, blindness and deafness, incontinence and confinement to a wheel chair, and he expired of bronchopneumonia.

The brain weighed 1,310 grams, showing a normal external appearance, but on section revealed almost complete demyelination of the white matter of frontal (Fig. 66a), temporal, parietal and occipital lobes, except for the U-fibers, sparing only the white matter of the motor areas.

Myelin stains revealed an almost complete disappearance of the myelin sheaths, except for the U-fibers (Fig. 66b) and there was corresponding gliosis (Fig. 66c). Axons were relatively preserved. Fat stains stained large amounts of sudanophilic lipid material (A) beneath the well preserved U-fibers (B), (Fig. 66d).

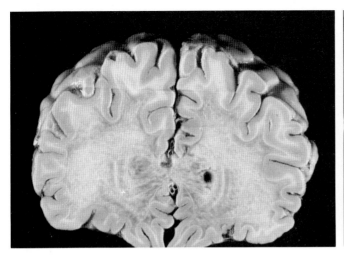

Fig. 66a. Schilder's disease

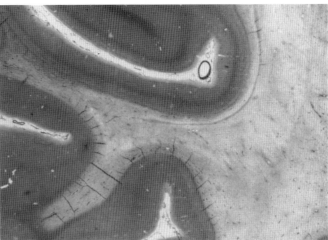

Fig. 66b. Weil method

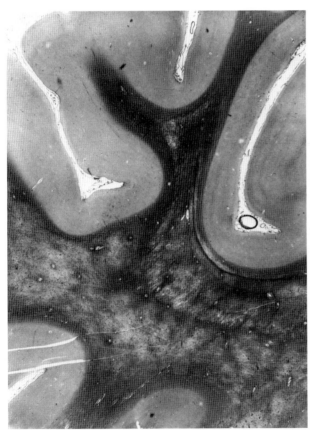

Fig. 66c. Holzer method

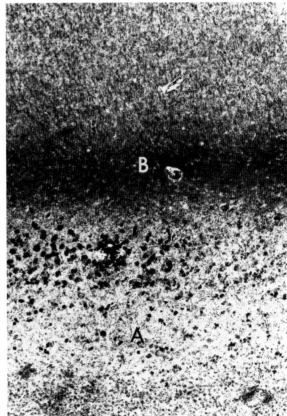

Fig. 66d. Oil Red O × 52

# IV

## Toxic, Anoxic, and Nutritional Disorders

A heterogeneous group of disorders, caused by a great variety of physical and chemical agents and nutritional deficiency factors, have in common a direct injurious effect on neural and at times vascular, tissues without evidence of inflammatory reaction. As such they may be designated as encephalopathies or neuropathies. Their morphologic differences often depend more on local susceptibility to the noxious agent than on histologic features. In any given case, either reversible or irreversible conditions may supervene, with which clinical recovery, sequelae, or fatal termination correlate.

### ENCEPHALOPATHY IN HYPERTHERMIA

The irreversible effects of heat are illustrated in the condition of heat stroke. The clinical manifestations and pathologic findings result from a complex combination of the direct effects of hyperthermia, indirect concomitants of shock and secondary complications. The high temperatures cause parenchymal lesions in brain, heart, bone marrow, lungs, liver, kidneys, and adrenals. The state of shock leads to hemorrhages from circulatory collapse in the nervous system, skin, and organs.

The encephalopathy has a special predilection for the Purkinje cells of the cerebellum, the cerebral cortex and basal ganglia in decreasing order of frequency. There are no demonstrable lesions in the hypothalamus including its heat regulating centers, although terminal hemorrhages in this region are common.

In fatal cases of less than twelve hours' duration, there are acute swelling, liquefaction, and shrinkage of the pyramidal cells of the cerebral cortex and of the Purkinje cells of the cerebellum, accompanied by edema, congestion, and hemorrhages.

In cases of several days' to weeks' duration, disintegration of neural tissue and glial activity become increasingly obvious.

> *Case:* A 25-year-old soldier collapsed while on a march in a Southern U.S.A. camp on a hot and humid day, and became unconscious. On examination the skin was hot and dry, the rectal temperature was 110° F., P 140, BP 80/40 mm Hg. Convulsions and vomiting of bloodly fluid occurred. Laboratory studies revealed increasing leukocytosis, an icterus index of 15–16, a $CO_2$ combining power of 38 vol. per 100 cc, and albumin, casts, and cells in the urine. He died in coma on the twelfth day of illness.

At autopsy the significant findings in the internal organs were hepatic necrosis, hemoglobinuric nephrosis, and bronchopneumonia.

The cerebral cortex showed diffuse depletion of nerve cells with shrinkage and hyperchromatosis of the few remaining ones; there was proliferation of microglia in the form of rod cells and of protoplasmic astrocytes (Fig. 67a). In the cerebellum there was almost complete disappearance of the Purkinje cells, the few remaining forms undergoing neuronophagia, accompanied by increased glia in the molecular and Bergmann layers (Fig. 67b).

*Reference*

Malamud, N., W. Haymaker, and R. P. Custer. Heat Stroke. The Military Surgeon. *99:* 397, 1946.

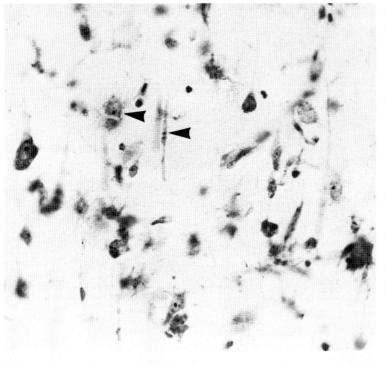

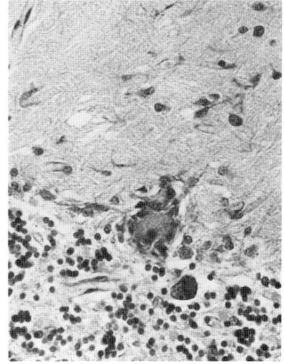

Fig. 67a.  Nissl × 475                    Fig. 67b.  Nissl × 450

Of the heavy metals that affect the nervous system, the most common are inorganic and organic arsenical preparations used both in industry and in drug treatment for syphilis and amebic dysentery.

Acute intoxication is manifested clinically by headaches, seizures, confusion, coma, and polyneuropathy.

Pathologically, the characteristic change in the brain is hemorrhagic encephalopathy, involving the cerebral white matter, that has been attributed to finding of large amounts of arsenic in walls of blood vessels.

In a fatal case following massive mapharsen therapy for lues, petechial hemorrhages were scattered through symmetrical parts of the semioval center, the corpus callosum, and internal capsules (Fig. 67c), that were predominantly in the form of ring hemorrhages (Fig. 67d).

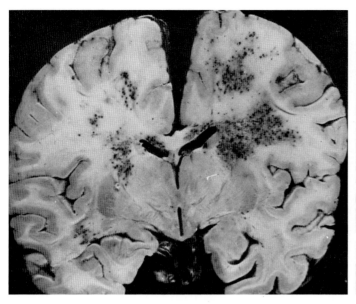

Fig. 67c. Arsenical hemorrhagic encephalopathy

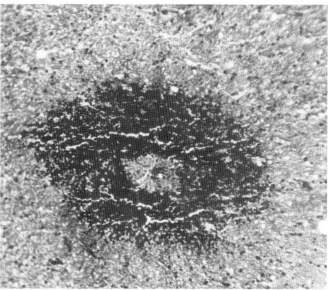

Fig. 67d. Heidenhain's aniline blue × 100

A great variety of conditions exert a toxic action on the nervous system by interfering with supply of oxygen or by removing substrate such as glucose, essential for oxidation processes. The brain is particularly vulnerable to a state of hypoxia because its normal consumption of oxygen is much greater than that of other organs and tissues. About 4–5 minutes of anoxia, on the average, is bound to result in irreversible damage.

The causes are numerous, including effects of anesthetics and hypnotics, carbon monoxide poisoning, high altitude anoxia, cardiac arrest and respiratory failure. The effects are due to the direct action on the neurons of oxygen lack, accompanied by vascular congestion due to accumulation of $CO_2$ and lactic acid.

The resulting encephalopathy is characterized by cellular changes in a fairly stereotyped manner of distribution which, regardless of cause, are referred to as *selective neuronal (parenchymal) degeneration.* The specific histologic features are: ischemic or homogenizing type of neuronal degeneration with eosinophilic staining of cytoplasm and pyknosis of nucleus that has a predilection for the gray matter in the following regions: cerebral cortex, commonly in a pattern of pseudolaminar necrosis especially around troughs of sulci, the hippocampus where fields $H_1$ (Sommer's sector) and $H_{3-5}$ (end plate) are selectively involved, and the cerebellum where the Purkinje cells are the most susceptible. Variations in accordance with specific causes and/or intensity of the hypoxia may determine additional changes in basal ganglia and white matter, with least involvement of brain stem and spinal cord. The explanation for such selective vulnerability has remained controversial, vascular or physico-chemical factors being considered.

### FATAL NITROUS OXIDE ANESTHESIA

One of the most common anesthetics to cause immediate or delayed death is nitrous oxide, brought about by respiratory or cardiac failure.

In a case, in which death occurred seventy-two hours following administration of the anesthetic, the degenerative changes progressed to a state of pseudolaminar necrosis of the cortex. A marked loss of neurons was noted in parts of the third, fourth, and fifth layers, accompanied by proliferation of microglia and newly formed capillaries (Fig. 68a). Also involved were striatum, hippocampus, and cerebellum.

### CARBON MONOXIDE POISONING

The toxicity of carbon monoxide is due to its affinity for hemoglobin resulting in formation of the stable compound of carboxyhaemoglobin. CO also has an affinity for the iron of cytochrome oxidase, resulting in a direct effect on cellular respiration. The pathologic changes are apt to be necrotic and hemorrhagic, although affecting much the same areas as in other conditions of hypoxia with special predilection for the globus pallidus and the reticular part of the substantia nigra. Consequently, Parkinsonism is one of the more noteworthy clinical sequelae.

In an acute case of carbon monoxide poisoning, necrosis of the medial segment of the globus pallidus stood out against the normal surrounding tissue (Fig. 68b). The hippocampus showed selective necrosis of Sommer's sector (S.S.), the dorsal cell band of the pyramidal layer (D.B.) and the dentate fascia being preserved, the lesions being characterized by anemic or hemorrhagic necrosis, in which capillary and gitter-cell proliferation occurred in the absence of vascular occlusion (Fig. 68c).

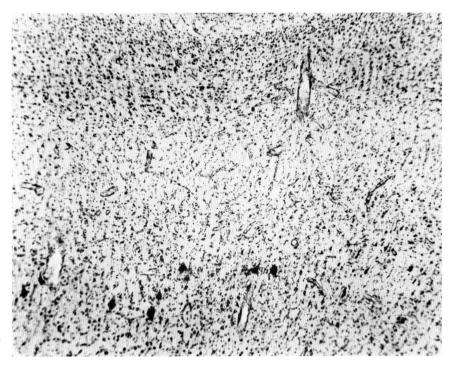

Fig. 68a. Nissl × 42

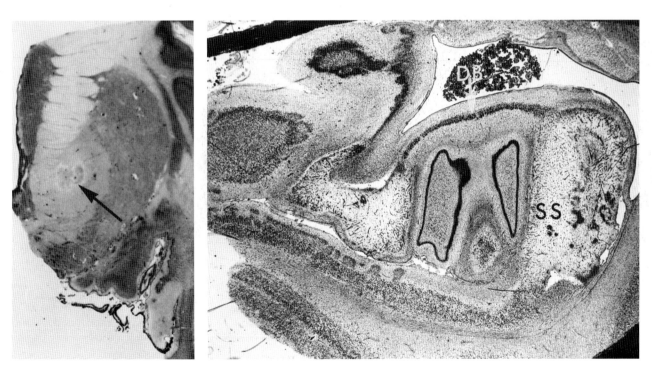

Fig. 68b. Nissl × 3

Fig. 68c. Nissl × 5

Although hypoglycemia is not a state of anoxia in the strict sense, the effects on the nervous system are similar because of nonutilization of oxygen. It is seen in cases of prolonged insulin coma that may develop during treatment of diabetes or in the course of insulin shock therapy for mental illness, as well as in hyperinsulinism associated with islet cell tumors of the pancreas.

## Insulin Shock Therapy

In the course of insulin shock treatment for mental illness a not infrequent complication of prolonged coma may end fatally. Under the circumstances the changes in the nervous system depend upon the duration of the irreversible coma.

> *Case:* A 21-year-old man was treated for an acute schizophrenic psychosis with a course of subshock doses of insulin. He received seven injections consisting of a total of 315 units, administered twice daily over a period of four days, the final treatment consisting of 60 units. Immediately after this injection he went into shock, followed by coma and convulsions. The blood sugar was 48 mg per 100 cc. Later, signs of decerebrate rigidity and increasing hyperthermia set in. Death occurred after sixty hours of persistent coma, in spite of the restoration of the blood sugar to normal and even hyperglycemic levels.

The brain showed widespread edema, liquefaction necrosis, and ischemic changes in the neurons of the cerebral cortex (Figs. 69a and b); hippocampus with predilection for Sommer's sector, basal ganglia, and cerebellum.

## Hyperinsulinism with Islet-cell Adenoma

Islet-cell tumors of the pancreas produce attacks of hyperinsulinism associated with neurologic signs that may ultimately result in a permanent organic brain syndrome.

> *Case:* A 30-year-old woman had had a history of six years of fainting spells and convulsive attacks, followed by signs of progressive mental deterioration. When she was admitted to a mental hospital in an advanced stage of her condition, the fasting blood sugar was found to be 35 mg per 100 cc. In spite of maintenance of the blood sugar at a normal level by dietary measures, there was no longer any change in her clinical picture; operation on the pancreas did not seem justified.

Autopsy disclosed a small tumor embedded in the tail of the pancreas. It consisted of proliferated islet cells of Langerhans (arrow) arranged in cords, separated by a fibrous capsule from the surrounding acinar tissue of the pancreas (Fig. 69c).

The brain was diffusely atrophic, especially the cerebral cortex. Microscopically, a chronic state of cortical degeneration showed a characteristic pseudolaminar pattern involving primarily the supragranular layers, with marked reduction in neurons and astroglial reaction (Fig. 69d).

*References*

Malamud, N. Fatalities Resulting from Treatment with Subshock Doses of Insulin. Am. J. Psychiat. 105: 373, 1948.
Malamud, N., and L. C. Grosh. Hyperinsulinism and Cerebral Changes. Arch. Int. Med. 61: 579, 1938.

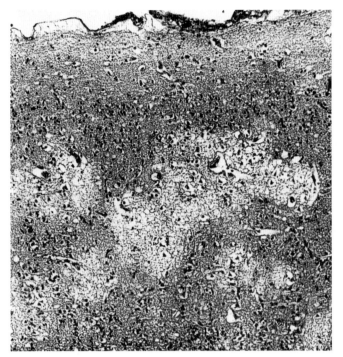

Fig. 69a. HVG × 90

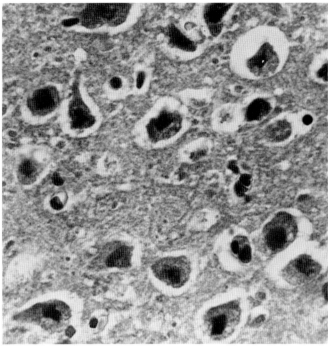

Fig. 69b. HE × 470

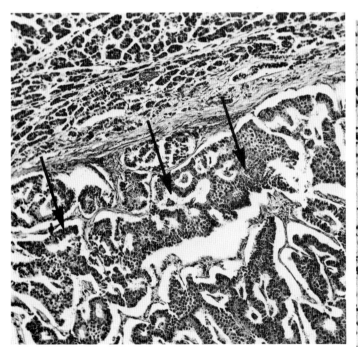

Fig. 69c. HE × 100

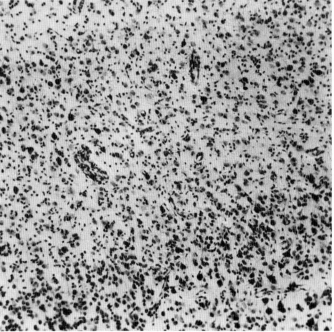

Fig. 69d. Nissl × 100

Cardiac and respiratory arrest, such as complicate surgical procedures, can lead to irreversible brain damage, if of sufficient duration before resuscitation is accomplished. Arrest, ranging from two to ten minutes may lead to immediate fatal termination or to severe sequelae. The resulting anoxic encephalopathy shows the classic morphologic changes previously outlined.

## Cardiac Arrest

*Case:* A 43-year-old man, while undergoing a sympathectomy for malignant hypertension, had a sudden cardiac arrest. The pericardium was rapidly opened, and the heart was massaged for an estimated four minutes before the cardiac beat was re-established. The patient remained in coma for the next seven days, during which time he exhibited focal seizures involving the right extremities and flaccid paralysis with pyramidal signs on both sides.

The cytoarchitecture of the cerebral cortex had disintegrated, with dropout of many neurons and diffuse proliferation of microglia and astroglia, especially in the third layer (Fig. 70a). In the cerebellum, there was almost total disappearance of Purkinje cells, with reaction by proliferation of the glia of the Bergmann layer (Fig. 70b). Sommer's sector of the hippocampus was equally severely involved. The surviving neurons showed typical anoxic changes.

## Respiratory Arrest

Changes similar to those of cardiac arrest occur in respiratory arrest following surgical procedures, strangulations, etc.

The following case illustrates the chronic sequelae of anoxic encephalopathy:

*Case:* A 60-year-old man underwent an operation for a perforated gangrenous appendix. Postoperatively, his condition remained satisfactory for about five days, at which time he developed acute pulmonary congestion requiring extensive tracheal suction. He then complained of blurring of vision, followed by increasing confusion and convulsions, and lapsed into coma. Later his condition was described as one of "akinetic mutism," with eyes open but with apparent blindness, and emotional lability. There were bilateral pyramidal tract signs in both upper and lower extremities. His condition remained unchanged for about a year when he succumbed to bronchopneumonia.

The brain weighed 1,140 grams and on section showed striking laminar necrosis in symmetrical parts of the cerebral cortex, especially of the occipital lobes, including the calcarine region, and in the dorsal parts of the corpus striatum (Fig. 70c).

Microscopically, chronic laminar degeneration, predominantly of layer III (Fig. 70d) was widespread, associated with tissue disintegration and reaction by macrophages and astroglia. Similar changes were observed in the hippocampus, caudate nucleus, putamen, globus pallidus, and cerebellum.

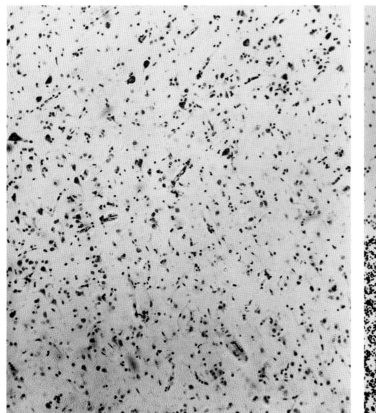

Fig. 70a. Nissl × 100

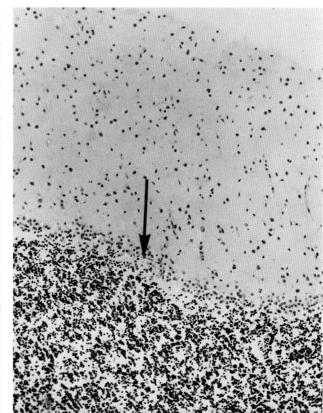

Fig. 70b. Nissl × 100

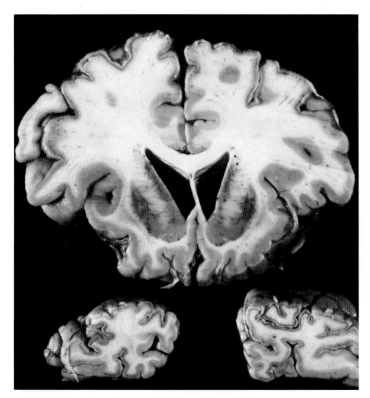

Fig. 70c. Anoxic encephalopathy

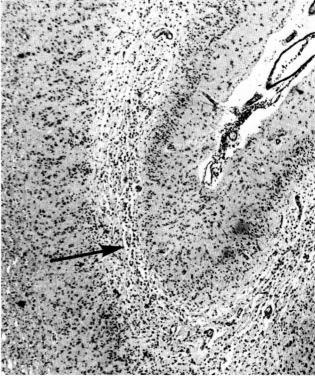

Fig. 70d. HVG × 44

## Status Epilepticus

Status epilepticus, whether developing on a background of acute febrile illnesses and toxic disorders, or in patients with "idiopathic" grand mal epilepsy, may lead to fatal termination. Under such circumstances, cerebral changes occur that are typical of anoxic encephalopathy resembling those outlined previously in cardiorespiratory arrest, hypoglycemia, etc. There is the same selective neuronal necrosis involving primarily the cerebral cortex, hippocampus, cerebellum, and thalamus with less tendency to involve such other structures as the striatum, and dentate and inferior olivary nuclei.

The pathogenesis has been variously attributed to reduction in oxygen supply, consumptive hypoxia due to increased metabolic activity, or changes in circulation due to alterations in blood pressure or angiospasm occurring during seizures.

A great variety of sequelae with clinical manifestations of mental retardation, quadriplegia, hemiplegia, and chronic epilepsy have been known to develop following an acute onset of severe seizures, especially occurring in early life.

> *Case:* A previously healthy 11-year-old boy, while playing in school, suddenly fell down with a convulsion, followed by repeated seizures. On admission to a hospital, skull x-rays, lumbar puncture, and pneumo- and electro-encephalography were negative, and the etiology remained unknown. Following cessation of convulsions, his state of consciousness progressively decreased. Within two weeks he developed coma and generalized spasticity. EEGs showed evidence of depressed cortical function. He remained in a state of coma until his demise six months following the onset.

The brain was grossly atrophic and showed on section almost total cortical necrosis, including the hippocampus, but not involving the basal ganglia; the lateral ventricles were markedly dilated (Fig. 71a).

Microscopically (Fig. 71b), the cerebral cortex was completely destroyed, showing variations in reaction from diffuse gliosis to microcystic degeneration, whereby large numbers of plump astrocytes were intermingled with small cysts that contained lipid-laden macrophages.

In this case, although of unknown etiology, the severe anoxic encephalopathy appeared to be the result of an acute status epilepticus.

## Chronic Epilepsy

In patients with recurring grand mal convulsions, no consistent structural changes in the brain have been reported with the exception of a high incidence of two types of lesions:

(a) Mesial temporal sclerosis, more often unilateral than bilateral, largely involving the hippocampal formation, in the form of so-called Ammon's horn sclerosis, and to a more limited degree the uncus-amygdaloid region, and

(b) Cerebellar atrophy, focal or diffuse, with more severe degeneration of the Purkinje than the granular layer.

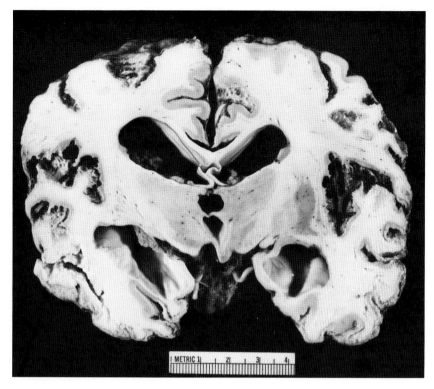

Fig. 71a. Anoxic encephalopathy

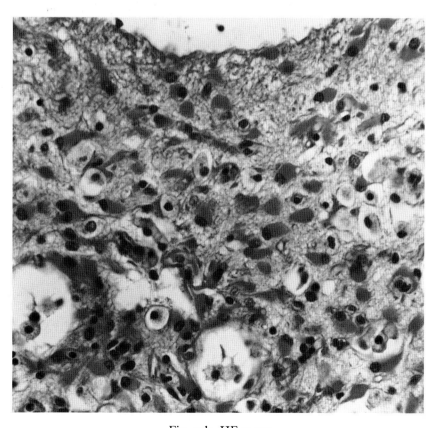

Fig. 71b. HE × 330

## Chronic Epilepsy (continued)

The pathogenesis of mesial temporal sclerosis has been much debated. Some, notably Spielmeyer and Scholz, have considered it to be a manifestation of the process of selective neuronal degeneration, characteristic of anoxic encephalopathy, whether on a vascular and/or pathoclitic basis. Others (Earle, et al.) regarded mesial temporal sclerosis as a complication of increased intracranial pressure usually attributed to perinatal trauma, resulting in so-called incisural sclerosis.

It is evident from a survey of a large series of cases that some are precipitated by febrile convulsions, some may follow perinatal trauma, and still others are of unknown cause or "idiopathic."

The clinical significance of mesial temporal sclerosis has received increasing attention in recent years because of its correlation with the syndrome of psychomotor or temporal lobe epilepsy.

> *Case:* A 12-year-old boy with negative family history and normal birth and early development had an onset at the age of two and one half years of grand mal seizures associated with an upper respiratory infection with high fever. Subsequently, convulsions continued with increasing frequency despite treatment with dilantin and phenobarbital. Some of the seizures were later described as running fits during which he would suddenly "scream, start to run, fall, kick and writhe and would be very weak when the seizure was over." He was also subject to "temper tantrums," and at the age of ten was brought to the attention of the juvenile court because he had made overt threats with a loaded rifle. He was then committed to a hospital for the retarded although tests revealed normal intelligence. Repeat EEGs disclosed a spike-wave focus in the mid and anterior regions of the left temporal lobe. His condition was diagnosed as mixed grand mal and psychomotor epilepsy. His death occurred when on a hike near the hospital reservoir, he had one of his running seizures, ran into the lake and drowned.

The brain was grossly normal with the exception of sclerosis of Ammon's horn on the left side (Fig. 72a), and of focal atrophy of the cerebellum.

Microscopically, a comparison of the normal hippocampal formation (Fig. 72b) with that of the case (Fig. 72c) showed an almost complete disappearance of the neurons from the end-plate (H 3-5) by contrast with the preservation of the fascia dentata, and of Sommer's sector ($H_1$) by contrast with the normal appearance of the dorsal cell band ($H_2$). A corresponding gliosis was demonstrated with the Holzer glial method (Fig. 72d).

The psychomotor seizures and the aggressive behavior appeared to be the clinical expressions of focal discharges originating in the region of the sclerotic hippocampus.

The cerebellar changes consisting of a dropout of Purkinje cells were not associated with any clinical symptoms.

*References*

Sano, K., and N. Malamud. Clinical Significance of Sclerosis of the Cornu Ammonis. Arch. Neurol. and Psychiat. 70: 40-53 (July) 1953.

Malamud, N. Some Observations on the Pathology of Epilepsy Following Birth Trauma and Postnatal Infection in the Light of Temporal Lobe Epilepsy. *Temporal Lobe Epilepsy.* Charles C. Thomas (Springfield, Illinois, 1958), pp. 149-165.

Malamud, N. The Epileptogenic Focus in Temporal Lobe Epilepsy from a Pathologic Standpoint. Arch. Neurol. and Psychiat. 14: 190, 1966.

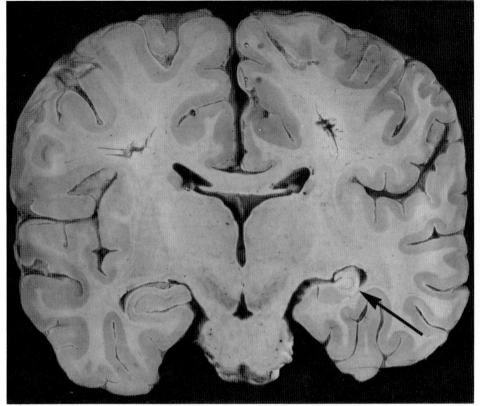

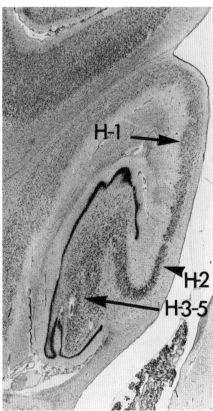

Fig. 72a. Sclerosis of the left Ammon's horn (sides reversed)

Fig. 72b. Nissl × 5

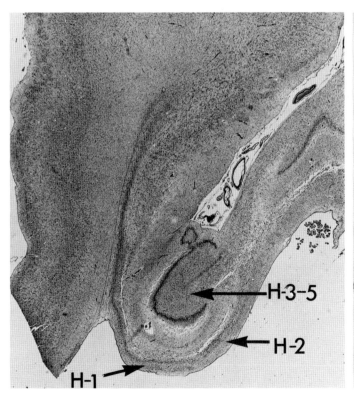

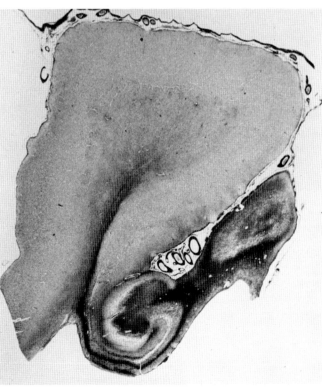

Fig. 72c. Nissl × 5

Fig. 72d. Holzer × 5

Among the disorders of the nervous system that are associated with vitamin deficiency, the most common are those related to deficiencies in the various factors of vitamin B.

## WERNICKE-KORSAKOFF'S SYNDROME

Following the separate descriptions in the 1880s of these two syndromes by Wernicke and Korsakoff, it has become increasingly clear that both are variants of the same fundamental disorder: deficiency in $B_1$ or thiamine hydrochloride.

The clinical manifestations are: variations from acute mental confusion to chronic amnestic-confabulatory psychosis, with or without ocular palsies, nystagmus, ataxia, and polyneuropathy. Both occur in association with chronic alcoholism and other causes of malnutrition.

The pathologic features vary accordingly from an acute ischemic-hemorrhagic state with prominent vascular proliferation to a chronic degenerative condition associated with astrogliosis. The changes have a characteristic distribution centered in the periventricular structures around the third ventricle, aqueduct of Sylvius, and fourth ventricle, and in the superior vermis, in addition to the peripheral neuropathy. Biochemically, deficiency in two thiamine dependent enzymes have been incriminated: pyruvate decarboxylase and transketolase although their precise role is still not established.

### Acute Wernicke's Syndrome

Although commonly developing in chronic alcoholics, the following case is noteworthy for its occurrence on the basis of starvation. It may be assumed that endogenous release of thiamine under such conditions does not satisfy the tissue needs despite minimal carbohydrate metabolism.

*Case:* A 39-year-old man was admitted to a hospital after being found comatose in his room by his landlord who had not seen him for three to four days. According to the history, the patient was attempting to reduce his body weight in a short time, resulting in decline from a high of 289 to 205 lbs. on admission, and suggesting that he was in a state of near complete fasting during the interval. On admission, he was in semicoma; there were internal and external ophthalmoplegias, papilledema, reduced to absent deep reflexes, bilaterally positive Babinski signs, and rapid clonus of the left arm. The cerebrospinal fluid was slightly xanthochromic with 84 crenated R.B.C. and no W.B.C. per cmm, the pressure was 320 mm $H_2O$, total protein was 230 mg % and glucose was 197 mg %. (Blood sugar was moderately elevated.) On the second hospital day patient developed periods of apnea requiring a tracheostomy. He expired five days following admission, of bronchopneumonia.

The brain weighed 1,650 grams. It was edematous but the most striking gross changes were small hemorrhages and focal softenings in the structures surrounding the third ventricle, aqueduct, and fourth ventricle.

Microscopically, there were acute ischemic and demyelinative lesions with marked proliferation of thin-walled congested blood vessels, rarely associated with perivascular hemorrhages, in the immediate vicinity of the third ventricle, including the dorsomedial nuclei of the thalamus, massa intermedia and periventricular hypothalamic structures (Fig. 73a), in the periaqueductal region, including the mesial tectal and tegmental regions (Fig. 73b) and the floor structures of the fourth ventricle. In higher magnifications, the proliferating blood vessels, with swollen endothelial cells, were embedded in a loose edematous matrix in which proliferation of microglia was the chief reaction (Fig. 73c).

*Reference*

Drenick, E. J., C. B. Joven, and M. E. Swendseid. Occurrence of Acute Wernicke's Encephalopathy during Prolonged Starvation of Obesity. New Eng. J. Med. 274: 937, 1966.

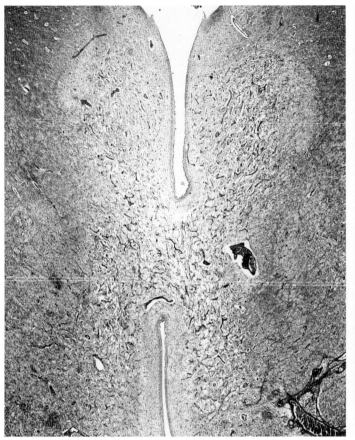

Fig. 73a. LFB-PAS × 8

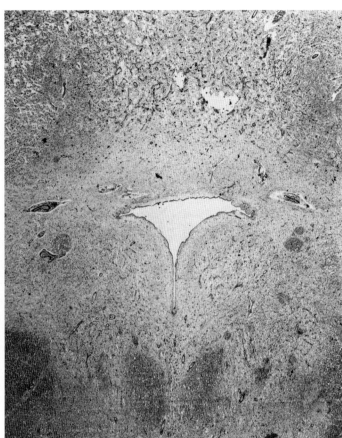

Fig. 73b. LFB-PAS × 8

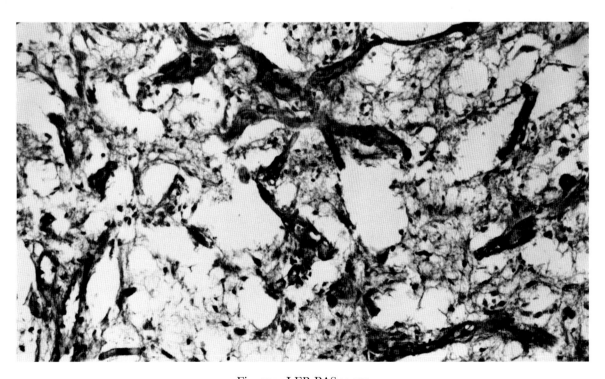

Fig. 73c. LFB-PAS × 150

## Chronic Wernicke's or Korsakoff's Syndrome

*Case:* A 67-year-old man, a chronic alcoholic, was admitted to a State mental hospital with a history of progressive mental deterioration over a period of several years. Examination revealed emotional apathy and impairment of memory for time with tendency towards confabulation. For example, he claimed that he talked to the governor that morning and that he went that day to look the situation over regarding employment. Neurologic examination showed a left peripheral facial weakness, sluggish reaction of both pupils to light, impaired coordination, and decreased knee jerks. Two years following admission, he developed a lymphosarcoma on the right side of the neck that later metastasized to bone marrow, liver, and lungs, and that led to his death within a month's time.

The brain weighed 1,460 grams, showing no gross abnormalities other than bilaterally severe atrophy and brownish discoloration of the mammillary bodies along with disproportionate dilatation of the third ventricle, suggestive of atrophy of the periventricular structures, including the massa intermedia (Fig. 74a).

Microscopically (Fig. 74b), the atrophy was reflected in the diffuse gliosis in the floor and walls of the third ventricle, including the mammillary bodies, dorsomedial nucleus of the thalamus and the massa intermedia. Nissl preparations of the same areas revealed reduction in nerve cells with replacement by numerous nuclei of astroglial cells as, for example, in the mammillary body (Fig. 74c).

Similar changes were present in the periaqueductal area including the Edinger-Westphal nuclei of the third nerve, the cranial nuclei in the floor of the fourth ventricle, especially the vestibular and the dorsal efferent nuclei of the vagus (Fig. 74d), and the folia of the superior vermis of the cerebellum. There were also degenerative changes in peripheral nerves associated with axonal reaction in anterior horn cells of the spinal cord.

The case thus demonstrated the chronic counterpart of the acute Wernicke's syndrome.

*References*

Malamud, N., and S. A. Skillicorn. Relationship between the Wernicke and the Korsakoff Syndrome. Arch. Neurol. and Psychiat. 76: 585, 1956.

Victor, M., R. D. Adams, and G. H. Collins. *The Wernicke-Korsakoff Syndrome.* F. A. Davis (Philadelphia 1971).

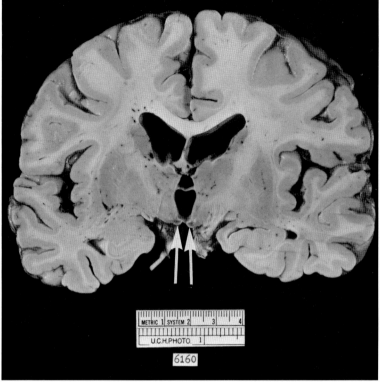

Fig. 74a. Bilateral atrophy of structures around third ventricle

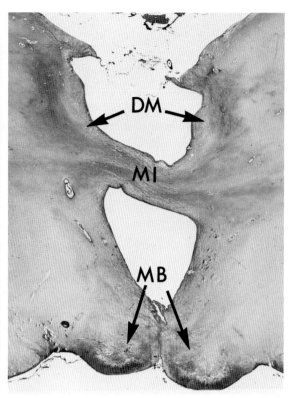

Fig. 74b. Holzer × 3

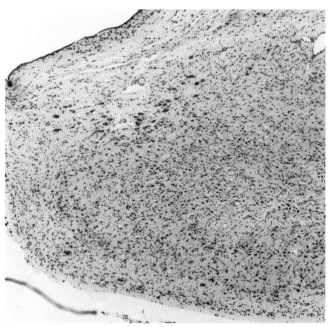

Fig. 74c. Nissl × 40

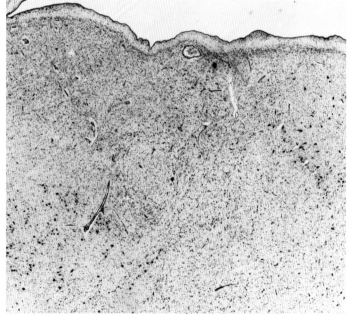

Fig. 74d. Nissl × 16

The cerebellar changes often encountered in cases with the Wernicke-Korsakoff's syndrome may exist independently, causing a syndrome of cerebellar ataxia, presumably on the basis of similar nutritional disturbances. The ataxia involves primarily stance and gait of leg movements because of the localization of the lesion in the anterior-superior aspects of the vermis and hemispheres.

> *Case:* A 49-year-old man was admitted to a hospital with a history of chronic alcoholism and development, in the past six months, of gait disturbances. Examination revealed good orientation and no memory deficit. Neurologically, he showed horizontal nystagmus and ataxia, predominantly of lower extremities. The liver was palpable four finger breadths below the right costal margin. His condition continued unchanged for the next ten days when he suddenly choked on food, became cyanotic, and expired.

The general autopsy revealed hepatic cirrhosis.

The brain was grossly remarkable only for atrophy restricted to folia of the superior vermis and of the immediately adjacent hemispheres (Fig. 75a).

In Nissl preparations the involved folia showed a complete loss of Purkinje cells associated with moderate rarefaction of the granular layer, contrasting with relatively normal adjacent folia (Fig. 75b).

*Reference*

Victor, M., R. D. Adams, and E. L. Mancall. A Restricted Form of Cerebellar Cortical Degeneration Occurring in Alcoholic Patients. Arch. Neurol. 1: 579, 1959.

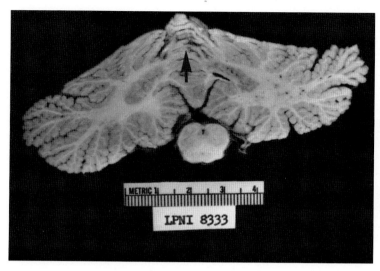

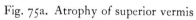

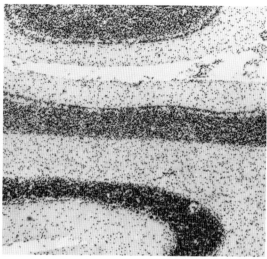

Fig. 75a. Atrophy of superior vermis                    Fig. 75b. Nissl × 40

Deficiency in nicotinic acid or the B₂ factor usually associated with pellagra, causes a specific encephalopathy characterized by so-called central neuritis involving the pyramidal cells of the cerebral cortex, especially the Betz cells, brain stem, and spinal cord, along with a polyneuropathy.

*Case:* A 36-year-old man with a history of chronic alcoholism, was admitted to the hospital in a confused and disoriented state. He exhibited brown pigmentation of the skin of the face, elbows, and chest; the tongue was coarse and furrowed. Deep reflexes were absent. The clinical diagnosis was psychosis with pellagra.

The Betz cells of the motor cortex showed characteristic swelling with central chromatolysis and eccentricity of the nuclei, associated with mild proliferation of oligo-, micro-, and macroglia (Fig. 75c).

## SUBACUTE COMBINED DEGENERATION

Deficiency in vitamin B₁₂, commonly associated with pernicious anemia, produces unsystematized degeneration of various tracts in the spinal cord, of which posterolateral column involvement merely indicates its most common clinical expression. The changes are characterized by a primary myelinolysis giving the lesions a spongy appearance (Fig. 75d). Later, axons may also become involved, accounting for development of Wallerian degeneration superimposed over the primary affection. Changes may also occur in peripheral nerves and cerebral white matter.

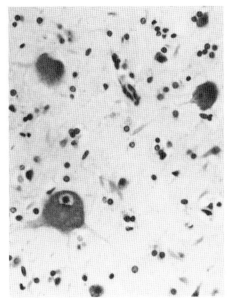

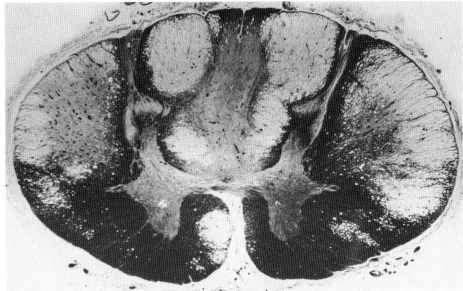

Fig. 75c. Nissl × 150

Fig. 75d. Weil × 15

Cerebral lesions in association with chronic hepatic diseases of various types have received increasing attention following the discovery of Wilson's disease (see Chapter IX). In fact, histologic changes in the brain, of a subclinical degree are commonplace. Less frequently the lesions are of sufficient intensity to result in clinical symptoms. These are subject to variation corresponding to the disseminated distribution of the changes and may consist of dementia, extrapyramidal, pyramidal, and cerebellar signs. Elevation of blood ammonia levels and no signs of disturbed copper metabolism differentiate hepatic encephalopathy from Wilson's disease.

The pathologic features are essentially of two types: 1. spongy areas of necrosis having a predilection for junctions between gray and white matter in the cerebral cortex, basal ganglia, brain stem, and cerebellum; and 2. Alzheimer's glia in the form of proliferation of enlarged and altered nuclei of astrocytes with intranuclear glycogen inclusions, known as Alzheimer's glia, type II. (Absence of Alzheimer's glia type I is one of the distinguishing features from Wilson's disease.)

The pathogenesis of the effects of impairment of liver function on the central nervous system is unclear, whether it is due to failure of ammonium metabolism or some other toxic factor.

*Case:* A 55-year-old woman, whose family history was negative, had exhibited signs of cirrhosis of the liver for approximately nine years. Two months before death she suddenly developed mental confusion, dysarthria, ataxia, rigidity, and pyramidal signs. There was laboratory evidence of marked impairment in liver function. Her course was progressively downhill, and she died in coma.

The principal autopsy finding was cirrhosis of the portal type (Fig. 76a).

In the cerebral cortex there were widespread areas of pseudolaminar spongy necrosis, predominantly in lower layers of both hemispheres (Fig. 76b); similar lesions were found in the basal ganglia (Fig. 76c), midbrain and cerebellum that were disseminated in both gray and white matter.

Microscopically, the vacuolated areas were devoid of any significant glial fiber reaction (Fig. 76d) but often showed proliferating reticulin fibers. Throughout the gray matter there was diffuse proliferation of large numbers of Alzheimer's glia of type II (Fig. 76e).

*References*

Victor, M., R. D. Adams, and M. Cole. The Acquired (Non-Wilsonian) Type of Chronic Hepatocerebral Degeneration. Med. 44: 345–396, 1965.

Waggoner, R. W., and N. Malamud. Wilson's Disease in the Light of Cerebral Changes Following Ordinary Acquired Liver Disorders. J. Nerv. and Ment. Dis. 96: 410–423, (Oct.) 1942.

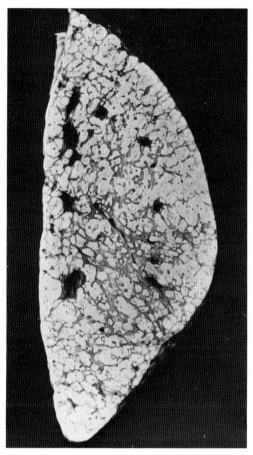

Fig. 76a. Cirrhosis of liver

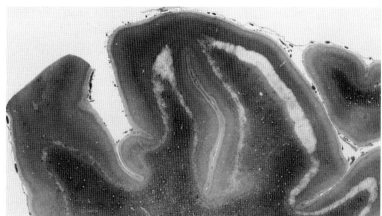

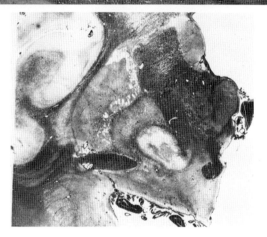

Fig. 76b. HVG × 2 (above)
Fig. 76c. HVG (below)

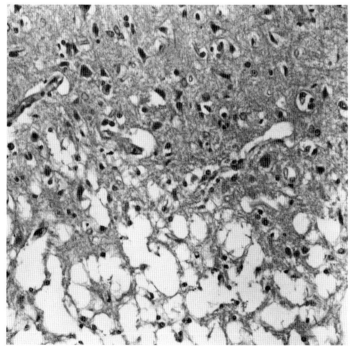

Fig. 76d. HE × 150

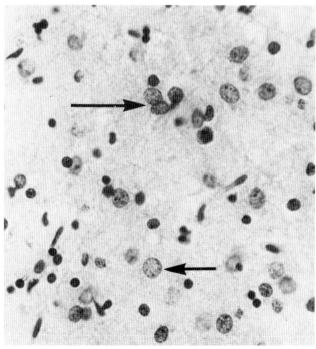

Fig. 76e. HVG × 600

Central pontine myelinolysis was first reported in 1959 by Adams, et al., as a rapidly progressing disorder, characterized by quadriplegia, dysarthria and dysphagia, in association with chronic alcoholism on the basis of presumable malnutrition. An increasing number of cases have since been reported with or without histories of alcoholism, raising doubts about a specific etiology. Some cases are associated with other causes of malnutrition, dehydration, electrolyte imbalance and renal transplantation. Also, the characteristic lesion is not uncommon in cases of Wilson's disease where it occurs along with the other classic findings.

The pathology appears to be unique in its consistent localization in the center of the pons, more often in its rostral than caudal part, and in its histologic features of a sharply circumscribed area of demyelination in which neurons and axons are relatively preserved.

*Case:* A 29-year-old woman developed four months prior to hospitalization an attack of "asthma," associated with recurrent vomiting of unknown cause. Later she developed paresthesias in her right side, followed by remission and relapse three weeks before admission. Since then there has been intermittent vomiting and several days before admission the left side of the body also became involved so that she was unable to keep her balance. On admission she was unable to move and complained of paresthesias and diplopia. Examination revealed a right sixth nerve palsy, bilateral mystagmus, right hemiparesis, bilaterally hyperactive deep tendon reflexes with Babinski signs. The cerebrospinal fluid contained 18 lymphocytes per cmm. but was otherwise negative. Shortly after admission she developed respiratory distress requiring a tracheostomy. A ventriculogram was performed but showed poor filling, and following an occipital trephination, the patient's condition deteriorated and she expired ten days after admission.

The general autopsy findings revealed only a terminal bronchopneumonia.

Grossly, the brain was not remarkable with the exception of softened consistency of the pons, without any evidence of occlusion of the basilar artery, associated with tonsillar herniation.

Microscopically, a circumscribed area of demyelination replaced almost the entire cross section of the caudal part of the pons, leaving only areas of intact myelin on its peripheral margins (Fig. 77a). A comparison of stained preparations for myelin (Figs. 77 b and c) and axons (Fig. 77d) disclosed relatively greater loss of myelin sheaths than axons and neurons. The glial reaction was moderate, more of microglia and scattered fat-laden macrophages than of astrocytes, while the oligodendroglia were greatly diminished.

Although the etiology remained obscure, it appeared that the intractable vomiting with progressive malnutrition led to the neurologic disorder.

*Reference*

Adams, R. D., M. Victor, and E. L. Mancall. Central Pontine Myelinolysis. Arch. Neurol. Psychiat. 81: 154, 1959.

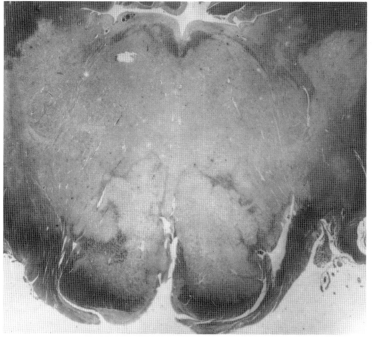

Fig. 77a. Weil × 3

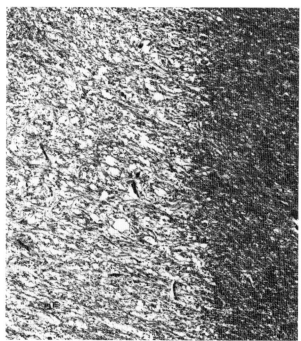

Fig. 77b. LFB-PAS × 40

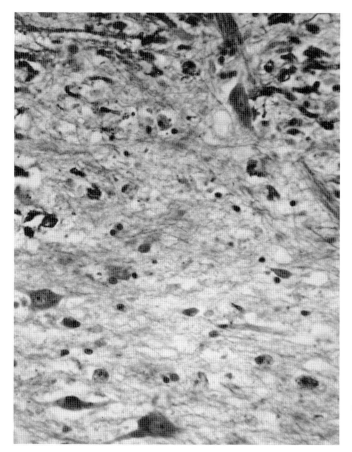

Fig. 77c. Weil × 250

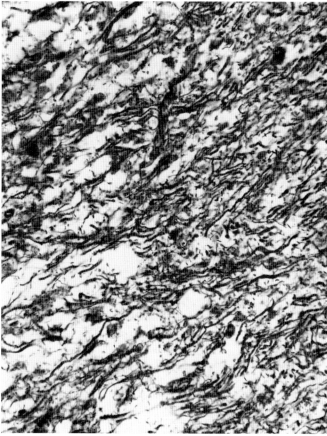

Fig. 77d. Holmes × 250

# V

# *Vascular Disorders*

Any vascular disorder must be considered with respect to causative vascular disease, and its effects on the nervous tissue. The most common vascular disease is arteriosclerosis followed by hypertension, aneurysm, various forms of angiitis, sinus-venous thrombosis and hemorrhagic diathesis. The effects are either infarcts induced by occlusive vascular disease or hemorrhages secondary to rupture, alteration in vascular permeability, and reduced coagulation of the circulating blood.

## Infarcts with Arterial Thrombosis

A number of factors determine the production of infarcts: 1) topographic arrangement of the cerebral arteries, their intracranial and extracranial anastomoses, 2) the hemodynamics governing the circulation, 3) occlusion, whether total by thrombo-embolism or partial by stenosis, and 4) maintenance of blood pressure.

Discrepancies between degrees of stenosis or thrombosis in cerebral arteries and infarct formation are common observations. Thus occlusion of an intracranial artery has been found only in about 25–30% of infarcts, other sources being extracranial, such as stenosis of the vessels in the neck, circulatory insufficiency in states of hypotension, and/or angiospasm.

The sites of thrombosis and/or infarct formation, in decreasing incidence, are the middle cerebral, internal carotid, anterior cerebral, posterior cerebral, basilar, and vertebral arteries.

Pathologically, the infarct undergoes three stages: 1) stage of necrosis, marked by edema, softening and ischemic or hemorrhagic tissue changes with absent to minimal glial or vascular reaction, 2) stage of resorption, characterized by tissue disintegration and active gliovascular reaction, and 3) stage of cyst formation, manifested by cystic cicatrization and cessation of glial and vascular reactivity. The duration of the first may be estimated in days, the second in weeks and the third in many months to years.

*Case 1:* A 54-year-old man had a sudden onset of a right hemiparesis. He soon became comatose, demonstrating bilateral Babinski signs, and died approximately thirty-six hours after the onset of the stroke.

The brain showed a recent infarct involving the left hemisphere in the vascular territory of the internal carotid artery (Fig. 78a). There was swelling due to edema of the cerebral cortex and basal ganglia with variations from pallor to hyperemia, softened consistency and ventricular displacement to the right.
Further posteriorly, there were signs of transtentorial herniation accompanied by terminal hemorrhages in the tegmentum of the upper brain stem.

The intracranial portion of the left internal carotid artery was distended by a recent thrombus in the presence of only minimal arteriosclerosis (Fig. 78b). It was possible to trace the thrombus to its origin in a severely atheromatous region at the bifurcation of the common carotid artery in the neck.

Histologically, edematous necrosis obliterated the cytoarchitecture of the cortex (Fig. 78c), the surviving neurons showing typical ischemic necrosis (see Fig. 1b). In some areas, there were accumulations of polymorphonuclear leukocytes (Fig. 78d) and small hemorrhages but there was no reaction by either glial cells or capillaries.

160

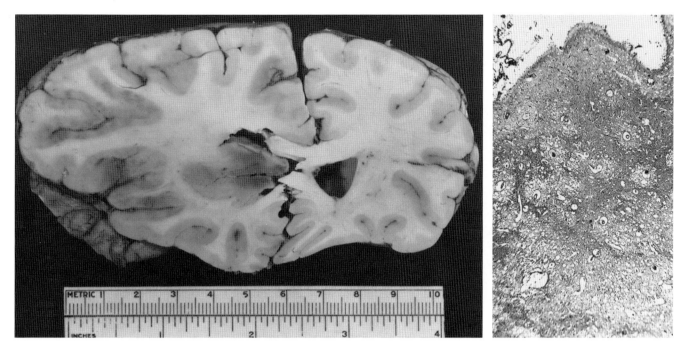

Fig. 78a. Acute infarct in left hemisphere

Fig. 78c. HE × 24

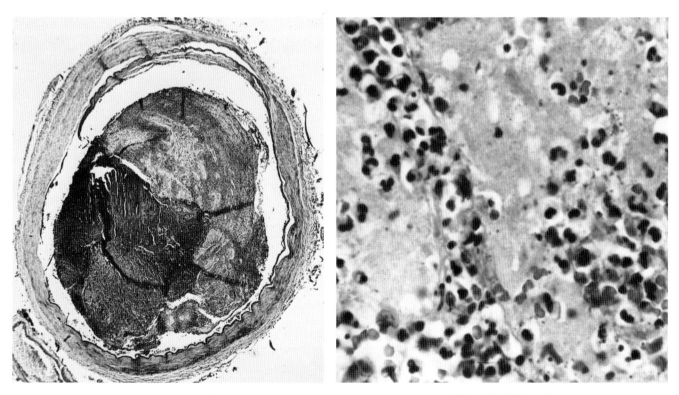

Fig. 78b. HE × 16

Fig. 78d. HE × 560

A somewhat later stage, characterized by early signs of resorption, is illustrated in the following case:

> *Case 2:* A 64-year-old man had a sudden onset ten days prior to hospitalization of bitemporal headaches, lightheadedness, staggering gait, and right hemianopsia. Examination on admission revealed a blood pressure of 130/95 and a right lower quadrantanopsia. The total protein of the cerebrospinal fluid was 67 mg %. EKG showed evidence of old myocardial infarcts. A week following admission the patient suddenly became comatose and developed rigidity of all extremities. The eyes tended to deviate to the right; the right pupil was larger than the left although both reacted to light; all tendon reflexes were hyperactive and both plantar reflexes were extensor. He never regained consciousness and expired a week following the onset of coma.

The brain showed severe atherosclerosis of the basal arteries, acute thrombosis of the basilar artery, and infarction of the pons involving the base and tegmentum, more extensive on the right side, where it also involved part of the overlying cerebellar hemisphere (Fig. 79a).

Histologically, there was early reaction by adventitial histiocytes and microglia showing a tendency to develop into macrophages (Fig. 79b).

In the above case there was clinical evidence of an earlier transient ischemic attack (t.i.a.) in the same basilar-posterior cerebral arterial territory before the permanent effects of a basilar artery thrombosis became established.

In a case with a history of two recurrent C.V.A.'s, one episode characterized by left hemiparesis occurring two months prior to demise following an episode of aphasia seventeen years earlier, corresponding subacute and chronic infarcts were present in the right and left parasylvian regions, respectively (Fig. 79c).

Histologically, the subacute infarct was characterized by a subpial zone of proliferating astrocytes overlying a necrotic cortex in which the parenchyma had disintegrated and been replaced by large numbers of macrophages (Fig. 79d). The chronic infarct consisted of a multiloculated cyst containing filaments of glial and collagen fibers, devoid of any cellular reaction (Fig. 79e).

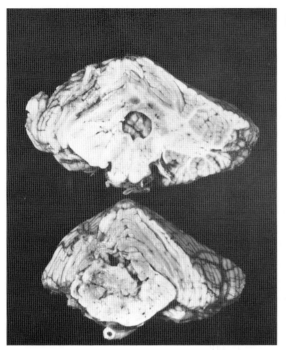

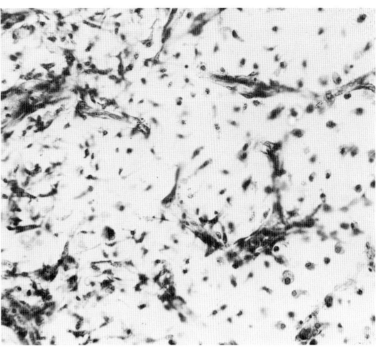

Fig. 79a.  Acute thrombosis of basilar artery
(sides reversed)

Fig. 79b.  Nissl × 200

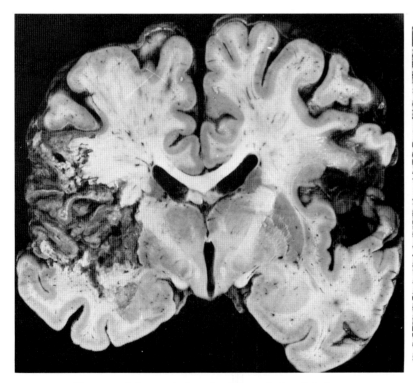

Fig. 79c.  Subacute infarct in right and chronic infarct
in left hemisphere (sides reversed)

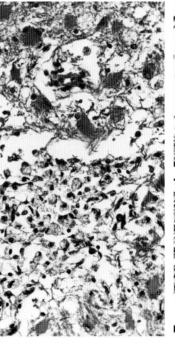

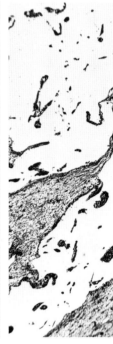

Fig. 79d.  HE × 200

Fig. 79e.  HE × 24

In a large number of cases, the effects of thrombosis and embolism are closely related and often indistinguishable. Thus thrombi developing at the site of atheromatous lesions in any part of the arterial system between the heart and brain can either propagate as continuous thrombi or become dislodged as emboli. Mural thrombi in association with auricular fibrillation or overlying myocardial infarcts are other sources of embolism. Embolic infarcts are often hemorrhagic because of fragmentation and migration of the embolus or because of cessation of angiospasm.

Thrombotic emboli may be aseptic or septic.

### ASEPTIC EMBOLISM

In the illustrated case (Fig. 80a) acute thrombosis of the right internal carotid artery led to the dislodgment of scattered emboli that plugged terminal branches in the territories of the middle and anterior cerebral arteries. Acute hemorrhagic infarcts resulted, which were disseminated in midfrontal and cingulate cortex and in parts of the caudate and putamen nuclei.

Microscopically, an acute thrombotic embolus is found plugging a small blood vessel in the meninges, producing a wedge-shaped focal area of acute ischemic necrosis in the underlying cortex (Fig. 80b).

### SEPTIC EMBOLISM

Septic embolism of the central nervous system generally occurs as a complication of bacterial endocarditis or pulmonary infections. Under such conditions aseptic infarcts may be intermingled with gross or miliary brain abscesses.

*Case:* A 59-year-old man with a history of rheumatic heart disease suddenly developed a right hemiplegia and aphasia. Examination revealed a temperature of 102.8° F., white blood count of 17,700, sedimentation rate of 25 mm per hour, albumin and casts in the urine, and a positive blood culture of Streptococcus viridans.

Autopsy disclosed chronic rheumatic endocarditis with mitral stenosis, subacute bacterial endocarditis, and focal glomerulonephritis.

Microscopically, scattered aseptic and septic emboli resulted in disseminated microinfarcts (Fig. 80c) and miliary abscesses (Fig. 80d) predominantly in the left hemisphere.

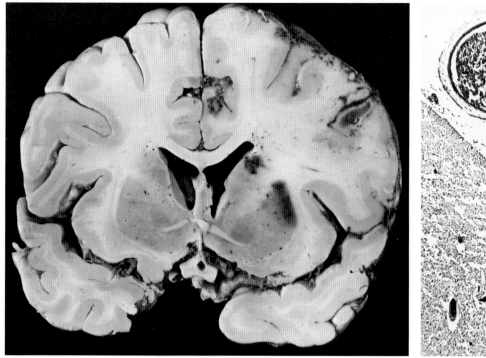

Fig. 80a. Scattered acute embolic infarcts

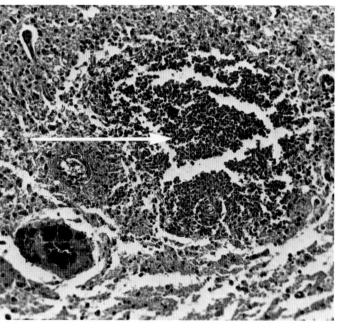

Fig. 80b. HE × 32

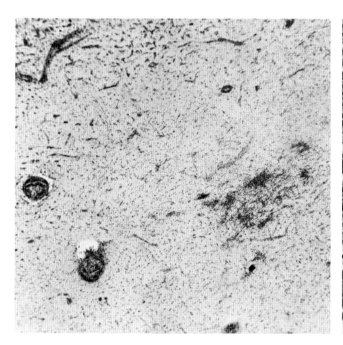

Fig. 80c. Nissl × 32

Fig. 80d. HE × 140

Fat embolism of the central nervous system may develop following fractures of long bones. Under such conditions, the emulsified fat globules pass through the pulmonary capillary filter to reach the cerebral circulation. The pathologic picture is one of hemorrhagic encephalopathy, virtually confined to the cerebral white matter.

*Case:* A man who was in an automobile accident was admitted to a hospital in coma. Examination disclosed multiple fractures of long bones of the extremities. Death occurred five days following the injury.

Large parts of the white matter of the brain were occupied by petechial hemorrhages (Fig. 81a) that surrounded fat globules plugging the capillaries and venules and extended into the perivascular tissue (Fig. 81b).

### AIR EMBOLISM

In rare circumstances air emboli may gain entrance into the central nervous system.

*Case:* A 37-year-old woman, with a long history of chronic pulmonary emphysema experienced recurrent attacks of dyspnea and cyanosis associated with rupture of emphysematous cysts that resulted in pneumo-thorax. In the last year of her life the episodes were complicated by recurrent states of mental confusion.

The brain showed no evidence of vascular disease, but there were disseminated infarcts in both gray and white matter, varying in age.

Microscopically, a chronic wedge-shaped infarct with early cyst formation is seen in the cerebral cortex, in the absence of any demonstrable emboli in the congested blood vessels of the meninges (Fig. 81c).

### EMBOLISM FOLLOWING CARDIAC SURGERY

A variety of complications may follow cardiac surgery, induced by emboli of particulate matter, fat, silicon, and air.

*Case:* A 40-year-old woman had a history of chronic rheumatic heart disease with mitral stenosis and insufficiency associated with bouts of pulmonary embolization in the past eighteen months. A mitral commissurotomy was performed. In the immediate postoperative period she developed a left hemiparesis and did not regain consciousness. She died twenty-four hours following surgery.

The brain showed grossly an acute thrombus in the right internal carotid artery with related infarct in its vascular territory.

Microscopically, fibrocalcific material associated with thrombosis plugged many meningeal branches of the right internal carotid and basilar arteries; the infarcts were in an acute ischemic phase without reaction (Fig. 81d).

### THROMBO-EMBOLISM ASSOCIATED WITH CARCINOMA

The association of thrombophlebitis migrans with carcinoma, especially of the pancreas, has been known to involve the central nervous system, either due to thrombosis in situ or from embolic fragments of nonbacterial thrombotic endocardial vegetations.

In a woman with carcinoma of the pancreas, an acute right hemiparesis and obtunded mental state developed in the last weeks of her life.

The brain contained multiple thrombi and related infarcts in the left cerebral hemisphere.

Microscopically, a thromboembolus undergoing early signs of organization is seen involving a meningeal artery, overlying a subacute infarct in the underlying cortex (Fig. 81e).

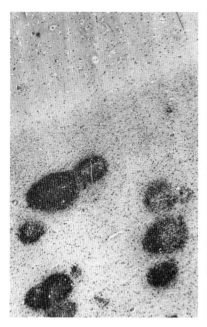

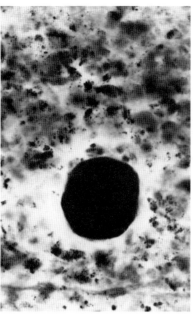

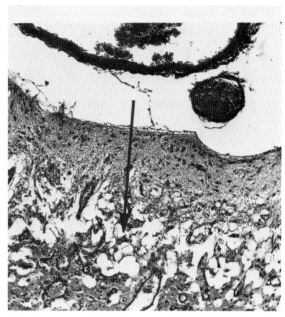

Fig. 81a. Weil × 32     Fig. 81b. Oil Red O × 560     Fig. 81c. HVG × 100

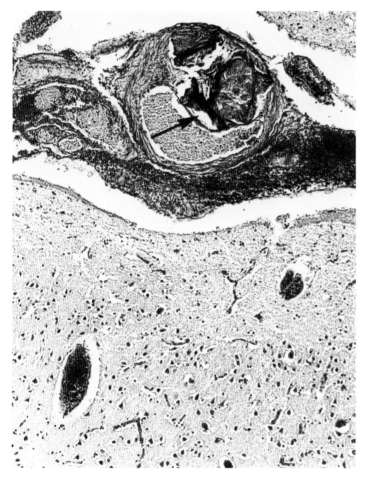

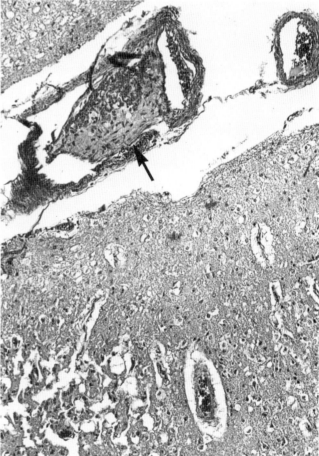

Fig. 81d. HVG × 90     Fig. 81e. HE × 90

Arteriosclerosis, whether cerebral or systemic, is the principal vascular disease in which thromboembolism occurs. It may take the form of athero- or arteriolo-sclerosis, either combined or independently, their effects differing accordingly.

In *atherosclerosis*, the large arteries forming the circle of Willis are the sites of predilection, producing focal eccentric plaques or diffuse fusiform dilatation.

The plaque is subendothelial in location, and presents a mixed picture of intimal fibrous hyperplasia and lipoidosis that encroaches on the lumen; the elastica interna may be frayed and delaminated, and the media compressed and degenerated.

The stenosed artery in combination with superimposed thromboembolism account for the infarct. A variety of syndromes result, depending on the location and size of the occluded vessel.

*Case 1:* A 40-year-old man had had a five-year history of hypertension. At the age of thirty-six he had suffered a stroke that resulted in a left-sided hemiplegia. This was followed by another stroke at the age of thirty-nine, causing a right-sided hemiplegia. When admitted to a hospital he presented symptoms of bilateral hemiplegia (more marked on the left side), dysarthria, dysphagia, emotional lability, and convulsions. He died in status epilepticus at the age of forty-three.

The brain showed grossly (Fig. 82a) a severe degree of atherosclerosis; an extensive old infarct destroyed the basal ganglia and internal capsule on the right side, and a small chronic lesion occupied the knee of the internal capsule on the left side; the base of the pons was atrophic due to Wallerian degeneration of the pyramidal tracts (involvement of cortico-bulbar fibers accounted for the pseudobulbar syndrome).

Microscopically, chronic cystic infarcts were present in the neighborhood of atherosclerotic vessels (Fig. 82b).

In *arteriolosclerosis*, commonly associated with hypertension, concentric thickening, hyalinization and calcification of the walls of arterioles, progressively reduce their lumens and result in small cysts with or without gliosis (état lacunaire and criblé). Such lesions are particularly common in basal ganglia and subcortical white matter, giving rise to a great variety of neurologic and mental signs.

*Case 2:* A 74-year-old man had had a two-year history of increasing irritability and episodes of confusion. In the hospital he exhibited explosive unmotivated crying and laughing, tremor and rigidity of the limbs, slowness of speech, a right Babinski sign, adiadokokinesis of the left hand and transient left hemiparesis. The blood pressure was 210/100, the heart was enlarged, and there was peripheral and retinal arteriosclerosis.

The brain showed grossly (Fig. 82c) mild atherosclerosis of the large arteries without infarct formation; there were scattered minute cysts in the basal ganglia and white matter, particularly in the putamen.

Microscopically, concentrically thickened and hyalinized arterioles were associated with scattered hemosiderin-laden phagocytes and astrogliosis (Fig. 82d), and/or perivascular rarefaction (Fig. 82e).

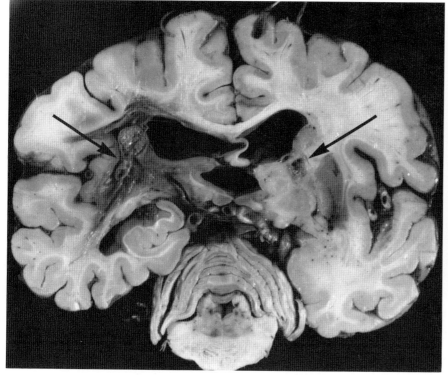

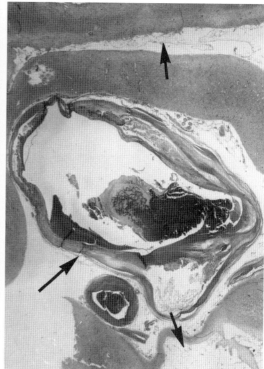

Fig. 82a. Cerebral atherosclerosis with chronic bilateral infarcts (sides reversed)

Fig. 82b. HVG

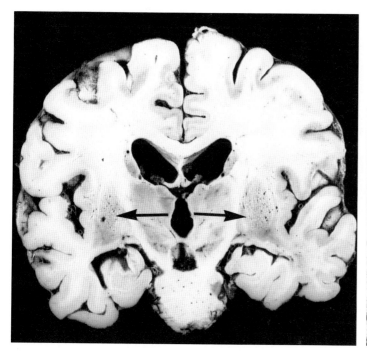

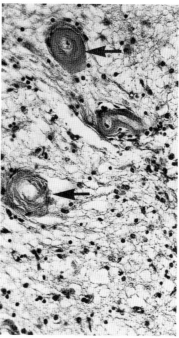

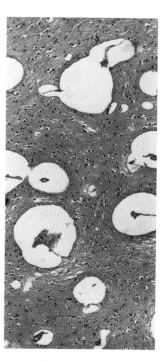

Fig. 82c. Cerebral arteriolosclerosis with minute cysts

Fig. 82d. HVG × 200

Fig. 82e. HE × 60

The most common condition causing massive intracerebral hemorrhage is hypertension. Several locations are favored in the following decreasing order of frequency: claustrum-putamen, thalamus, cerebellum, pons and cerebral white matter. Although the lenticulo-striate arteries are said to be the sites of origin of the common claustrum-putamen hemor-rhage, there is no clearcut topographic relationship to specific vascular territories in this or other sites.

The pathogenesis of massive hemorrhage remains obscure although several factors have been considered: increased intravascular pressure, decreased pressure of surrounding tissue, and alterations in the walls of blood vessels in the form of angionecrosis, hyalinosis, and ectasia or "aneurysms."

Massive hemorrhage most often leads to death through intraventricular rupture or complications of herniation. In fewer instances, resolution or encapsulation may take place.

*Case 1:* A 62-year-old woman with a past history of hypertension had several episodes of dizzi-ness and syncope during the past year. She was admitted to the hospital after having been found comatose in her room. On admission she had a right-sided hemiplegia and her blood pres-sure varied from 200/100 to 260/102. Her coma deepened, her previous bilateral extensor plantar responses became unobtainable, and she died twelve hours after admission.

The brain contained a massive hemorrhage originating in the claustrum-putamen region on the left side that had ruptured into the ventricular system (Fig. 83a).

Microscopically, the hematoma was surrounded by edema and petechial hemorrhages, the nearby blood vessels showing hyalinosis (Fig. 83b).

In recent years, there have been reports of anticoagulant therapy for occlusive vascular disease, acting as a precipitating factor in massive hemorrhage, especially in the presence of hypertension. In the following case, this may have been a contributing factor:

*Case:* A 79-year-old man had a past history of hypertension, arteriosclerotic cardiovascular disease, and a cerebrovascular accident, six years previously, with residual aphasia and mild right-sided weakness. He had been receiving anticoagulant therapy since that time. Twelve hours prior to his last admission he suddenly developed nausea and vomiting. On admission the blood pressure was 210/130 on the right and 190/126 on the left side. Neurologic examination revealed, in addition to the residual signs, nystagmus on lateral gaze bilaterally and deviation of the tongue to the right. A few hours following admission, he suddenly developed an acute respiratory arrest and expired.

The brain weighed 1,450 grams, showing moderate atherosclerosis, a chronic subcortical infarct in the left inferior frontal region and adjacent basal ganglia, and a massive recent hemorrhage in the right cerebellar hemisphere that penetrated the fourth ventricle (Fig. 83c), surrounded by edematous tissue and petechial hemorrhages (Fig. 83d).

*Reference*

Barron, K. D., and G. Ferguson. Intracranial Hemorrhage as a Complication of Anticoagulant Therapy. Neu-rol. 9: 447, 1959.

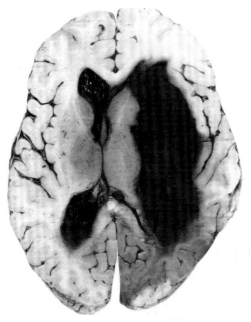

Fig. 83a. Massive hemorrhage in left claustrum-putamen region (sides reversed)

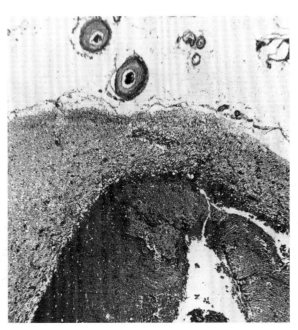

Fig. 83b. HE × 32

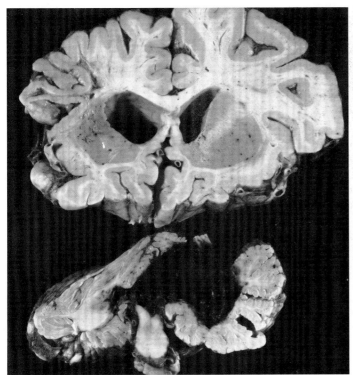

Fig. 83c. Recent hemorrhage in right cerebellar hemisphere;
chronic infarct in left frontal lobe

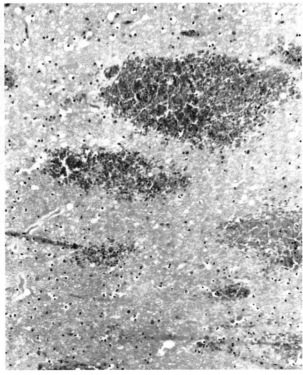

Fig. 83d. HE × 150

In the event of resolution, the massive hemorrhage undergoes gradual resorption and through the organizational process ultimately ends up as a slit-like cystic scar that possesses a yellowish capsule. In a case of hypertension with recurrent "strokes" an old encapsulated yellowish cyst replaced the caudate-putamen nuclei on the left, and an acute hemorrhage obscured the claustrum-putamen area on the right (Fig. 84a). The cyst contained hemosiderin-laden phagocytes (A) and the wall consisted of astrocytes, many of which also contained blood pigment, and of glial fibers (B) (Fig. 84b).

Rarely, a massive hemorrhage may encapsulate and lead to clinical signs of a space-consuming mass.

*Case:* A 66-year-old woman had an old history of rheumatic heart disease with episodes of auricular fibrillation that had recently become exacerbated. Two months before demise, she gradually developed clumsiness of her right side and was admitted to a hospital in a somnolent state. Examination revealed a blood pressure of 170/90, impairment of left lateral and upward gaze, narrowing of the right palpebral fissure, right hemianesthesia and right hemiparesis with bilateral Babinski signs. A lumbar puncture revealed a straw colored fluid under a pressure of 130 mm of $H_2O$ and contained 4,160 R. B. C./cmm, a total protein of 240 mg %, and a sugar of 25 mg %. Left carotid angiography showed no abnormality but a combined ventriculogram and pneumoencephalogram disclosed a mass in the region of the midbrain that displaced the third ventricle superiorly and to the right. X-ray therapy was recommended for a suspected tumor but patient expired before this was instituted.

The left thalamus was completely replaced by a massive hematoma, displacing to the right and obstructing the third ventricle; there were also scattered small infarcts and hemorrhages in the right temporal lobe (Fig. 84c).

Microscopically, the hematoma was walled off by a collagenous capsule (A) surrounded by a narrow zone of hemosiderin-containing macrophages (B) (Fig. 84d).

It is possible that the hematoma developed either on the basis of hypertension and/or from hemorrhagic infarcts caused by embolism related to auricular fibrillation, that accounted also for the small acute infarcts.

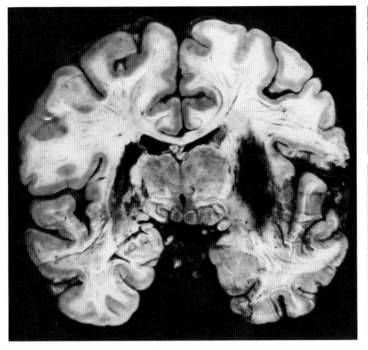

Fig. 84a. Bilateral claustrum-putamen hemorrhages, chronic on left and acute on right side

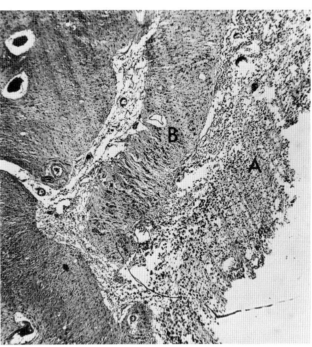

Fig. 84b. HE × 32

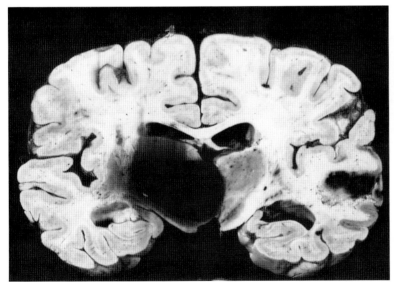

Fig. 84c. Encapsulated hematoma, left thalamus

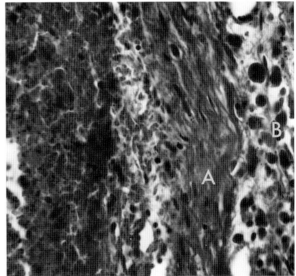

Fig. 84d. HVG × 250

## CEREBRAL ANEURYSMS

Aneurysms result from localized abnormal dilatation of blood vessels, of either saccular or fusiform shape, and may be classified as congenital, arteriosclerotic, mycotic, and dissecting varieties.

### CONGENITAL ANEURYSMS

The congenital variety is by far the most common. It is believed to be caused by medial defects at the bifurcation of the cerebral arteries in which hypertension and possibly other unknown factors may play a role. Though congenital, few occur in early life, the majority having a peak incidence at thirty to sixty years of age. Pathologically, they consist of a fibrous sac, single or lobulated, of 3–7 mm in average diameter, although at times reaching giant size. The wall varies in thickness from very thin and tenuous to cushion-like thickening, and consists of connective tissue and endothelial layers, lacking muscle fibers and often elastic fibers. They are usually single (Fig. 85a), at times multiple (Fig. 85b). Their effects differ: about 25–30% remain asymptomatic; the majority rupture, resulting in recurring episodes of subarachnoid hemorrhage; a few undergo progressive thrombosis, preventing rupture, resulting in either infarcts or space-consuming lesions.

Aneurysms most commonly involve the anterior portions of the circle of Willis, such as the junctions of the internal carotid and the posterior communicating branch, the anterior communicating and the anterior cerebral arteries, and at various branching sites of middle cerebral arteries. A much lesser number are related to the posterior circulation: junction of the basilar artery with either the posterior cerebral arteries or with the vertebral artery, or the latter with its branches (Fig. 85c).

*Case 1:* A 44-year-old man had a sudden onset of orbital pain followed by increasing visual impairment (especially on the right side), frontal headaches, and mental confusion. Five months later he developed recurring episodes of shock with hypertension, associated with stiffness of the neck. The spinal fluid was xanthochromic. An arteriogram disclosed a large aneurysm in the right internal carotid artery and three small aneurysms in the left artery. Eleven hours after angiography the patient developed respiratory difficulty and died.

The brain showed a large saccular aneurysm (A) (3 × 2 × 2 cm) in the right internal carotid artery, which had ruptured superiorly, the hemorrhage dissecting into the base of both frontal lobes but more so on the right side, obliterating the optic chiasm; there were three small berry aneurysms in the left internal carotid artery (B) (Fig. 85d).

Microscopically, the aneurysm consisted of a collagenous wall with alternating thin and cushion-like thickened parts; it had ruptured superiorly and the adjacent branches showed varying degrees of atherosclerosis (Fig. 85e).

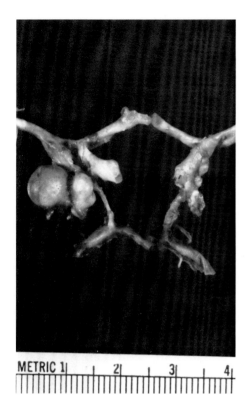

Fig. 85a. Lobulated aneurysm, junction of left internal carotid and posterior communicating arteries

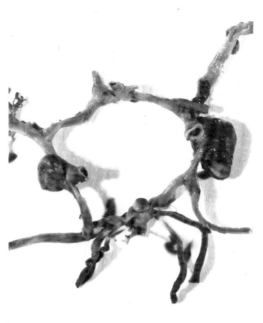

Fig. 85b. Bilateral aneurysm, junction internal carotid and posterior communicating arteries

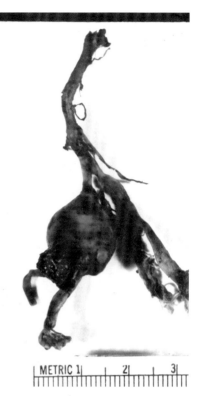

Fig. 85c. Aneurysm, junction of left vertebral and posterior inferior cerebellar arteries

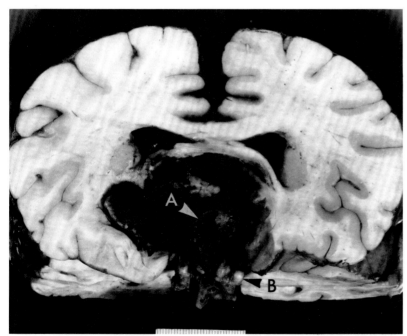

Fig. 85d. Ruptured aneurysm, right side (sides reversed)

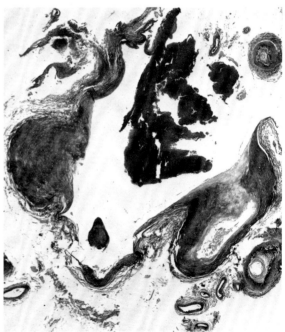

Fig. 85e. HVG-elastica stain

One of the principal complications of ruptured aneurysms is the tendency to ischemic infarct formation that is attributed to angiospasm; the pathogenesis of the latter is not clearly understood.

*Case:* A 57-year-old woman had an acute episode of headaches and confusion over a period of ten days, then became comatose and was admitted to a hospital. On admission she was in coma and had a left hemiparesis; papilledema was present on the right; the neck was rigid; carotid pulses were full without bruits. There was bilateral sixth nerve palsy and Babinski signs. The cerebrospinal fluid was under a pressure of 480 mm, was xanthochromic and contained 237 R.B.C./cmm. A right carotid arteriogram revealed two questionable saccular aneurysms of the right internal carotid artery at its junction with the middle and anterior cerebral branches, and spasm of the internal carotid vasculature with minimal shift of the pericallosal artery to the left. Two days later, the patient suddenly became hypertensive and developed a decerebrate posture with dilatation and fixation of the right pupil. She responded somewhat to hypothermia and Mannitol, but expired ten days following admission.

The brain showed a large aneurysm (Fig. 86a) of over 1 cm in diameter, that had its origin in the left internal carotid artery; it was largely occluded by old organized laminated thrombi, except for a small area on its inferior aspect where the wall was very thin and had recently ruptured, giving rise to minimal subarachnoid hemorrhage. There were bilateral areas of acute infarction in the vascular territories of both internal carotid arteries, more extensive on the right that through transtentorial herniation had ultimately resulted in terminal thalamic and brain stem hemorrhages. It was apparent that the clinical course was determined primarily by the extensive infarct formation that was secondary to angiospasm and led to fatal termination through herniation.

Giant aneurysms pursue a progressive clinical course, not unlike that of space-consuming tumors.

*Case 3:* A 43-year-old woman was admitted to a hospital with a history of recurrent right-sided headaches and progressive decrease in visual acuity for over two years. Examination revealed left homonymous hemianopsia; visual acuity was 20/50 in the right eye and 20/30 in the left eye. A brain scan revealed an abnormal focus to the right of the midline in the suprasellar region. Right carotid and vertebral angiography disclosed a large aneurysm, the size of a golfball, arising from the right carotid artery that crossed the midline and that failed to fill either anterior cerebral arteries but partly filled the right middle cerebral artery. A ventriculogram revealed displacement of the third ventricle to the left with incomplete obstruction of the foramen of Monro, and a Selverstone clamp was applied to the right carotid artery. Postoperatively, patient remained lethargic. On the tenth day there was an acute rise in intracranial pressure followed by episodes of high blood pressure, when both pupils were in a mid-dilated position and nonreactive. Bilateral Torkildsen shunts were without benefit, and she died two months following admission.

A large unruptured aneurysm, measuring 3.5 × 4 cm, was found adherent to the right internal carotid artery at its junction with the posterior communicating branch, replacing the optic chiasm except for part of the left nerve (Fig. 86b). It was completely filled with laminated clot, its wall varying in thickness and consisting of an endothelial and a collagenous layer without showing any muscle or elastic fibers (Fig. 86c).

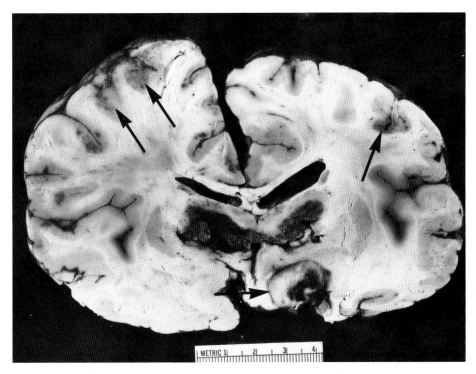

Fig. 86a. Aneurysm on right side; bilateral acute cerebral infarcts and diencephalic hemorrhages (sides reversed)

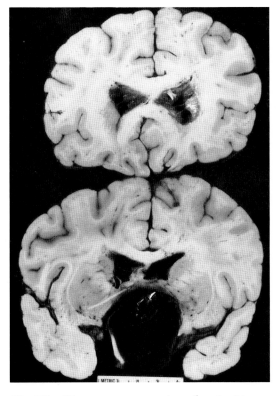

Fig. 86b. Giant aneurysm, region of optic chiasm

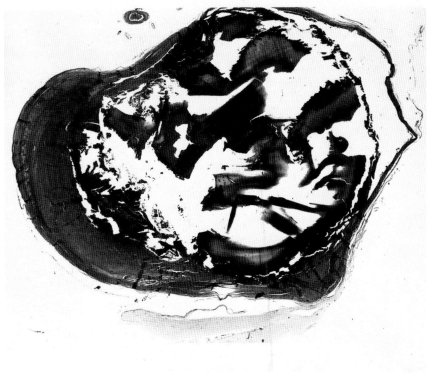

Fig. 86c. HVG stain

Syphilis usually involves large and medium-sized arteries of the brain and spinal cord, resulting in panarteritis that affects all the coats of the blood vessel, generally referred to as Heubner's syphilitic endarteritis. The condition may exist independently of, or be associated with, meningitis. Occlusion of the diseased blood vessels results in infarcts.

> *Case:* A 60-year-old black man had a one-year history of recurring "strokes" resulting in paralysis of the extremities. He was admitted to a hospital showing evidence of a right hemiplegia, bilateral Babinski signs, ankle clonus on the left, lateral nystagmus, and dysarthria. Blood and spinal fluid showed a strongly positive Kolmer reaction and a first-zone rise in the gold curve. Patient died of an intercurrent bronchopneumonia.

Grossly, all major arteries at the base of the brain were concentrically thickened and grayish-white in color, associated with multiple small cysts in the cerebral tissue of both hemispheres (Fig. 87a).

Microscopically, the vascular changes varied from acute phases of infiltrations with lymphocytes and plasma cells in all layers (Fig. 87b) to chronic stages with concentric intimal thickening and minimal inflammatory reaction.

## GIANT CELL ARTERITIS

Giant cell arteritis, also known as temporal arteritis, may involve arteries of all sizes, the most characteristic changes consisting of a granulomatous angiitis. The temporal and ophthalmic arteries are the most frequently involved with corresponding clinical signs, associated with inconstant fever and elevated protein in the cerebrospinal fluid. It occurs usually in advanced age, predominates in females and often terminates in an acute cerebrovascular accident, due to thrombosis or obliterating endarteritis. The etiology remains unknown but a hyperergic state has been suggested.

> *Case:* A 77-year-old man was admitted to a hospital because of blurring of vision of two to three weeks' duration associated with episodic pains in the temporal region, more pronounced on the left side. On examination, blood pressure was 170/78. The temporal arteries were tortuous and dilated. There were diminished ability to look up, mild right-sided ptosis and a large defect in the right lower visual field. Later, ataxia and depression of biceps and supinator reflexes with wasting of the small muscles of the right hand were noted. A right retrograde brachial arteriogram showed no filling of the intracranial ramifications of the vertebral artery. A biopsy of the right temporal artery was diagnosed as a granulomatous temporal arteritis. Anticoagulants and steroid hormones were administered without benefit. The patient became comatose with fixed pupils and died one month following admission.

At autopsy there was granulomatous arteritis involving the temporal arteries, aorta, and the coronary and iliac arteries, with thrombosis of the left circumflex branch and infarction of the left lateral ventricle wall, embolization to the spleen, kidney, and brain, and thrombosis of the right common iliac artery.

Microscopically, the adventitia of the temporal arteries was infiltrated with lymphocytes, the media contained scattered giant multinucleated cells while the lumen was occluded by proliferation of the intima (Fig. 87c).

In the brain there was no evidence of the granulomatous angiitis. The left posterior cerebral artery and many meningeal and intracortical arterioles were acutely or subacutely thrombosed associated with corresponding stages of coalescing infarcts, composed of variable macrophage and capillary proliferation (Fig. 87d).

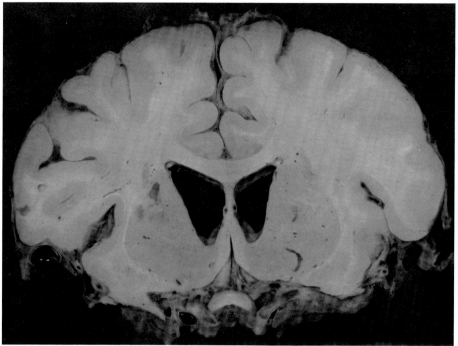

Fig. 87a. Syphilitic arteritis

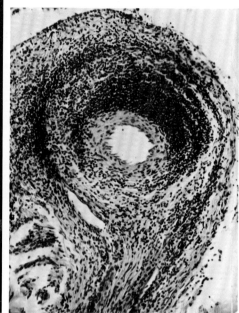

Fig. 87b. HE × 65

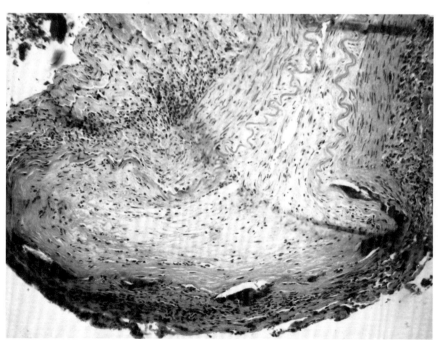

Fig. 87c. Temporal arteritis

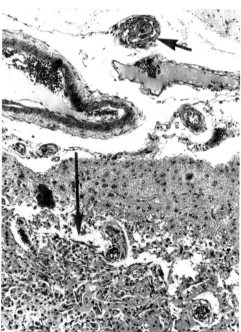

Fig. 87d. HE × 70

Systemic lupus erythematosus is generally classified as a "collagen" disease because of widespread alterations of extracellular components of connective tissues. It is considered to be an autoimmune disorder, with damage to small blood vessels induced by excess of autoimmune antibodies. It occurs predominantly in females, in the second to fourth decades of life. The nervous system is involved in about one-third to one-half of the cases. Neurologic symptoms consist of convulsions, psychoses, focal signs, and polyneuropathy. The diagnosis is based on demonstration of phagocytosed nuclear material by leukocytes—the so-called LE cells.

Pathologically, the vascular lesions generally involve small and medium-sized meningeal arteries, most commonly in the cerebral and cerebellar cortex. They are characterized by fibrinoid necrosis without inflammatory reaction in the acute phases, and of intimal proliferation in the chronic stages; superimposed thrombosis results in infarcts.

*Case:* A 43-year-old woman had had a two-year history of recurring "schizophrenic" psychotic episodes accompanied by mild neurologic signs and slight changes in the colloidal gold reaction of the spinal fluid. In the last year of her life she developed an erythematous rash on the face, arthritis, albuminuria, hypertension, a systolic cardiac murmur, and flame-shaped hemorrhages in the fundi. Her mental picture changed from the initial psychosis to an organic syndrome, characterized by disorientation and lethargy. Administration of cortisone was of no benefit, and she died from congestive heart failure.

The general autopsy confirmed changes of disseminated lupus erythematosus.

The brain showed a gross picture of "granular" atrophy of the cortex, particularly in the frontal lobes (Fig. 88a).

Microscopically, vascular lesions of different ages were noted. Some of the meningeal arteries showed a diffuse eosinophilic fibrinoid necrosis of the wall (Fig. 88b), associated with thrombi that resulted in acute infarcts (Fig. 88c) while others had undergone chronic endothelial proliferation with recanalized thrombosis associated with focal gliosis in the underlying cortex (Fig. 88d).

*Reference*

Malamud, N., and G. Saver. Neuropathologic Findings in Disseminated Lupus Erythymatosus. Arch. Neurol. and Psychiat. 71: 723–731 (June) 1954.

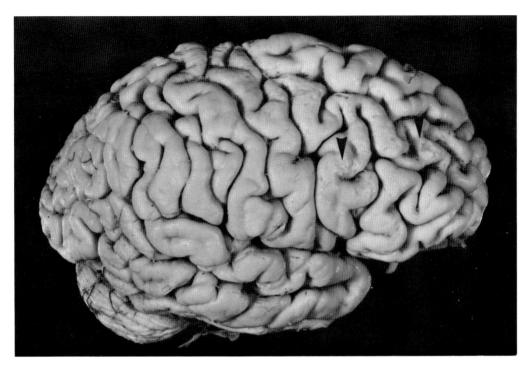

Fig. 88a. Granular atrophy of cortex in lupus erythematosus

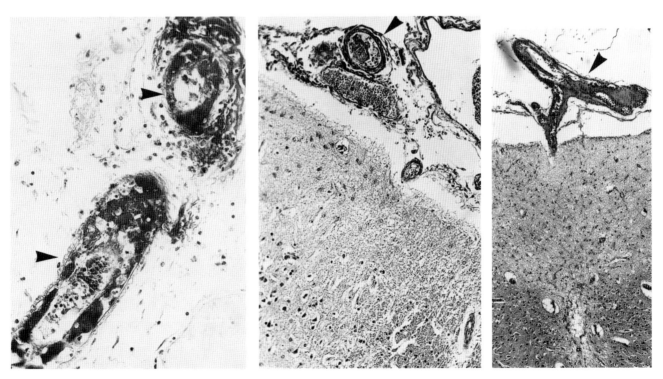

Fig. 88b. HE × 100          Fig. 88c. HVG × 75          Fig. 88d. HVG × 50

# POLYARTERITIS NODOSA

Poly- or periarteritis nodosa is another form of multi-system "collagen" disease. It more commonly affects males, either young or of middle age. The peripheral nervous system is involved in about 20% and the central nervous system in about 10% of cases. It is considered to be a hyperergic arteritis caused by infection, allergy, and various drugs and chemicals. Pathologically, the vascular lesions predominate in small arteries and are characterized by an initial subendothelial fibrinoid necrosis, followed by an inflammatory reaction, and ending in intimal proliferation. Infarcts result from occlusion of nutrient arteries and hemorrhages from less common aneurysms. Diffuse infiltration of meninges with lymphocytes is reflected in pleocytosis and raised protein in the cerebrospinal fluid.

> *Case 1:* A 43-year-old man developed, over a period of eight months, weakness, pain in the legs, blurred vision, diplopia, nocturia, and ankle edema. When admitted to the hospital he had a low-grade fever and showed paralysis of the third and fourth cranial nerves, lateral nystagmus, pyramidal signs, and muscle tenderness. The spinal fluid contained 18–56 lymphocytes per cmm., and increased protein. A muscle biopsy was diagnostic of periarteritis nodosa. The clinical course was marked by remissions and exacerbations. Ultimately, mental confusion, dysarthria, dysphagia, and pyramidal and meningeal signs became established. He died one year following the onset of symptoms.

There were disseminated vascular lesions throughout all organs and the central and peripheral nervous systems.

Only the smaller arteries were affected. Some contained rings of "fibrinoid" material in the subintimal and medial layers, surrounded by lymphocytic infiltrations in the adventitia (Fig. 89a). Others exhibited chronic changes, in which the layer of fibrin had been replaced by intimal fibrous proliferation, surrounded by lymphocytes (Fig. 89b).

Lymphocytic meningitis, coalescing small infarcts and arteritis were found throughout the central nervous system (Fig. 89c), in the peripheral nervous system, muscles, and many organs.

Involvement of the peripheral nervous system usually presents clinically as a mononeuritis multiplex.

> *Case 2:* A 70-year-old man noted prickly sensations and weakness in his hands and feet over a three-months' period. Examination revealed splenohepatomegaly, decreased sensation in all fingers of the right hand and in the second and third digits of the left hand, and generalized muscle weakness. Laboratory studies showed HCT range of 27–36, platelet counts from 52,000 to 149,000/cmm; W.B.C. of 2,200 per cmm; reticulocyte count of 0.9% to 1.9%, and total serum protein of 8 with hypergammaglobulinemia. The total protein in the spinal fluid was 110 mg % but was otherwise normal. A liver biopsy showed infiltrates of lymphocytes and muscle biopsy evidence of denervation atrophy. He later became comatose, and expired of a pontine hemorrhage.

General autopsy findings were those of disseminated polyarteritis nodosa. In the brain there were occasional changes of arteritis, the terminal pontine hemorrhage being attributed to the thrombocytopenia.

In the peripheral nervous system, the nerve fascicles showed focal demyelination (Fig. 89d) along with axonal loss, related to various stages of arteritis involving the nutrient blood vessels (Fig. 89e).

*Reference*

Malamud, N., and D. B. Foster. Periarteritis Nodosa. Arch. Neurol and Psychiat. 47: 828–838 (May) 1942.

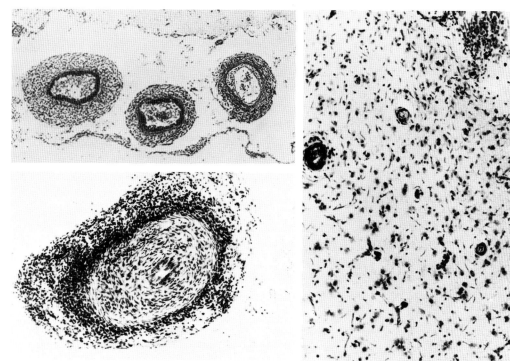

Fig. 89a. Heidenhain's aniline blue × 75
Fig. 89b. Nissl × 100

Fig. 89c. Nissl × 100

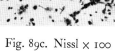

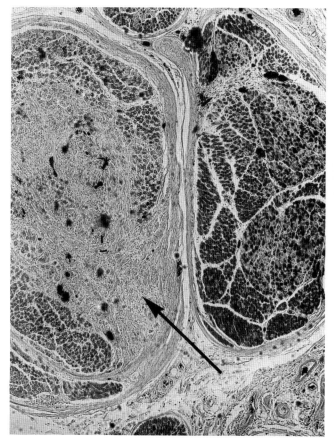

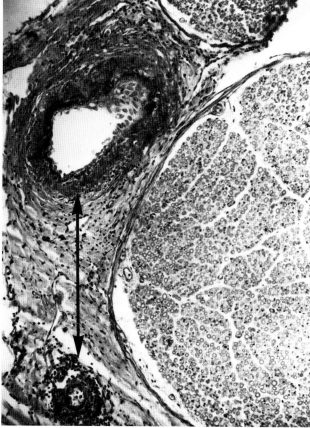

Fig. 89d. Weil × 50

Fig. 89e. LFB × 80

Sinus and venous thrombosis results from a variety of causes such as infection of adjacent structures, trauma, and disturbed circulation as in polycythemia, sickle cell anemia, or states of malnutrition and dehydration ("marantic" thrombosis). Their effects depend on the specific sinus involved and its tributaries.

Pathologically, the thrombi tend to extend from the sinus into the draining tributaries, often in a discontinuous fashion. Subarachnoid hemorrhage and hemorrhagic necrosis of the nervous tissue result.

> *Case 1:* A 6-year-old girl, with cerebral palsy and severe malnutrition, had an acute onset of fever and respiratory difficulty, followed the next day by tremors of the right arm, stiffness of neck, and increasing stupor. A lumbar puncture revealed blood in the cerebrospinal fluid; smear and cultures were negative for microorganisms. Coma ensued, and death occurred five days following the onset of symptoms.

Autopsy revealed an acute otitis media and thrombosis of the left lateral sinus that extended into the superior longitudinal sinus.

The convexity of the temporo-parieto-occipital region of the brain was diffusely hemorrhagic on both sides, particularly on the left side, and some of the superior cerebral veins were thrombosed (Fig. 90a).

Microscopically (Fig. 90b) acutely distended and thrombosed meningeal veins stood out in contrast with the normal appearance of adjacent arteries; the underlying cerebral cortex showed ischemic necrosis and contained numerous perivenous hemorrhages.

> *Case 2:* A severely malnourished child with cerebral palsy became acutely comatose and expired shortly following the onset.

The brain showed grossly bilateral, fairly symmetrical, hemorrhages in parasagittal cortical areas and in the thalamus, corresponding to drainage territories of the superficial and deep veins respectively (Fig. 90c).

Microscopically, changes in the basal ganglia resulted from thrombi in the internal veins of Galen that extended into their tributaries draining the caudate nucleus, the thalamus, and putamen, resulting in either hemorrhagic or ischemic infarcts (Fig. 90d).

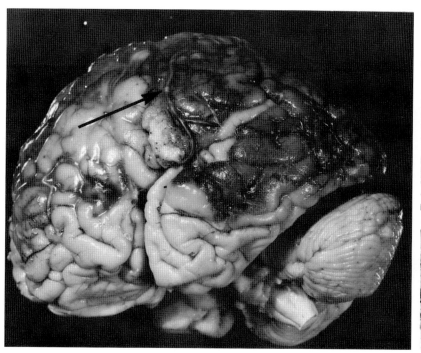

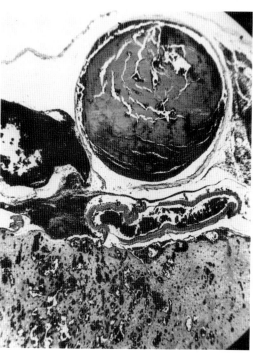

Fig. 90a. Venous thrombosis and hemorrhagic infarction

Fig. 90b. HE × 16

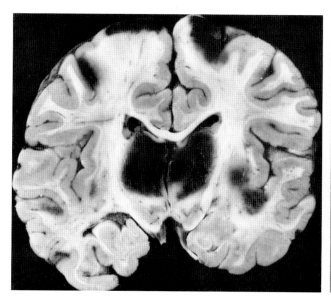

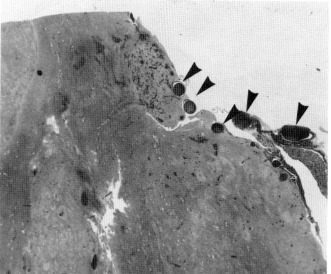

Fig. 90c. Hemorrhagic infarcts in superficial and deep venous territories

Fig. 90d. HVG

Sickle-cell anemia, a disorder of the black race, is caused by inheritance from parents with sickle cell traits of an abnormal hemoglobin that results in transformation of the red blood cells to filamentous or crescentic shapes under conditions of reduced oxygen tension. Diagnosis is established through identification of homozygous Hemoglobin S by electrophoresis. Due to insolubility of Hemoglobin S, increased blood viscosity takes place leading to infarct formation through stasis and thrombosis both of arteries and veins. Patients with sickle cell disease undergo acute hemolytic crises with anemia, icterus, cardiac and liver enlargement, and often with various neurologic symptoms.

*Case 1:* A 9-year-old black boy developed at the age of four years an episode diagnosed as a sickle cell crisis, at which time his hemoglobin was 5.5 g % and the hematocrit was 14%. He recovered and remained well for the next five years. Five days before his demise he developed headaches, vomiting, and lethargy and was hospitalized. At this time his hemoglobin was 8.6 g % and the hematocrit was 26; the cerebrospinal fluid was under a pressure of 480 mm and was grossly bloody with 20,000 R.B.C. and 5,000 W.B.C. per cmm, a total protein of 78 mg % and sugar of 70 mg %. There was a harsh systolic murmur at the apex. Sickle cell preparations were positive. Neurologically, there was nuchal rigidity and later generalized seizures, deepening coma, and a decerebrate state. The blood pressure continued to rise. Towards the end, the pupils became dilated and fixed, and he expired.

The brain showed grossly diffuse acute subarachnoid hemorrhage, an intracerebral hematoma of 2 x 3.5 cm in the right frontal lobe and generalized edema and congestion (Fig. 91a).

Microscopically (Fig. 91b), there was marked stasis of blood in the arterioles, venules, and capillaries of the meninges and brain tissue, associated with numerous ischemic infarcts, the local hemorrhage in the white matter representing a hemorrhagic infarct. The congested blood vessels and the hemorrhagic areas showed sickling of the red blood cells (Fig. 91c).

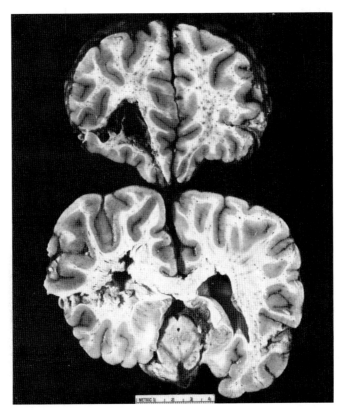

Fig. 91a. Acute cerebral changes in sickle-cell anemia (sides reversed)

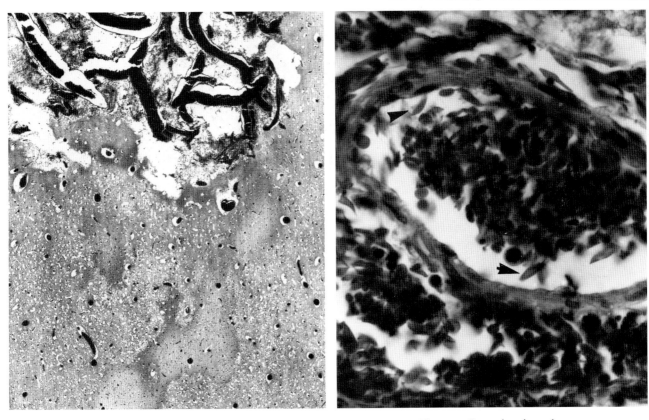

Fig. 91b. HE × 20

Fig. 91c. Gomori stain × 640

The chronic neurologic sequelae of sickle-cell anemia are less well known in the literature.

*Case 2:* An 11-year-old black girl was diagnosed as having SS hemoglobinopathy (sickle-cell disease) at age five months. Her parents carried sickle-cell trait but four siblings were clinically normal. The patient was well until age four years when she rapidly developed left hemiplegia, slurred speech, and impaired vision, followed by partial remission. Over the ensuing sixteen months, she had four other episodes, during hemolytic crises, of either right or left hemiparesis, became unable to speak, barely able to see, was severely spastic in the right extremities, incontinent, and moderately retarded in all mental and motor functions. At the age of five and one-half years, she rapidly became semicomatose. Examination revealed a temperature of 103° F. rectally. Hemoglobin at this time was 5.2 gm%, hematocrit 14%, W.B.C. 24,900, and blood smear contained numerous nucleated erythrocytes. She gradually became more alert with red cell infusions but never regained the ability to move her extremities. On admission to a State hospital at the age of seven years, she was totally helpless, unable to roll over or speak, and showed bilaterally hyperactive reflexes with severe contractures. At the age of eight years generalized seizures began, and an EEG showed left temporal seizure discharges. She developed pneumonia and died following a generalized convulsion.

The general autopsy findings were pulmonary and renal thromboemboli and infarcts, and cardiomegaly associated with sickle-cell disease.

The brain weighed 720 grams. It showed severe bilateral chronic areas of necrosis, resulting in atrophy of both gray and white matter, primarily in the dorsal parts of the hemispheres, with corresponding ventricular dilatation (Fig. 92a).

Microscopically, chronic infarcts characterized by cyst formation and dense collagenous and glial fibrosis were associated with distended meningeal blood vessels that contained sickle cells (Fig. 92b). There were old organized thrombi in both internal carotid arteries and in some of their branches (Fig. 92c). That the veins were likewise occluded seemed probable from the frequent dense fibrosis of the walls of veins and from the pattern of gliosis in the caudate and putamen on the left in the form of typical status marmoratus (Fig. 92d) (see Chapter X).

*References*

Baird, R. L., D. L. Weiss, A. D. Ferguson, J. H. French, and R. B. Scott. Pediat. 34: 92, 1964.
Hughes, J. J., L. W. Diggs, and C. E. Gillespie. The Involvement of the Nervous System in Sickle Cell Anemia J. Pediat. 17: 166, 1940.

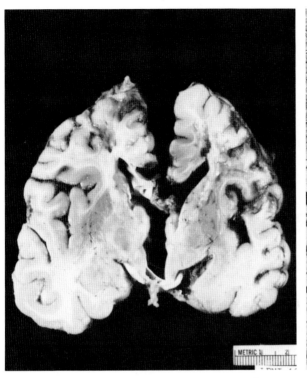

Fig. 92a. Chronic cerebral changes in sickle-cell anemia

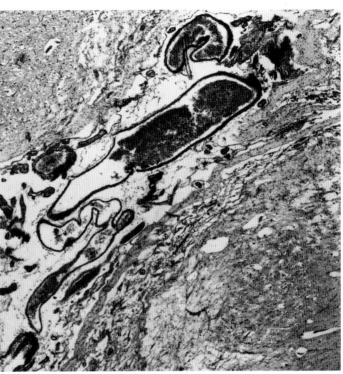

Fig. 92b. HVG × 80

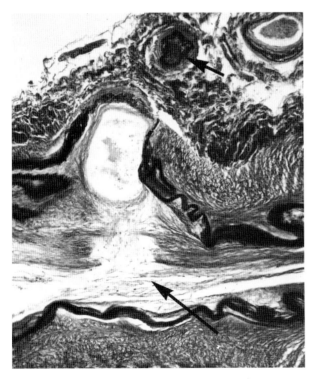

Fig. 92c. HVG × 28

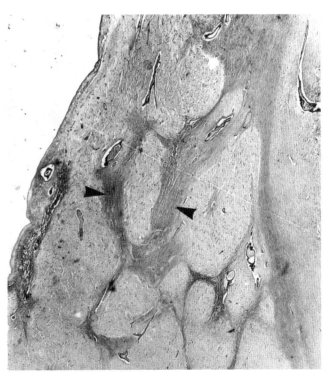

Fig. 92d. Holzer × 12

# VI

## *Traumatic Disorders*

The effects of trauma to the head or spine differ depending on the manner, tempo, and degree of intensity with which the injury is sustained and whether it is closed or open.

### CLOSED HEAD INJURIES

In injuries that are not associated with fractures, a number of pathologic lesions result, either singly or in combination, as a result of movements of acceleration and deceleration brought about by the force of mechanical impact. They may be classified as subdural hemorrhage, acute or chronic; subarachnoid hemorrhage; concussion, contusion, and laceration. In either case, one of the most serious complications is herniation, especially through the incisura of the tentorium.

#### ACUTE SUBDURAL HEMORRHAGE

Subdural hemorrhage takes place when the shearing force of impact causes rupture of the bridging veins as they cross the subdural space to enter the sinuses. Such a condition is particularly apt to occur in infants or the aged even with relatively moderate trauma.

It is usually located on the convexity in the frontoparietal region, uni- or bilaterally, and acts as a space-occupying mass locally by compression and at a distance through displacement of structures and threatened herniation.

> *Case:* A 64-year-old man, chronic alcoholic, sustained a fall and became unresponsive. X-rays of the skull failed to disclose any evidence of fracture. Examination revealed coma and a dilated fixed pupil on the right side. In his further course he vomited, the blood pressure fluctuated, the pulse rate became rapid, and he developed dilatation and fixation of both pupils and respiratory irregularities, and expired approximately twenty-four hours following the injury.

The brain showed (Fig. 93a) an acute subdural hematoma on the right side (the clot having fallen out at the time of autopsy), compressing the underlying frontoparietal cortex, displacing the ventricles and midline structures to the left, and causing trans-tentorial herniation of the entire hippocampal gyrus. Slit-like hemorrhages occurred in the latter at the site of direct contact with the sharp edge of the tentorium, while indirectly, through circulatory disturbance, hemorrhages developed in the midline of the midbrain and tegmentum of the pons.

Microscopically, the mass of R.B.C. (A) adhered to the undersurface of the dura (Fig. 93b). The indirect effects of herniation were seen as confluent petechial hemorrhages in the floor of the aqueduct of Sylvius (Fig. 93c).

Diffuse subarachnoid hemorrhage, while a common independent complication of head injuries, is often associated with subdural hemorrhage.

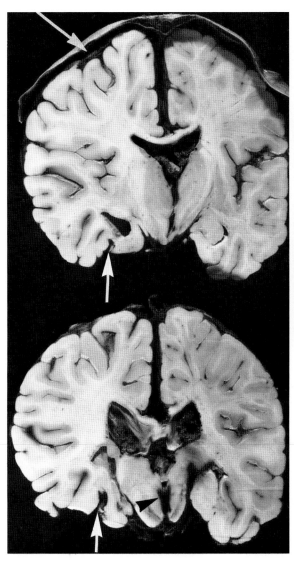

Fig. 93a. Acute subdural hematoma on right side
(sides reversed)

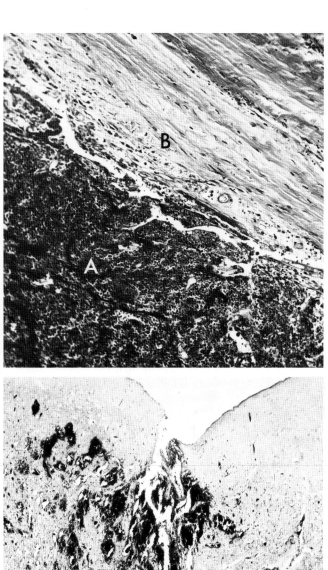

Fig. 93b. HE × 40

Fig. 93c. Hemorrhages in midbrain

A chronic subdural hematoma develops insidiously as a result of venous oozing, often after trivial head injuries, especially in the aged. It is usually unaccompanied by intracranial displacements of structures but acts by compressing the underlying brain tissue. A special feature is its tendency to encapsulation by the formation of outer and inner membranes, respectively from the dura and arachnoid. The outer membrane is the first to develop through invasion of the clot by fibroblasts, accompanied by dissolution of the blood with reaction by phagocytes, lymphocytes and capillaries. It is followed after a few weeks by a similar process developing in the arachnoid. The mass continues to expand for several months by intermittent bleeding and imbibition of fluid through osmosis.

> *Case:* A 57-year-old woman, diagnosed as having an involutional psychosis, sustained repeated injuries to the head through falls. Several months before her death, she showed mental confusion and increasing weakness of the right side of her body.

The lateral surface of the left cerebral hemisphere was compressed by a large encysted subdural hematoma; the outer membrane of the hematoma could be stripped from the under surface of the dura, and the inner membrane lay freely over the underlying pia-arachnoid (Fig. 94a).

Microscopically, layers of fibrous tissue (A), enclosing hemosiderin-laden phagocytes and scattered lymphocytes, adhered to the undersurface of the dura (B). Unorganized blood clots (C) occupied the more central parts of the hematoma (Fig. 94b).

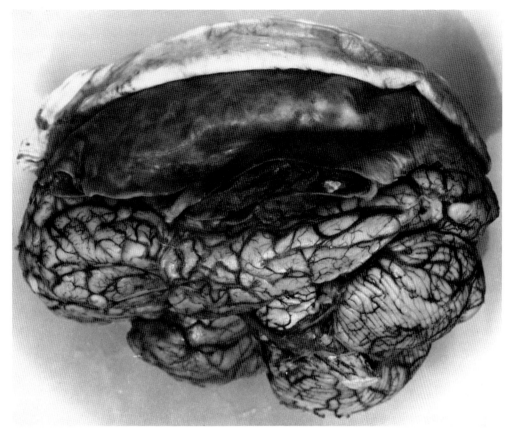

Fig. 94a. Chronic subdural hematoma

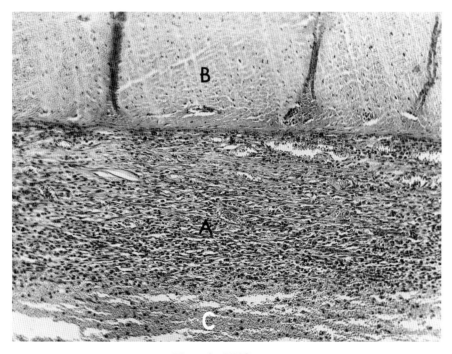

Fig. 94b. HVG × 100

While cerebral concussion is generally regarded as a transient functional disorder without demonstrable morphologic changes, contusions and lacerations are well defined lesions. They may be coup or contrecoup, the former being usually located on the lateral aspects of the hemispheres while the latter tend to involve basal cortex near the bony ridges of the base of the skull.

Histologically, they are characterized by focal wedge-shaped areas of necrosis and petechial hemorrhages with predilection for the cortical surface over the crests of gyri, often accompanied by diffuse subarachnoid hemorrhage.

> *Case:* A 22-year-old man, said to have fallen off a moving truck, was admitted to a hospital in a state of coma. He died shortly without regaining consciousness. There was no evidence of skull fracture.

Acute hemorrhage involved the inferolateral surface and the entire base of the left frontal lobe, the right rectus gyrus, and the anterior part of the left temporal lobe; subarachnoid hemorrhage filled all the cisterns around the brain stem, and there was bilateral uncal herniation (arrows), (Fig. 95a).

Coronal sections revealed multiple petechial hemorrhages, bilaterally but more on the left side, chiefly in the basal cortex of the frontal and temporal lobes (including the hippocampal gyri) and in the tegmentum of the upper brain stem (Fig. 95b).

Microscopically (Fig. 95c) diffuse subarachnoid hemorrhage surrounded foci of intracortical coalescing petechial hemorrhages and ischemic necrosis.

The complicating transtentorial herniation accounted for the hemorrhages in the upper brain stem (so-called Duret hemorrhages).

The phenomenon of transtentorial herniation is one of the most significant complications of supratentorial space-consuming lesions, whether due to trauma, massive infarcts, hemorrhages, abscesses, or neoplasms with their attendant edema. The distribution of such lesions corresponds to vascular territories supplied by either arteries or veins whose circulation has been interfered with by sudden compression or displacement at the incisura. Thus vascular lesions in the midbrain and pontile tegmentum are related to paramedian and short circumferential branches of the basilar artery and/or to corresponding venous tributaries; lesions in the medial and inferior aspects of the temporal and occipital lobes, thalamus, hypothalamus, lateral geniculate body and third nerve to branches of the posterior cerebral arteries; and lesions in the globus pallidus and parts of the uncus and hippocampus to branches of anterior choroidal arteries. Their clinical significance is the impairment of function of the various regions, especially that of the vital centers in the brain stem and diencephalon.

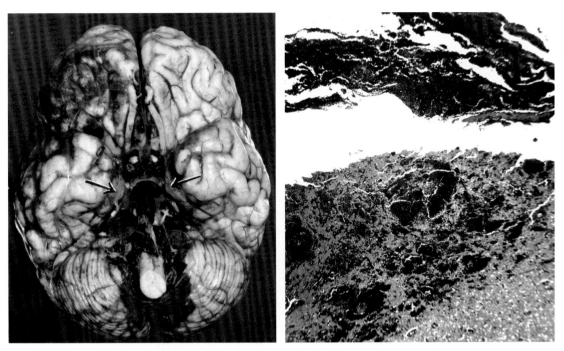

Fig. 95a. Acute cerebral contusions (basal view)          Fig. 95c. HE × 24

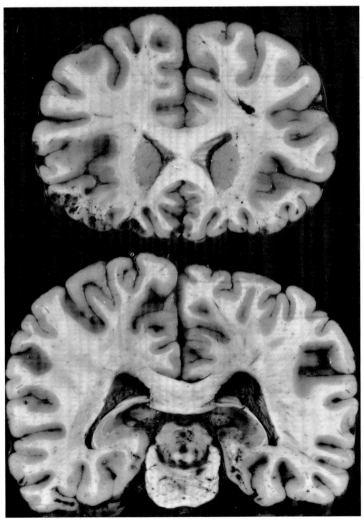

Fig. 95b. Acute cerebral contusions (coronal sections)

The chronic residuals of head injuries correspond to the topography of the acute lesions.

Acute subdural hemorrhages may resorb and organize into a rust-colored membrane, often of no clinical significance. Diffuse subarachnoid hemorrhage may organize into an adhesive arachnoiditis, especially at the base around the foramina of Magendie and Luschka, resulting in communicating hydrocephalus.

Cerebral contusions, with their coup and contrecoup localization, present a characteristic appearance of "plaques jaunes," manifested by worm-eaten pigmented gyri, showing cystic-atrophic changes, adherent to surrounding fibrotic meninges. Their clinical symptoms are often dominated by personality changes and convulsive disorder, because of predominant fronto-temporal localization.

> *Case:* A 38-year-old man sustained a head injury, and was unconscious for several weeks. He subsequently remained mentally confused, and showed personality changes of heightened irritability and irrational behavior. He died at the age of forty-two.

"Plaques jaunes" involved the poles and base of both frontal and temporal lobes, being more extensive on the left side (Fig. 96a).

Microscopically, the involved cortex was replaced by partly cystic fibrous tissue (Fig. 96b).

Under higher magnification, the meninges and gray matter were fused into meningo-cortical scars consisting of zones of collagen fibers, containing hemosiderin-laden phagocytes (A), and zones of fibrillary astrocytes (B) (Fig. 96c).

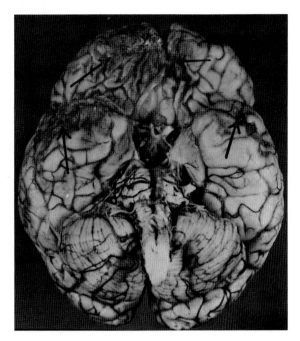

Fig. 96a. Chronic cerebral contusions

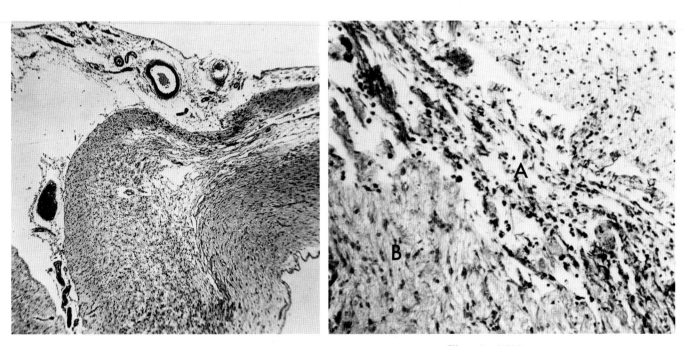

Fig. 96b. HVG × 24

Fig. 96c. HVG × 120

Complications of transtentorial herniation, when occurring in the form of brain stem hemorrhages, are usually fatal, however in a small percentage of cases may be survived although with severe sequelae.

*Case:* A 31-year-old man was in a motorcycle accident followed by coma. Examination showed no evidence of a skull fracture or subdural hematoma. He gradually developed a state of decerebrate rigidity, little response to painful stimuli, bilaterally fixed and unequal pupils, spastic quadriplegia with right-sided pyramidal signs and equivocal signs on the left, and a marked grasp reflex of the left hand. He died fifteen months following the head injury.

The brain showed grossly, generalized dilatation of all ventricles and a chronic area of necrosis restricted to the uncus and adjacent hippocampal gyrus on the left side (Fig. 97a).

Microscopically, scattered cysts with sparse glial fiber content and intervening linear foci of gliosis, extended across the uncus and hippocampal gyrus (Fig. 97b), while the adjacent posterior cerebral artery had a normal appearance.

In the region of the aqueduct there was diffuse demyelination and gliosis that extended into the oculomotor nuclei, associated with small perivascular cystic lesions that contained hemosiderin pigment in macrophages lying free in the tissue (Figs. 97c and d). There were similar focal lesions in the cerebral peduncles, substantia nigra, thalamus, splenium of the corpus callosum and optic radiation, bilaterally but more extensive on the left side.

The significant findings thus appeared to be chronic sequelae of transtentorial herniation following initial focal necrosis with·minimal hemorrhage at the time of the head injury. The ventricular dilatation could be attributed to a basal arachnoiditis resulting from a subarachnoid hemorrhage.

*Reference*

Malamud, N. The Effects of Trauma on the Brain Stem. Clinical Neurosurgery 6: 177, 1959.

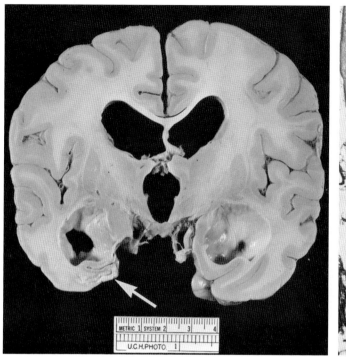

Fig. 97a. Chronic sequelae of transtentorial herniation

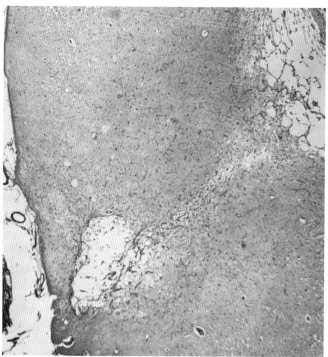

Fig. 97b. Holzer × 21

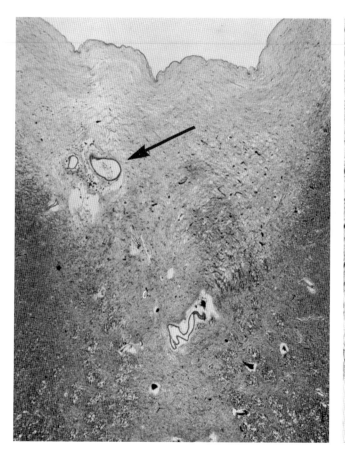

Fig. 97c. Weil × 21

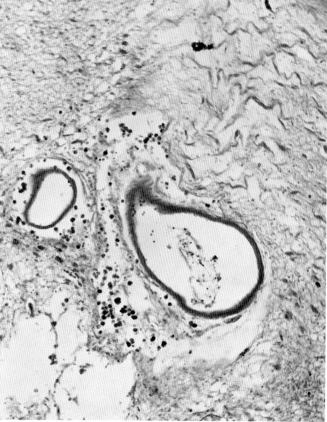

Fig. 97d. Weil × 140

Head injuries associated with fractures may lead to extradural hemorrhage, especially in association with fracture of the temporal bone when bleeding results from tears of the middle meningeal arteries. If sufficiently massive, it may be complicated by the effects of transtentorial herniation.

Penetrating injuries, caused by a variety of missiles, generally penetrate into the parenchyma and cause more extensive damage to deep than superficial structures. They frequently become infected from carrying inside contaminated clothing, hair, skin, and fragments of bone.

*Case 1:* A 56-year-old woman developed a left hemiplegia and epileptic attacks after an injury sustained at the age of nine, when she was accidentally shot in the head.

Autopsy revealed a defect in the right frontal region of the skull. In the right frontal lobe a ragged cavity communicated with the ventricles and the surrounding tissue was atrophic, necrotic, and was associated with fibrous thickening of the meninges (Fig. 98a).

The lesion penetrated deeply and caused extensive demyelinization of the cerebral white matter in the vicinity, even in areas where the cortex was intact (Fig. 98b), thus disrupting the fibers of the pyramidal tract.

*Case 2:* A 63-year-old man sustained a self-inflicted gunshot wound of the head. After this he exhibited signs of delirium, ptosis, and pupillary dilatation on the right; a Chaddock sign on the left; and signs of meningeal irritation. X-rays of the skull revealed a fistulous tract connecting the air sinuses with the ventricles, so that the latter became visible as in a ventriculogram (spontaneous pneumoencephalos). There was progressive enlargement of the ventricles in the frontal areas. The patient's course was downhill, with signs of right opthalmoplegia, bilateral forced grasping, bilateral Babinski signs, and flexion contractures of the extremities on the right side. He died in coma thirty-eight days after the injury.

There was extensive trauma to the frontal lobes, associated with fractures of the base of the skull. Bilateral cysts, lined by necrotic tissue, replaced the basal and adjacent inferolateral cortex and white matter and communicated directly with the enlarged ventricles (Fig. 98c). The location of the lesions was strikingly similar to that seen in prefrontal lobotomy. As in the latter circumstance, there was retrograde degeneration of the dorsomedial nucleus of the thalamus, whose nerve cells were depleted, shrunken, and partly replaced by reactive glia (Fig. 98d).

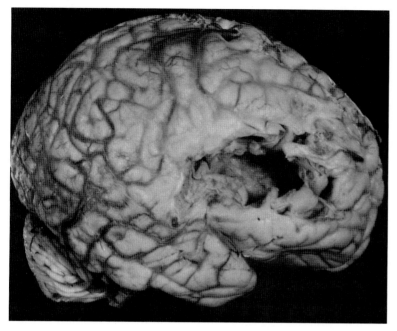

Fig. 98a. Chronic penetrating injury to right frontal lobe

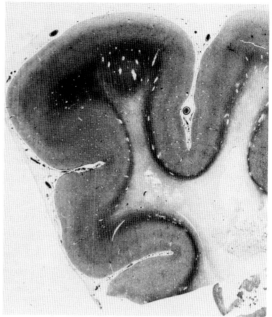

Fig. 98b. Weil stain

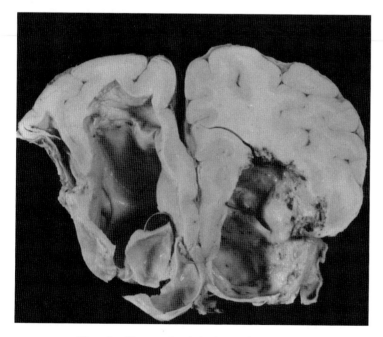

Fig. 98c. Penetrating injuries to frontal lobes

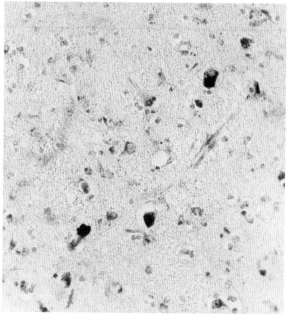

Fig. 98d. Nissl × 200

## Prefrontal Lobotomy

In the treatment of mental disorders and intractable pain with prefrontal lobotomy, the operative trauma produces pathoanatomic changes that resemble those caused by penetrating wounds. The cerebral changes seen at autopsy are determined by the particular operative method employed, by the duration of the postoperative period, and by the presence or absence of postoperative complications.

> *Case:* A 53-year-old woman had had a catatonic form of schizophrenic psychosis for at least eight years before recourse to prefrontal lobotomy. Following the operation she gradually became more accessible and tractable, finally returning to her prepsychotic personality. Three years later she died of a coronary thrombosis.

Coronal sections through the frontal lobes outlined the operative tracts as bilaterally symmetrical cystic scars that extended from the trephine openings toward the enlarged ventricles just anterior to the level of the head of the caudate nuclei (Fig. 99a).

By thus severing the thalamofrontal pathways, retrograde degeneration could be traced through the anterior thalamic radiation in the anterior limb of the internal capsule to the dorsomedial nuclei of the thalamus where there was bilaterally symmetrical gliosis (Fig. 99b) in reaction to disappearance of the neurons.

## Posttraumatic Abscess

Open injuries, whether accidental or postoperative, are subject to infection in the form of pachymeningitis or brain abscess.

> *Case:* A 55-year-old woman underwent an open prefrontal lobotomy for chronic paranoid schizophrenia. She maintained a satisfactory recovery during the first week postoperatively. Subsequently, she developed increasing lethargy to coma without fever. Examination revealed generalized muscle twitchings and bilateral flaccid paralysis with Babinski signs. A lumbar puncture revealed a xanthochromic fluid under pressure of 450 mm. of water. She expired two weeks following surgery.

Coronal sections through the frontal lobes at the level of the genu of the corpus callosum revealed symmetrical operative cavities with mixed hemorrhagic, necrotic, and purulent content that extended from the trephine openings down through the white matter to the base (Fig. 99c).

Microscopically, abscesses characterized by early encapsulation with fibroblasts around central accumulation of polymorphonuclear leukocytes (Fig. 99d) were intermingled with areas of hemorrhagic necrosis.

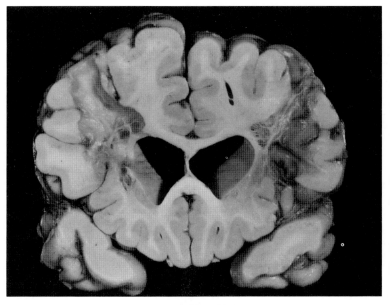

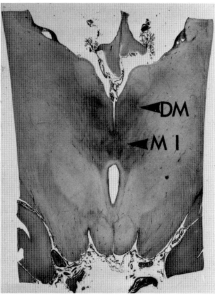

Fig. 99a. Prefrontal lobotomy

Fig. 99b. Holzer stain

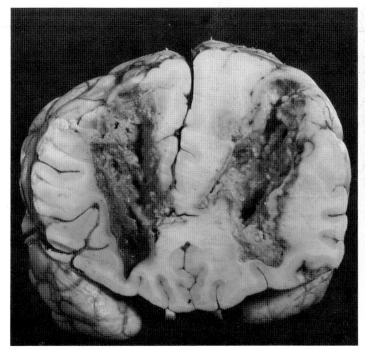

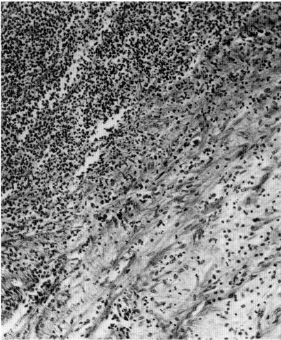

Fig. 99c. Abscesses complicating prefrontal lobotomy

Fig. 99d. HE × 100

# VII

## *Neoplastic Disorders*

A discussion of tumors of the nervous system calls for theoretical considerations of etiology, biologic growth, and manner of classification as well as practical considerations of diagnosis, prognosis, and therapy, depending on sites of predilection, age incidence, tempo of growth, and degree of accompanying increased pressure.

Tumors may be classified under these general headings: primary intrinsic; primary extrinsic, and secondary or metastatic.

### PRIMARY INTRINSIC TUMORS

Tumors that take their origin from the neuroectodermal elements of the central nervous system form the largest group of the primary intracranial neoplasms and much less so of the intraspinal tumors.

Various classifications of the gliomas have been proposed; the more generally accepted classification is that of Bailey and Cushing, which is based on histogenesis of the cells that differentiate from the medullary epithelium (Fig. 100a). According to this concept, each type of glioma corresponds to a specific stage of differentiation of the embryonic cell, and its malignancy is inversely proportional to the degree of differentiation. Since, however, many of the gliomas cannot be proven to arise from embryonic cells, others consider dedifferentiation or anaplasia of mature glial cells as a more likely pathogenesis in the majority of instances.

The primary intrinsic tumors may be classified into eight types: 1. Astrocytoma, 2. Glioblastoma Multiforme, 3. Oligodendroglioma, 4. Ependymoma, 5. Papilloma of the Choroid Plexus, 6. Medulloblastoma, 7. Pinealoma, and 8. Ganglioglioma.

### ASTROCYTOMA

Astrocytomas, the most common type of glioma in the brain, may be classified on the basis of the predominant cell type into protoplasmic, gemistocytic, fibrillary and pilocytic, forms. They may be considered from the standpoint of sites of predilection as cerebral, pontine, third ventricular, and cerebellar.

When well differentiated they are relatively slow growing. They are, however, prone to undergo varying degrees of dedifferentiation or anaplasia.

### Cerebral Astrocytoma

Astrocytomas of the cerebral hemispheres are predominantly tumors of adults. They occur in different sites but most frequently in the white matter of frontal and temporal lobes and in the corpus callosum. The growth is usually diffuse, blending with normal nervous tissue and tending to microcystic rather than macrocystic degeneration. Histologically, they are more commonly composed of fibrillary astrocytes (100b), less frequently of gemistocytic (Fig. 100c), and rarely of protoplasmic astrocytes while midline tumors often show the pilocytic variety. Admixtures of several cell types are common. The rate of growth is slower in the fibrillary form and more rapid in the gemistocytic type. The latter may contain areas showing large cells with stout foot plates attached to walls of blood vessels forming a pseudorosette pattern, diagnostic of astroblastoma (Fig. 100d).

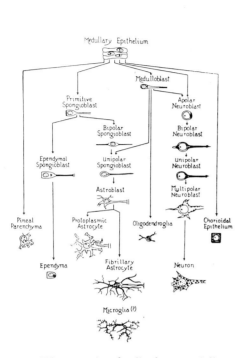

Fig. 100a. Histogenesis of cells from medullary epithelium

(*courtesy of Percival Bailey*)

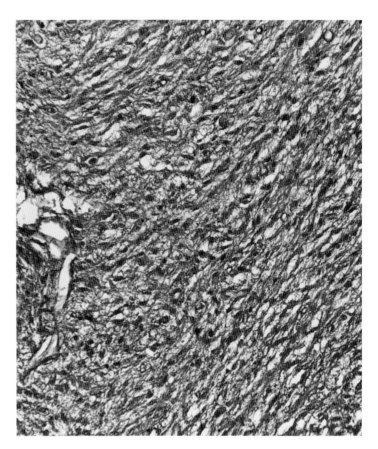

Fig. 100h. Holzer × 80

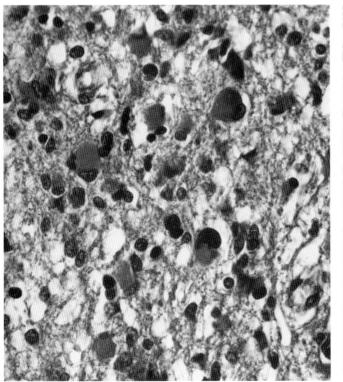

Fig. 100c. HE × 475

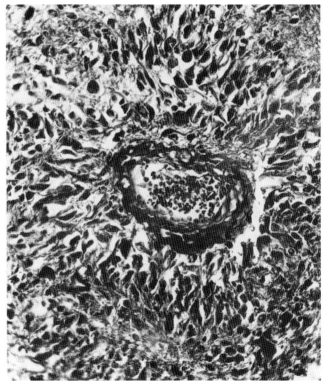

Fig. 100d. PTAH × 280

## Cerebral Astrocytoma (continued)

*Case 1:* A 34-year-old woman gave a history of dizzy spells, associated with disorientation and confusion, over a period of three years that had become more frequent in the past several months, leading to her admission to a hospital. Examination revealed facial asymmetry due to right seventh nerve paresis; general muscle weakness but symmetrical reflexes; emotional apathy and impairment of memory. The cerebrospinal fluid contained a total protein of 14 mg %, glucose of 67 mg %, and no pleocytosis. EEG showed a slow wave focus in the left precentral, lateral-frontal, and anterior temporal areas. A brain scan demonstrated increased activity in the left frontal lobe. Pneumoencephalogram and carotid arteriogram showed a calcified mass in the left frontal region. A needle biopsy was reported as a well differentiated astrocytoma. Postoperatively, the patient became comatose with dilated fixed pupils, despite administration of Decadron, and expired. The immediate cause of death was brain stem hemorrhages due to transtentorial herniation.

A diffusely infiltrating avascular tumor, containing minute cysts, occupied the entire right orbitofrontal region and extended into the rostrum of the corpus callosum; it obliterated and displaced superiorly the right lateral ventricle while dilating the left lateral ventricle (Fig. 101a).

Microscopically, the tumor consisted of an avascular tissue composed of stellate astrocytes with long fibrillary processes and glial fibers, separated by microcysts (Fig. 101b). There were scattered calcareous deposits. The diagnosis was fibrillary astrocytoma.

*Case 2:* A 47-year-old man had recurrent episodes of mental depression and infrequent grand mal seizures. The predominant psychotic picture apparently obscured any underlying clinical evidence of a tumor process, until a terminal state of somnolence led to his death about a year following the onset.

A large tumor occupied the major part of the left temporal lobe, causing displacement of the basal ganglia and ventricles superiorly and to the right; the lesion was grayish white, of soft, rubbery consistency, poorly circumscribed and contained scattered small cysts (Fig. 101c).

Microscopically, most of the cells were plump astrocytes with an eccentric single nucleus and ample homogeneous cytoplasm (Fig. 101d). The cell bodies and their short branching processes were uniformly impregnated with the use of Cajal's gold sublimate method, but there were relatively few glial fibers.

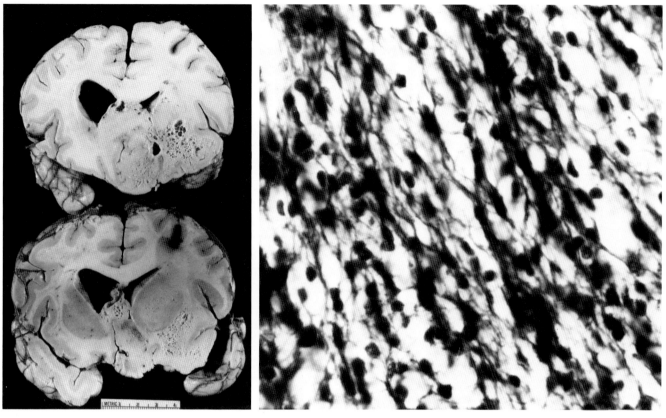

Fig. 101a. Astrocytoma, left orbitofrontal region (sides reversed)

Fig. 101b. PTAH × 560

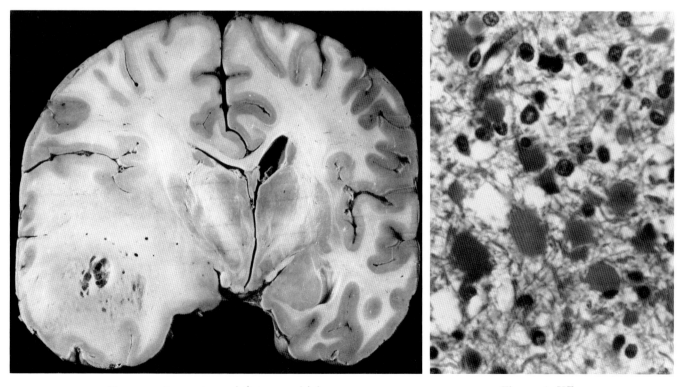

Fig. 101c. Astrocytoma, left temporal lobe

Fig. 101d. HE × 440

## Astrocytoma in the Region of the Third Ventricle

Gliomas developing in the floor of the third ventricle, in the region of the infundibulum and optic chiasm, are characterized as a "juvenile" form of pilocytic astrocytoma because they occur in early life and are histologically composed of a simpler form of piloid astrocyte. These tumors grow to large size, are vascular, microcystic, and are prone to a form of degeneration of neuroglial fibers known as "Rosenthal fibers." These are characterized by their elongated shape and homogeneous structure.

> *Case:* A 6-year-old girl developed at the age of thirteen months recurring episodes of nausea and vomiting followed by gradually increasing visual difficulties, and failure in mental development. Several months before her death, she became irrational and hostile, was unable to swallow, and developed prolonged seizures. On admission to a hospital, she was blind, showing bilateral vertical and horizontal nystagmus, sluggish response of pupils to light and optic atrophy; there was a suggestion of precocious sexual puberty. Bilateral carotid arteriograms revealed evidence of a large suprasellar mass, associated with lateral ventricular dilatation. A frontal craniotomy was performed and the biopsy diagnosis was astrocytoma. On the twenty-second postoperative day a bilateral ventriculovenous shunt was performed. However, she became hyponatremic, developed a consumption coagulopathy, and expired.

A gray tumor mass, largely replaced by massive hemorrhage, filled the third ventricle and obliterated all of the surrounding structures (Fig. 102a).

Histologically, the tissue was composed of uniformly small elongated cells, separated by cysts and greatly distended and congested thin-walled anomalous blood vessels (Fig. 102b). Under higher magnification, the tumor cells had a vague stellate shape with round to oval nuclei and tapering glial processes (Fig. 102c) that in some areas had altered into homogeneous round to elongated bodies (arrows) or Rosenthal fibers (Fig. 102d).

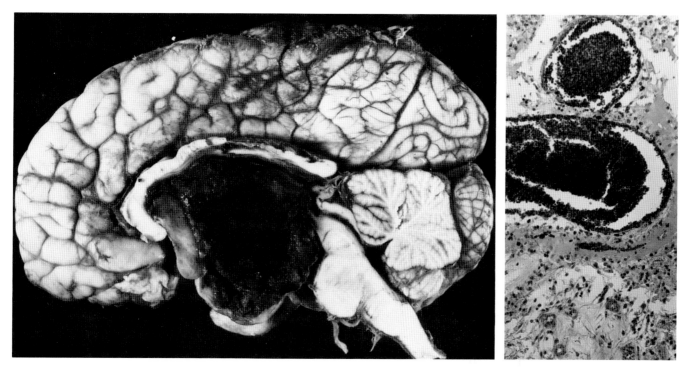

Fig. 102a. Astrocytoma, region of third
ventricle

Fig. 102b. HVG × 100

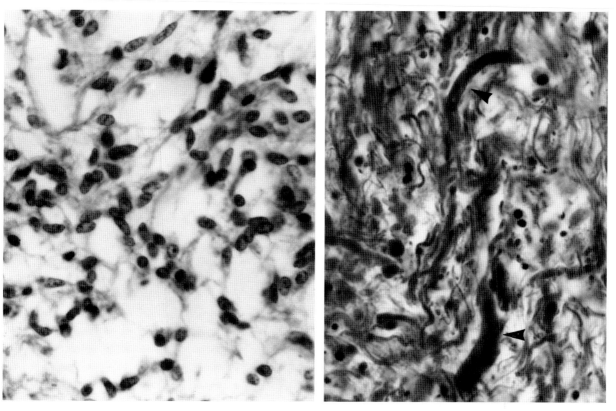

Fig. 102c. HVG × 440

Fig. 102d. PTAH × 720

## Cerebellar Astrocytoma

The astrocytoma of the cerebellum is the most common glioma to occur in the posterior fossa, and is primarily a tumor of childhood. It usually develops in one or other hemisphere, rarely in the midline. The classical appearance is one of a mural nodule projecting into a large cyst, the wall of which may or may not be composed of tumor tissue. Because of its circumscribed growth, it responds more favorably to surgical treatment than other types of glioma. Histologically, it is usually composed of pilocytic astrocytes arranged in alternating compact and loose areas but may be of a "juvenile" variety resembling the astrocytomas of the third ventricle.

*Case:* An 11-year-old boy complained of weakness, dizziness, headaches, vomiting, and staggering gait seven months before admission to a hospital. Neurologic examination disclosed a wide-based ataxic gait, dyssynergia, and adiadokokinesis on the right side, and nystagmus with slow component on gaze to the right. A ventriculogram revealed uniform dilatation of the lateral and third ventricles. Patient died suddenly after ventriculography.

A cyst with a mural nodule projecting into it (arrow), occupied the right cerebellar hemisphere and displaced the enlarged fourth ventricle to the left (Fig. 103a).

Microscopic examination revealed that the tumor nodule and the wall of the cyst consisted of whorls (arrow) of glial fibers interspersed by an edematous, loose, fibrillary tissue (Fig. 103b). Higher magnification showed uniform small spindle shaped cells with elongated processes associated with varying densities of glial fibers (Fig. 103c), prone to formation of Rosenthal fibers (arrows) like the astrocytomas of the third ventricle (Fig. 103d).

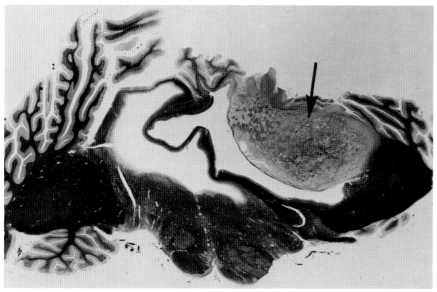

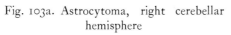

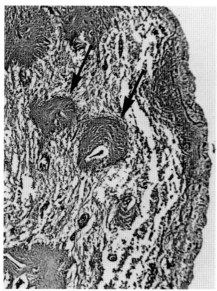

Fig. 103a. Astrocytoma, right cerebellar hemisphere

Fig. 103b. Holzer × 32

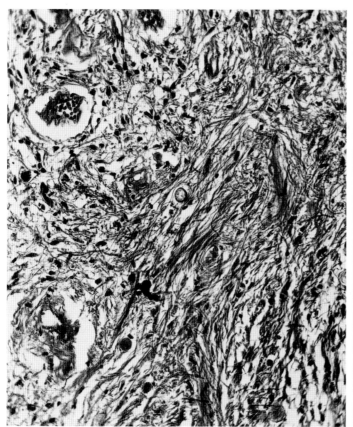

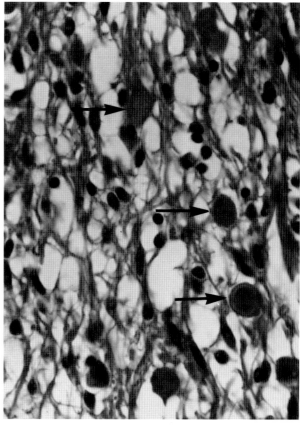

Fig. 103c. HE × 200

Fig. 103d. HE × 475

## Astrocytoma of Pons

The most common glioma of the brain stem is the astrocytoma that develops in the pons of children and relatively young adults. It begins as a diffuse enlargement of the pons, either uni- or bilaterally, in the base or tegmentum, whence it often extends asymmetrically and for a limited distance rostrally to involve the midbrain, caudally to the medulla and upper cervical cord, and laterally, the cerebellum. It is usually a firm and avascular neoplasm, although prone to anaplasia; obstructive hydrocephalus is a relatively late complication.

Microscopically, it is characterized by infiltration of tumor tissue between the normal fiber tracts and nuclear groups of the brain stem, to which it adapts itself by the cells becoming elongated uni- or bipolar forms, thus classified as a pilocytic astrocytoma. It is this feature that has led to an earlier classification as a polar spongioblastoma, implying a more primitive cell type which with rare exceptions is not borne out. Because of its location, the tumor shortens life by affecting vital centers of the brain stem and is inoperable.

> *Case:* A 20-year-old man was admitted to a hospital with a one-month history of occipital headaches, vomiting, and diplopia. Examinations revealed bilateral papilledema, nystagmus on lateral and upward gaze, an ataxic gait with tendency to fall to the right, bilateral dysdiadokokinesis, dysmetria and muscle-rebound phenomenon, and hyperactive reflexes on the left. A ventriculogram disclosed dilatation of all ventricles except the fourth, which was not visualized. A suboccipital craniotomy revealed tumor in the right cerebellar hemisphere, which was partly removed. Postoperatively, the patient's condition rapidly declined as dysphagia and dyspnea set in. He died eight months after the onset of symptoms.

The pons was diffusely enlarged (Fig. 104a) by a firm, avascular, nodular tumor that infiltrated the tegmentum and basis pontis, more on the right side, extending into the adjacent cerebellar hemisphere; the tumor also involved the upper part of the medulla and the cerebral peduncles and partly encircled the basilar artery.

Microscopically, parallel rows of elongated cells and nuclei with unipolar and bipolar processes were arranged in intersecting bundles, running either longitudinally or transversely (Fig. 104b). With glial stains, large numbers of glial fibers emanated from easily identified astrocytic cells among preserved neurons (Fig. 104c).

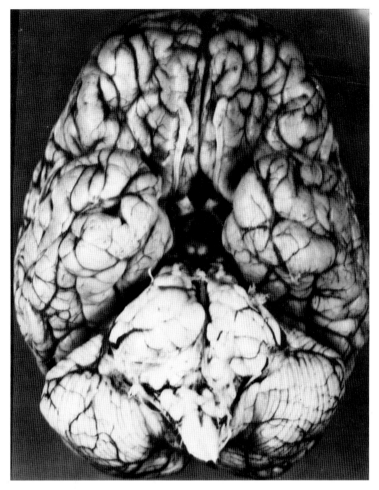

Fig. 104a. Astrocytoma of pons

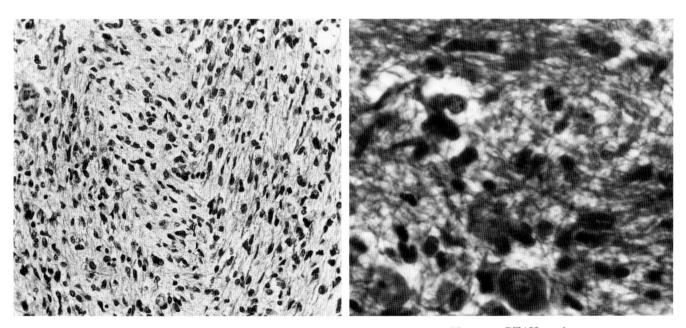

Fig. 104b. HE × 200

Fig. 104c. PTAH × 560

## Astrocytoma in Electron Microscopy

The electron microscopic study of astrocytoma has confirmed, in general, the results obtained with the light microscope. The tumor cells have many features characteristic of nonneoplastic reactive astrocytes. Most obvious are the accumulations of glial filaments (f) (Fig. 105). Sometimes these accumulations are associated with Rosenthal fibers. Glycogen granules, dense-core vesicles, and desmosomes are often present.

The tumors differ from normal tissue, or even reactive tissue in that the cells form masses. On the other hand, relationships between the tumor cells and either blood vessels or pia are essentially similar to those seen between nonneoplastic astrocytes and these structures. Another difference between tumor cells and normal mature astrocytes is the presence of relatively frequent microtubules in some tumor cell processes. Finally, in some cases, the nuclei may contain dense fibrillary material and other nuclear inclusions.

*References*

Duffeel, D., L. Farber, S. Chou, J. F. Hartmann, and E. Nelson. Electron Microscopic Observations on Astrocytomas. Amer. J. Path. 43: 539, 1963.

Sumi, S. M., and E. Reifel. Unusual Nuclear Inclusions in Astrocytomas. Arch. Neurol. 92: 14, 1971.

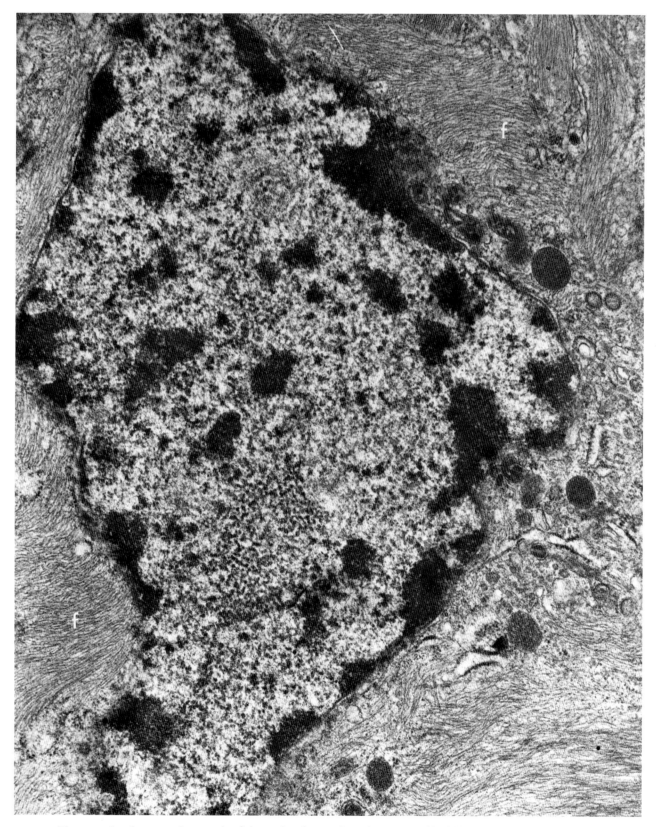

Fig. 105. An electron micrograph of the perinuclear region of a tumor cell within an astrocytoma × 33,000

## Rosenthal Fibers in Electron Microscopy

Rosenthal fibers may be seen within reactive astrocytes under a variety of conditions, especially certain chronic degenerative disorders and in certain neoplasms. In the electron microscope (Fig. 106), they are seen to consist of closely-packed masses of electron dense granules embedded in a matrix of compactly arranged glial filaments.

*References*

Herdon, R. M., L. J. Rubinstein, J. M. Freeman, and G. Mathieson. Light and Electron Microscopic Observations on Rosenthal Fibers in Alexander's Disease and in Multiple Sclerosis. J. Neuropath. and Expt. Neurol. 29: 524, 1970.

Schlote, W. Rosenthalsche "Fasern" und Spongioblasten im Zentralnervensystem. I. Vorkommen in ventrikelfernen Reparationsgliosen; Darstellbarkeit der "Fasern" im Zellbild. Beitr. path. Anat. 133: 225, 1966.

Schochet, S. S., P. W. Lampert, and K. M. Earle. Alexander's Disease. A Case Report with Electron Microscopic Observations. Neurology. 18: 543, 1968.

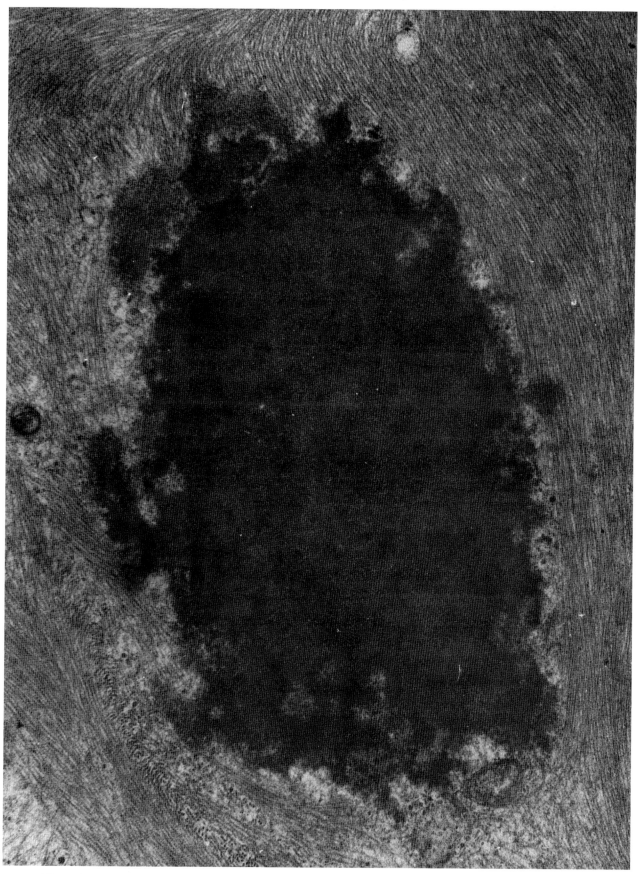

Fig. 106. An electron micrograph of a Rosenthal fiber in a reactive astrocyte adjacent to a craniopharyngioma
× 50,000

A rare tumor, characterized by widespread glial overgrowth throughout the central nervous system, has been described in the literature as diffuse gliomatosis, glioblastosis or Schwannosis. It has been considered by some as akin to neurofibromatosis of von Recklinghausen, and by others as a diffuse astrocytoma or polar spongioblastoma.

It presents diagnostic difficulties because of diffuse symptomatology, associated with signs of increased intracranial pressure indicative of a neoplastic process.

The histologic features are: widespread infiltrations, especially along subpial surfaces of cortex, cerebellum, brain stem, and spinal cord, often invading roots of cranial and spinal nerves, and by variations of the tumor cells from spongioblasts to astrocytes.

*Case:* A 17-year-old boy had a history of nausea, vomiting, and diplopia, which within eight months advanced to complete immobility of the right eye. Examination at that time revealed bilateral papilloedema, external ophthalmoplegia on the right, horizontal nystagmus to the left, and left hemiparesis. A ventriculogram showed slight enlargement of the lateral ventricles. A subtemporal decompression was performed, followed by a course of x-ray therapy, which led to remission of symptoms for one year. A relapse then occurred, characterized by more diffuse signs of decreased hearing and peripheral facial palsy on the left, bilateral oculomotor paresis, hypalgesia of the left side of the face, deviation of the uvula to the right, hemiparesis of the extremities on both sides, generalized and Jacksonian convulsions, aphasia, and mental blunting. In spite of another course of x-ray treatment, the patient died, approximately three years following the onset of his symptoms.

The brain showed generalized flattening of the convolutions and bulging of the right hemisphere in the region of the subtemporal decompression, but there were no distinct gross signs of tumor (Fig. 107a). There was, however, a nodular enlargement of the spinal cord in the region of the conus medullaris (Fig. 107b) that in myelin stains revealed tumor infiltration of the leptomeninges and nerve roots, and pressure necrosis of the underlying cord tissue (Fig. 107c).

Microscopically, there was widespread infiltration of the brain and spinal cord, with concentration on outer surfaces, by small cells varying from slender polar spongioblasts to stellate fibrillary astrocytes, as illustrated in sections from the cerebral cortex (Fig. 107d), and meninges around the conus medullaris (Fig. 107e).

*Reference*

Malamud, N., B. L. Wise, and O. W. Jones. Gliomatosis Cerebri. J. Neurosurg. 9: 409, 1952.

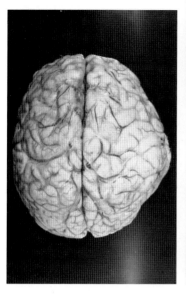

Fig. 107a. Gross appearance of brain

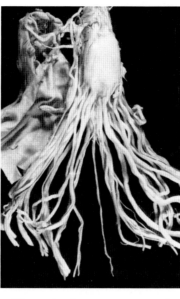

Fig. 107b. Gross appearance of conus medullaris

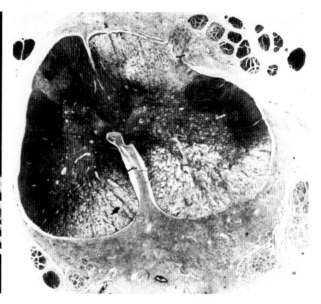

Fig. 107c. Weil stain of spinal cord

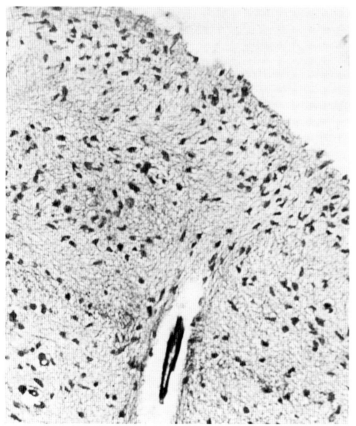

Fig. 107d. Holzer × 100

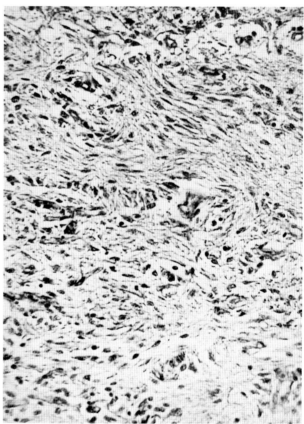

Fig. 107e. Heidenhain's aniline blue × 100

## Anaplastic Astrocytoma

As stated previously, astrocytomas in any location show a marked tendency to anaplasia, which is reflected clinically in a more malignant course and histologically by signs of rapid growth, associated with vascular changes and attendant necrosis or hemorrhages. Such features may be evident from the very outset and follow a rapid clinical course, often indistinguishable from that of glioblastoma multiforme, or develop as an exacerbation after a long period of insidious symptoms and signs.

> *Case:* A 19-year-old man developed at the age of nine years a chronic convulsive disorder. The seizures were initially described as "of petit mal type," followed later by grand mal attacks accompanied by jerking of the left extremities, inability to speak, right-sided headaches, and occasional vomiting. At the age of thirteen, his seizures became complex semipurposeful automatic acts that were regarded as psychomotor in type, for which he received a variety of anticonvulsant medications. Personality changes later developed with increasing withdrawal, aggressive behavior, and negativism. Neurological examination, including that of the spinal fluid, was normal. Repeated EEGs showed generalized paroxysmal dysrhythmia and right-sided foci of decreased voltage with spike and slow wave bursts that were centered about the right temporal region. Although depth electrode studies for possible stereotactic surgery were recommended, he was committed to a State mental hospital because of his mental state, diagnosed schizophrenia. His condition continued unchanged until he suddenly developed a state of coma and died within forty-eight hours.

The brain contained a small cystic grayish tumor that infiltrated the gray and white matter of the right hippocampal gyrus, compressed the hippocampal formation on its mesial side, and was intimately associated with massive fresh hemorrhage on its lateral side (Fig. 108a).

Microscopically (Fig. 108b), the medial part of the tumor was very fibrous, being composed of streaming uniform well differentiated fibrillary astrocytes (A); on its lateral aspect the fibrillary cells became transformed into pleomorphic forms associated with multinucleated giant cells (B) and proliferated thin walled, congested blood vessels that bled and became confluent as massive hemorrhages (Fig. 108c).

It was evident that the small well differentiated astrocytoma acted over a period of years as the discharging focus for the psychomotor seizures and that the ensuing anaplastic change in the tumor ultimately led to demise from massive cerebral hemorrhage. The involvement of limbic structures could explain both the psychomotor seizures and the personality change.

*Reference*

Malamud, N. Psychiatric Disorder with Intracranial Tumors of Limbic System. Arch. Neurol. 17: 113, 1967

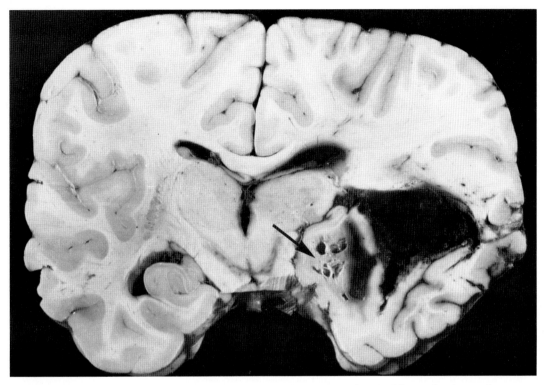

Fig. 108a. Small astrocytoma in right hippocampal gyrus associated with massive hemorrhage

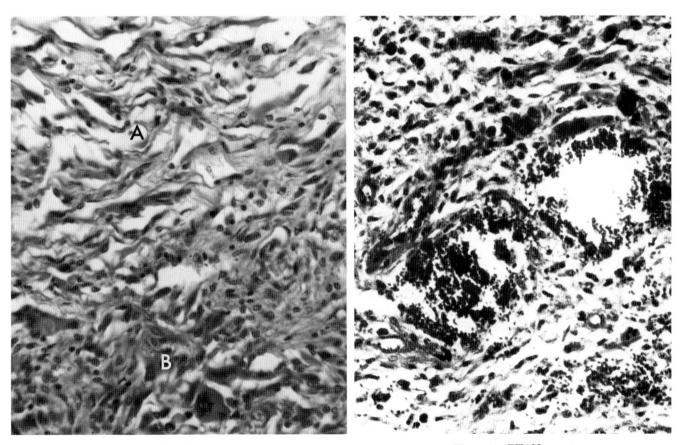

Fig. 108b. HE × 100

Fig. 108c. PTAH × 225

Glioblastoma multiforme derives its name from the pleomorphic pathoanatomic features. However, its separation from anaplastic astrocytoma has remained controversial. It seems reasonable to accept the view that while many of these tumors are fundamentally astrocytomas because they are composed predominantly of astrocytes, despite anaplastic transformation, others show a complex variety of glial cells, both of precursor and mature forms, that justifies the designation of glioblastoma multiforme.

The tumors occur predominantly in the cerebral hemispheres of adults during middle and advanced age, in a variety of locations with predilection for frontal, temporal, and callosal regions; less frequently, in basal ganglia, brain stem, cerebellum, and spinal cord in decreasing order.

Grossly, they are characterized by a variegated appearance with grayish soft tumor tissue being interspersed with focal necrosis and hemorrhage, old and recent, associated with marked vascularity. Although their borders are indistinct, they are often fairly well circumscribed from the surrounding edematous nervous tissue.

Histologically, they are compactly cellular in preserved parts and pleomorphic in any given field, with variations in different areas. The cells vary from spindle shapes to round or oval undifferentiated forms to some that can be identified as astrocytes; nuclei are characterized by hyperchromatism, variation in size, multinucleation, and scattered mitotic figures. Further complexity of structure is due to vascular changes, in the form of increased numbers of blood vessels with either thickened walls due to endothelial proliferation or as malformed thin-walled channels. Necrosis due to endarteritic changes and/or superimposed thrombosis, and hemorrhages from telangiectasias are associated with reactive phagocytosis, astrogliosis, and fibrosis by connective tissue. A distinctive feature is the pattern of pseudopalisade necrosis in which parallel disposed rows of cells and their processes are directed toward central areas of necrosis.

The tumor generally spreads from the white matter into the overlying cortex, showing a tendency to creep along the subpial surface but only occasionally infiltrating locally the meninges. Widespread metastasis through cerebrospinal fluid channels is rare, while remote extracranial metastasis probably occurs only following repeated surgery.

*Case 1:* A 46-year-old woman complained of recent onset of dizziness and weakness of the left side. A right carotid arteriogram revealed a tumor in the right frontoparietal region, which was operated and followed by a course of x-ray therapy. The patient felt well until fifteen months later, when a relapse occurred, this time characterized by hemiplegia, hypalgesia, and impairment of two-point discrimination on the left side. She died eighteen months after the onset of her symptoms.

The right cerebral hemisphere contained a fairly circumscribed grayish-yellow, partly necrotic, and slightly hemorrhagic tumor surrounding the scarred operative tract. The tumor replaced the cortex and subcortex of the inferior frontoparietal region, filling the Sylvian fissure, and was surrounded by edema; the ventricles were displaced to the left and there was subfalcial herniation of the cingulate gyrus (Fig. 109a).

Microscopically, the cells were pleomorphic, varying from round to oval forms with sparse cytoplasm and hyperchromatic nuclei of different sizes to scattered small astrocytes to large multinucleated forms (Fig. 109b). Vascular changes with marked endothelial proliferation were widespread (Fig. 109c); pseudopalisade necrosis was noted in some areas (Fig. 109d).

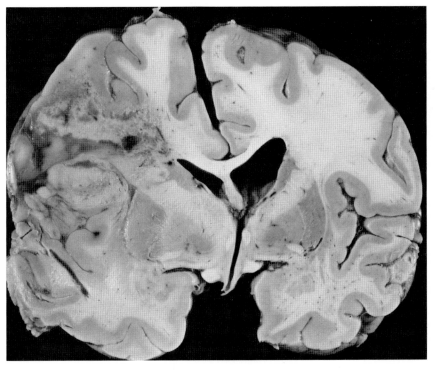

Fig. 109a. Glioblastoma multiforme, right hemisphere (sides reversed)

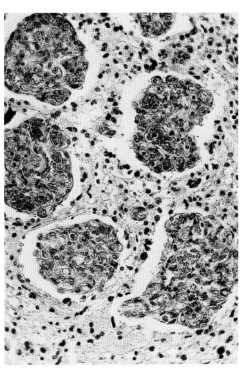

Fig. 109c. HVG × 200

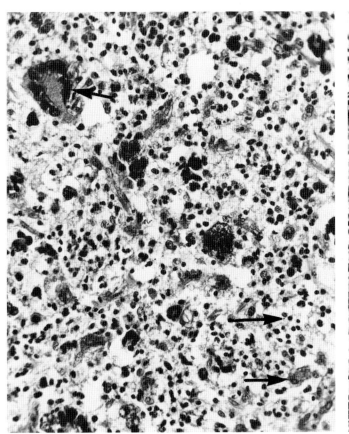

Fig. 109b. HE × 300

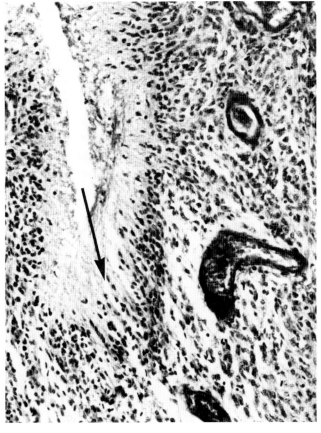

Fig. 109d. HVG × 160

## GLIOBLASTOMA MULTIFORME (CONTINUED)

*Case 2:* A 68-year-old man had a two months' history of increasing mental deterioration, tremulousness, and unsteadiness. Examination revealed mental confusion, somnolence, sluggish reaction of both pupils, right convergent strabismus, and paresis of the right leg associated with Babinski sign and ankle clonus. EEG was grossly abnormal with generalized and focal slowing, the latter in the left occipitotemporal area. The spinal fluid was xanthochromic and contained 48 white cells/cmm and a total protein of 204 mg %. A pneumoencephalogram showed dilatation of the lateral ventricles. Carotid and vertebral arteriography revealed an abnormal collection of vessels in the region of the pineal gland without displacement, thought to represent a tumor in that area. He pursued a rapidly downhill course and expired of pneumonitis, one month following admission.

A butterfly-shaped extremely hemorrhagic and necrotic tumor occupied the splenium of the corpus callosum, whence it extended almost symmetrically around the body of the lateral ventricles near the trigone, partially obliterating them (Fig. 110a).

Histologically, the pleomorphic tumor contained numerous thin-walled dilated and congested malformed vascular channels, associated with multiple hemorrhages (Fig. 110b).

### MULTICENTRIC GLIOMA

Multicentric gliomas refer to development, simultaneously or at various times, of widely separated tumors located in different lobes or hemispheres that cannot be explained either by local metastasis through satellite formation, spread by continuity via anatomic pathways, or through seeding by way of cerebrospinal fluid channels. Pathologically, they are glioblastomas or anaplastic astrocytomas. Their pathogenesis remains obscure. According to the literature, their incidence is approximately 2–3% of all intracranial gliomas. Because of their multiplicity, they present special problems in diagnosis and therapy.

*Case:* A 44-year-old man experienced his first symptoms approximately two-and-a-half years prior to death. These consisted of right-sided Jacksonian seizures followed by increasing listlessness, failing memory, blurred vision, and a right hemiparesis. Arteriography and ventriculography were suggestive of a left-sided parasagittal tumor. However, a biopsy failed to confirm it. Patient received x-ray therapy postoperatively, followed by some improvement. About two years later, left-sided weakness and ataxia developed. Examination at this time disclosed a left hemiparesis, bilateral extensor plantar responses, and diminution of sensory perception on the left side of his body. The cerebrospinal fluid contained a total protein of 170 mg %. It was now felt that a right cerebrosvascular accident was responsible for the left-sided signs. His condition continued to deteriorate, he became stuporous and died of bronchopneumonia.

The brain contained two distinct tumors, one in the inferomesial part of the left frontal lobe, and the other in the superior periventricular region of the right frontal lobe (Fig. 110c); the latter extended posteriorly into the basal ganglia, cingulate gyrus, and corpus callosum without however crossing through the latter to invade the opposite hemisphere.

Microscopically, both tumors had a similar structure, marked by pleomorphism and numerous giant cells, characteristic of glioblastoma multiforme (Fig. 110d).

There was neither gross nor microscopic evidence of connection between the two tumors, nor of seeding in either meninges or ependyma.

*Reference*

Batzdorf, U. and N. Malamud. The Problem of Multicentric Gliomas. J. Neurosurg. 20: 122, 1963.

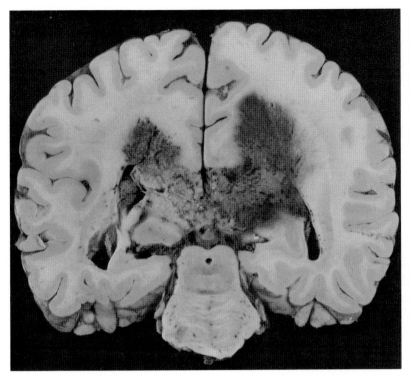

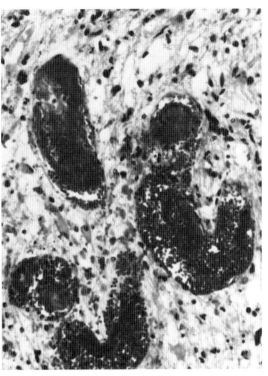

Fig. 110a. Glioblastoma multiforme of splenium of corpus callosum

Fig. 110b. HE × 175

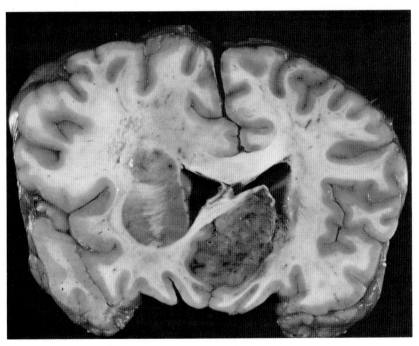

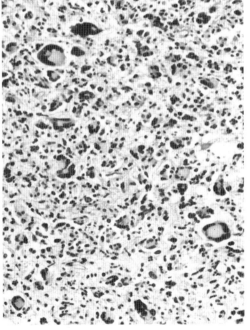

Fig. 110c. Multicentric glioma (sides reversed)

Fig. 110d. HE × 120

## Remote Metastases of Glioblastoma Multiforme

Remote or extracranial metastases of glioblastomas are rare. In the majority, if not all, such cases, there is a history of repeated surgical intervention. But while the pathogenesis is controversial, it has led to the assertion that previous surgery and/or radiation favors metastases through disruption of the dura, permitting spread via extracranial venous and lymphatic channels. The rare occurrence of such complications relates to the natural barrier of the cerebral blood vessels to tumor involvement, to the absence of intracranial lymphatics, and to the short survival from maligant primary tumors.

*Case:* A 22-year-old man developed progressive symptoms of right frontal headaches and generalized weakness. Investigations led to a diagnosis of a right cerebral tumor that was diagnosed as glioblastoma following a craniotomy. A second operation was performed four months later with subtotal removal of a right parietal mass, followed by radiotherapy. He was readmitted ten months later because he developed swelling in the region of the old scalp incision and in the left side of the neck. Examination now revealed increased papilledema, left homonymous hemianopsia, unsteadiness of gait, tremor of the head and hands, elevation of the bone flap, and large, firm palpable lymph nodes on the left side of the neck. Later he also developed two elevated tumors in the occipital area beneath the scalp of about 6 cm. in diameter, as well as enlarged nodes on the right side of the neck and behind both ears. Chest x-ray was negative. A biopsy of a lymph node was diagnosed as metastatic glioma. He was given a further course of radiotherapy but his condition deteriorated and he expired about two years following the onset of his symptoms.

The brain contained a large necrotic and hemorrhagic tumor mass, measuring 6 x 5 x 5 cm, adherent to the dura, that had replaced the major part of the superior and parasagittal region of the right parietal and occipital lobes (A); tumor nodules were present in the scalp (B), cervical and hilar lymph nodes (C) and in the lower lobe of the left lung (D) (Fig. 111a).

Microscopically, the cerebral tumor that had the structure of glioblastoma multiforme penetrated the dura and invaded the epidural tissues where it was composed predominantly of gemistocytic astrocytes (Fig. 111b).

Likewise, the tumor tissue in the scalp, lymph nodes, and lung (Fig. 111c) consisted exclusively of gemistocytic astrocytes.

*Reference*

Labitzke, H. G. Glioblastoma Multiforme with Remote Extracranial Metastases. Arch. Path. 73: 223, 1962.

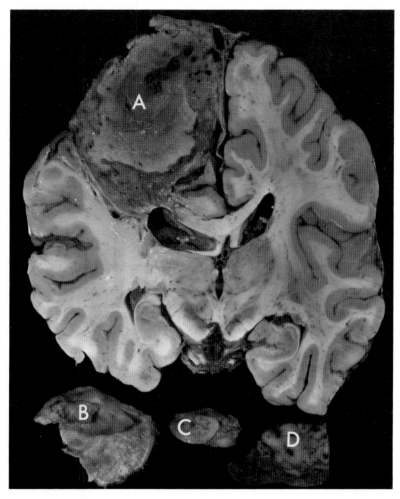

Fig. 111a. Glioblastoma multiforme (A) of right parietal lobe (sides reversed) with metastases to scalp (B), lymph node (C) and lung (D)

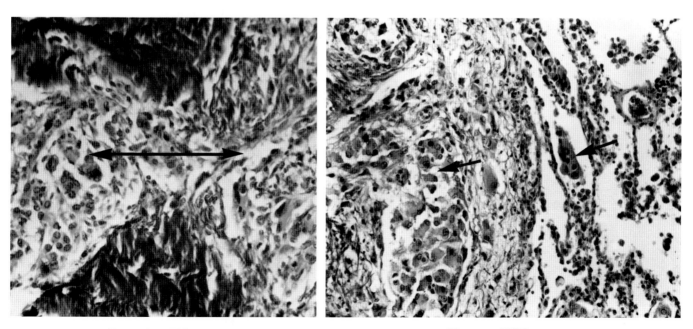

Fig. 111b. HVG × 175                    Fig. 111c. HVG × 175

## Glioblastoma Multiforme in Electron Microscopy

As might be expected, the fine structures of many of the tumor cells in glioblastoma multiforme display the morphologic features characteristic of glial cells, especially astrocytes. Thus, glial filaments, glycogen granules, and occasional desmosomes, either full or half, are present. The abundance of glial filaments varies from none to large accumulations reminiscent of those seen in reactive astrocytes.

On the other hand, the tumor cells differ from ordinary glial cells in several important respects. They display pronounced pleomorphism with regard to the outline and amount of the cytoplasm and the shape and size of their nuclei. The irregular shape of many of the nuclei results in an intranuclear cytoplasmic invagination which are the "inclusions" seen in the optical microscope. Furthermore, in contrast to normal brain, large extracellular (E) spaces are common (Fig. 112). For example, wide, debris-laden extracellular spaces are found in necrotic areas within the tumor mass. In addition to cellular debris, these spaces may also contain hematogenous fluid and even cells. Collagen-containing, widened extracellular spaces are common around blood vessels whereas collagen is quite scanty in the normal central nervous system.

*References*

Luse, S. A. Electron Microscopic Studies of Brain Tumors. Neurology. 19: 881, 1960.
Robertson, D. M., and J. D. MacLean. Nuclear Inclusions in Malignant Gliomas. Arch. Neurol. 13: 287, 1965.
Zulch, K. J., and W. Wechsler. Pathology and Classification of Gliomas in Progress in Neurological Surgery, Vol. 2 (H. Krayenbühl, P.E. Maspes, and W. H. Sweet, eds.) Karger, (Basel, 1968), p. 1.

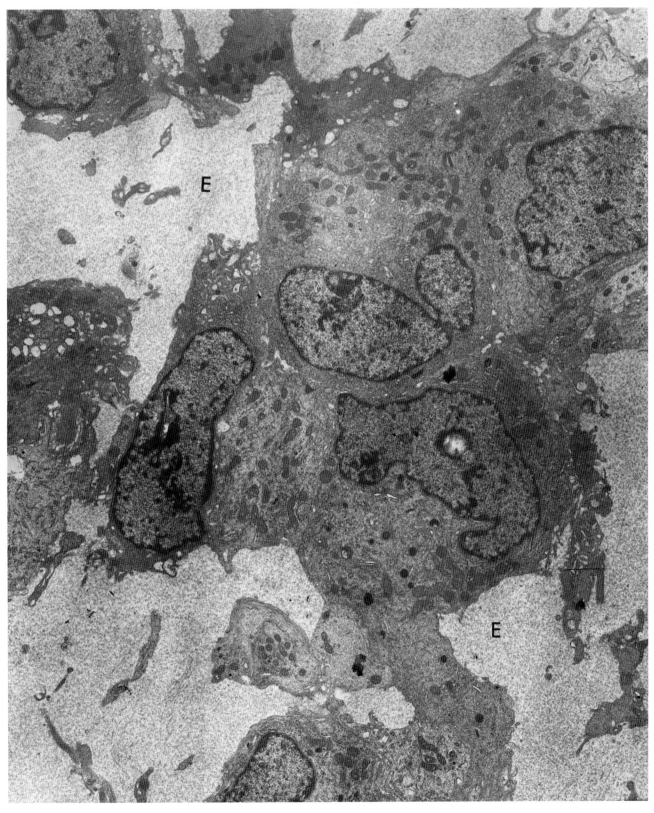

Fig. 112. An electron micrograph of a glioblastoma multiforme × 5,000 (Hirano, in The Structure and Function of Nervous Tissue, Vol. II, (G. H. Bourne, ed.). Academic Press (New York, 1969), p. 69.)

Oligodendrogliomas are next in order of frequency to astrocytomas and glioblastomas although much less common. It is a tumor primarily of young and middle-aged adults, following a relatively slow clinical course. Predilection sites are convexities of cerebral hemispheres and the septal region but very seldom the posterior fossa structures or spinal cord.

Grossly, it has the appearance of a grayish-pink solid mass, often showing mucinous change but little evidence of necrosis or cyst formation. Special features are calcification in the majority, and spontaneous hemorrhage and seeding into the cerebrospinal fluid channels in a number of instances. Microscopically, the characteristic structure is a honeycomb arrangement of uniform lymphocytic-like nuclei surrounded by perinuclear halos of sparse cytoplasm, showing no distinct processes. There is little tendency to anaplasia but mitotic figures are common, yet bearing no relationship to malignancy of clinical course. The stroma of the tumor consists of astroglial and/or connective tissue with variable proliferation of blood vessels though to a much lesser degree than in astrocytomas.

*Case 1:* A 52-year-old man had a seven-year history of Jacksonian seizures affecting the left side of his face and body. Repeated neurologic examinations revealed impairment of two-point discrimination in the left leg. A pneumoencephalogram was negative, but electroencephalograms showed a focus of slow activity in the right frontotemporal region. Toward the end, hemiparesis and hemianesthesia to pain and touch were noted in the entire left side.

The brain showed enlargment, grayish discoloration, and slight nodularity of the superior parts of the precentral and adjacent superior frontal gyri (Fig. 113a).

Microscopic examinations revealed infiltration of the cortex and subcortex by uniform small cells, consisting of round hyperchromatic nuclei, scant cytoplasm, and perinuclear clear spaces, accompanied by scattered calcium deposits (Fig. 113b). In Holzer glial preparations, the cells lacked glial processes and only a fine glial fiber network formed the stroma of the tumor (Fig. 113c).

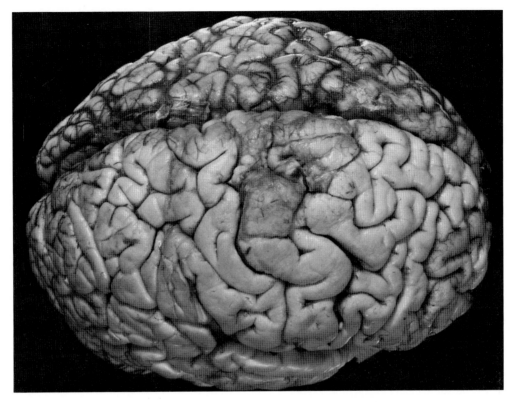

Fig. 113a. Oligodendroglioma of right central region

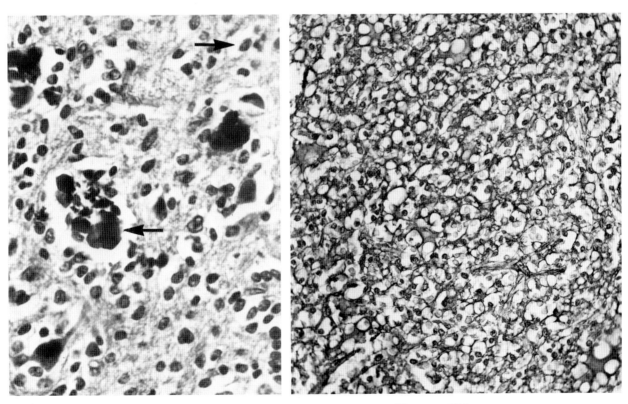

Fig. 113b. HE × 460

Fig. 113c. Holzer × 200

*Case 2:* A 33-year-old man had a history of grand mal and psychomotor seizures over a period of several months. On admission to a hospital, studies led to a craniotomy for a tumor of the right temporal lobe. Postoperatively, he received radiation therapy and was maintained on anticonvulsant medication, but complained of vague spells, characterized by subjective sensations of fullness, tastelessness, and weakness. Four years later, a second admission became necessary when he developed severe bifrontal headaches. Examination now revealed facial weakness and difficulty with finger-to-nose movement on the left side. Following pneumo-encephalography, a craniotomy was performed and recurrent tumor was partially resected. Postoperatively, patient developed a left hemiparesis. He subsequently continued to deteriorate and died four and one-half years following the onset of symptoms.

A large solid gray tumor with focal hemorrhages and sprinkled with fine granules of calcium extended from the old operative site inferiorly to occupy the gray and white matter of the right temporal and frontal lobes, involving also the insula and adjacent basal ganglia, and distorting and displacing the lateral ventricles; there were disseminated small tumor nodules in the left lateral ventricle and in the basal meninges (arrows), (Fig. 114a).

Microscopically, the tumor was composed of round nuclei, showing varying amounts of chromatin and frequent mitoses, with indistinct cytoplasm and no processes or glial fibers, both in the main mass (Fig. 114b) and in the meningeal (Fig. 114c) and subependymal seeds. The hemorrhages could be traced to proliferated blood vessels.

It is not uncommon to find mixed tumors that are composed of a mixed population of neoplastic oligodendroglia and astrocytes, each following its own independent type of growth behaviour. This is illustrated in the following case, in which an area of predominantly oligodendroglia (A) tumor cells is located next to a purely fibrillary astrocytoma (B), (Fig. 114d).

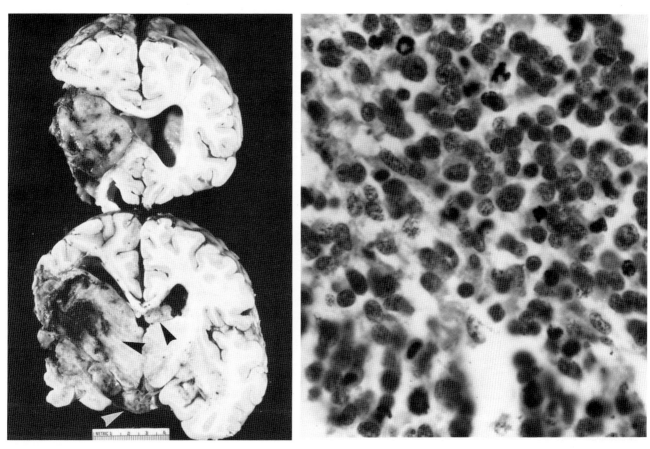

Fig. 114a. Oligodendroglioma, right temporal and
frontal lobes (sides reversed)

Fig. 114b. PTAH × 560

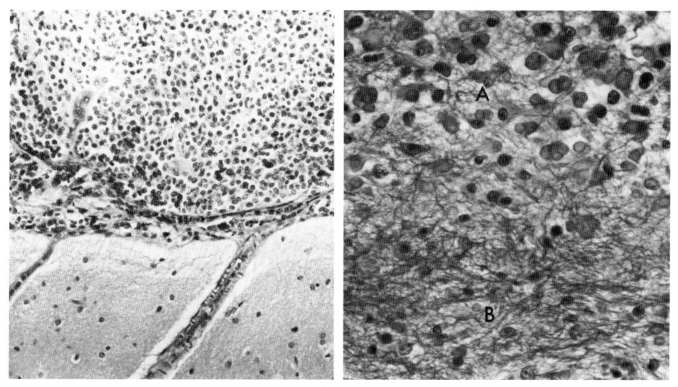

Fig. 114c. HE × 190

Fig. 114d. Holzer × 375

Tumors that take their origin from ependyma may be found in any part of the ventricular system of the brain and in relation to the central canal of the spinal cord down to the filum terminale. Ependymomas of the brain constitute about 5% of all gliomas, where they occur most frequently in the fourth ventricle, including the region of the cerebellopontine angle. By contrast they are the single most common glioma in the spinal cord and filum terminale, in the range of about 50%. They predominate in children and young adults. The clinical course is relatively slow, especially in the tumors of the spinal cord.

Pathologically, they have been classified by Kernohan, et al., as cellular, epithelial, and myxopapillary varieties, although admixtures are frequent. The cellular type is characterized by abundant vascularity and a pseudorosette pattern around blood vessels. The epithelial form contains true rosettes about central canals and blephoroplasts which are microscopic intracytoplasmic round to rod-like structures, that are normal constituents of ependymal cells. The myxopapillary form possesses a structure of cuboidal or columnar ependymal cells lining central cores of connective tissue showing a tendency to myxomatous change; it is virtually restricted to tumors of the conus and filum terminale. In general, ependymomas show little tendency to anaplasia, necrosis, or calcification. Seeding through cerebrospinal fluid channels is found in about one-third of the cases.

### Ependymoma of Fourth Ventricle

*Case 1:* A 2½-year-old boy developed in the course of one month headaches, vomiting, staggering gait, convulsions, and lethargy. Examination disclosed ataxia of gait, stiffness of neck, paresis of the abducens nerves, and papilledema. A ventriculogram demonstrated internal hydrocephalus and a block in the fourth ventricle. The patient died of hyperthermia three days after ventriculography.

The fourth ventricle was filled by a recent hemorrhage (A) that had destroyed all but a solid grayish-white part of a tumor (B) projecting from the floor and elevating the roof of the fourth ventricle (C), to which it was not adherent (Fig. 115a).

Microscopic examination revealed pseudorosettes composed of uniform ependymal cells with hyperchromatic round nuclei surrounding unstained zones around blood vessels (Fig. 115b).

*Case 2:* A 30-year-old woman had a one-year history of dizziness, vomiting, headaches, bilateral tinnitus, deafness on the left side, and staggering to the right. Examination revealed a dilated left pupil, deafness on the left side, nystagmus in all directions, bilateral papilledema, rigidity of neck, bilateral Babinski signs, and ataxia. Patient lapsed into stupor and died before further studies could be accomplished.

A large gray, partly hemorrhagic, circumscribed tumor extended from the roof of the compressed fourth ventricle chiefly into the inferior part of the left cerebellar hemisphere, presumably, arising from the ependyma of the lateral recess and foramen of Luschka (Fig. 115c).

The histologic structure of the tumor was similar to that of Case 1.

The myxopapillary type (Fig. 115d) shows a papillary pattern with columnar epithelium lining inner cores of vascular connective tissue (A) that undergoes a myxomatous change (B).

*Reference*

Kernohan, J. W., H. W. Woltman, and A. W. Adson. Intramedullary Tumors of the Spinal Cord. Arch. Neurol. & Psychiat. 25: 679–699, 1931.

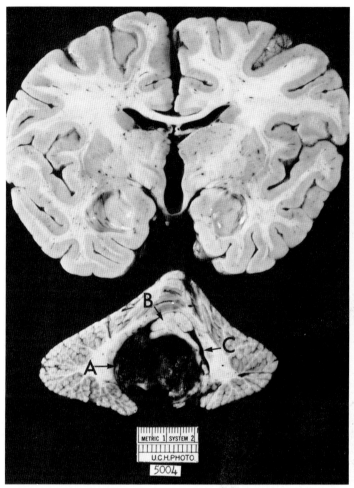

Fig. 115a. Ependymoma of fourth ventricle

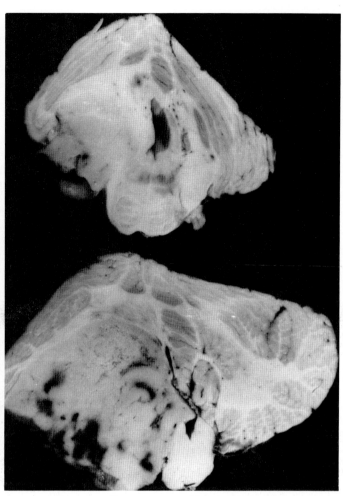

Fig. 115c. Ependymoma of left cerebellopontine
angle

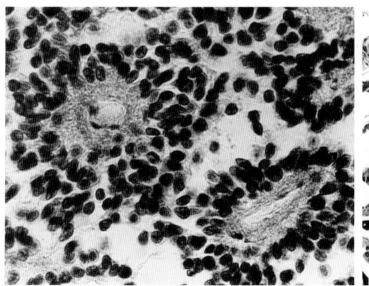

Fig. 115b. HVG × 475

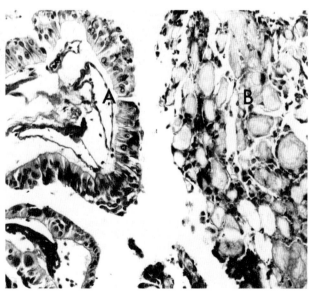

Fig. 115d. PTAH × 125

## Ependymoma in Electron Microscopy

Instead of the precisely arranged single layer of cells which comprises the ependymal lining of normal brain, ependymomas consist of large masses of tumor cells. At the fine structural level, the cells appear relatively undifferentiated. Nevertheless, certain distinct similarities between the tumor cells of ependymomas and normal ependymal cells have, on occasion, been seen in the electron microscope. Sometimes, for example, a small space is found within the tumor mass and the cells lining the space may display both microvilli (MV) and cilia. Such cell protrusion may sometimes obliterate the miniscule space (Fig. 116). Furthermore, the borders of adjacent cells may be joined by a junctional apparatus (arrows) similar to that found between normal ependymal cells, resulting in the so-called "ependymal rosettes" described by the light microscopists. In other respects, the tumor cells differ significantly from normal ependyma. Sometimes they contain large numbers of glial filaments and sometimes, in presumably younger cells, microtubules, may be found scattered throughout the cytoplasm in contrast to normal ependyma where they are confined to the apical region of the cell. Tumor cell processes extend toward blood vessels resulting in a so-called "pseudo-rosette" formation.

Very few detailed reviews devoted to ependymoma are available so that the bulk of the bibliography appended here includes several papers concerned with normal ependyma.

*References*

Brightman, M. W., and S. L. Palay. The Fine Structure of Ependyma in the Brain of the Rat. J. Cell Biol. 19: 415, 1963.

Goebel, H. H., and H. Cravioto. Ultrastructure of Human and Experimental Ependymomas. A Comparative Study. J. Neuropath. and Expt. Neurol. 31: 54, 1972.

Hirano, A., and H. M. Zimmerman. Some New Cytological Observations of the Normal Rat Ependymal Cell. Anat. Rec. 158: 293, 1967.

Tennyson, V. M., and G. D. Pappas. An Electron Microscopic Study of Ependymal Cells of the Fetal, Early Postnatal, and Adult Rabbit. Z. Zellforsch. 56: 595, 1962.

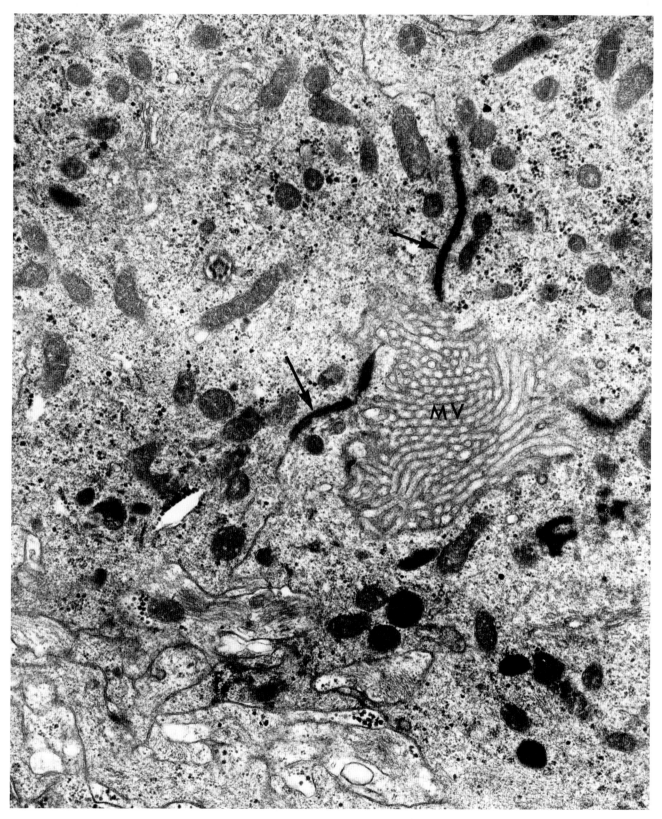

Fig. 116. An electron micrograph of an ependymoma
× 30,000 (Hirano, in Progress in Neuropathology,
Vol. I (H. M. Zimmerman, ed.). Grune and Stratton
(New York, 1971), p. 1.)

## Subependymoma

Small lobulated intraventricular tumors, also called subependymal glomerate astrocytoma, are occasionally found incidentally at autopsy in the fourth ventricle, less commonly in lateral and third ventricles. They are generally clinically asymptomatic. However, they may grow to sufficient size to block the cerebrospinal fluid circulation, requiring surgery.

The following tumor was found at autopsy to be attached to the floor of the fourth ventricle as a discrete and globular nodule (Fig. 117a).

Microscopic examination revealed nests of cells with uniform nuclei resembling ependymal cells embedded in a dense fibrillary network originating from intervening astrocytes (Fig. 117b).

Such tumors appear to be mixed forms, combining features of ependymoma and astrocytoma.

### PAPILLOMA OF CHOROID PLEXUS

Papillomas of the choroid plexus are rare intraventricular tumors, closely related to ependymomas. The most common sites are the fourth ventricle of adults and the lateral ventricles of infants.

The characteristic gross appearance is one of a cauliflower growth with papillary filaments, often associated with hydrocephalus, that is generally attributed to excessive secretion by the tissue of choroid plexus. Microscopic structure consists of vascular connective tissue cores lined by columnar epithelial cells, that contain mucus but lack cilia or blepharoplasts, by contrast with ependymomas. Seeding through cerebrospinal fluid channels is common.

*Case:* A 2-month-old girl developed progressive hydrocephalus. Examination at three and one-half months revealed a fairly alert child with a head circumference of 47 cm, a tense anterior fontanelle, spreading sutures, and asymmetry of the skull, which was thinner and larger on the right side. A ventriculogram and injections of dye failed to reveal a block, but there was a shift of the enlarged ventricles to the left. Exploration revealed multiloculated cysts in the right hemisphere. The further course was one of increasing hydrocephalus and mental deterioration. Death occurred at the age of fifteen months.

The brain showed marked hydrocephalus involving the entire ventricular system and pressure atrophy of the nervous tissue. A tumor occupied the enlarged right lateral ventricle, consisting of an encapsulated solid granular tissue surrounded by numerous cysts separated by membranes that adhered to the capsule of the tumor (Fig. 117c).

Microscopically, the tumor reproduced the papillary structure of the choroid plexus, consisting of cores of vascular connective tissue lined by high columnar epithelium (Fig. 117d).

Both the cystic changes and the hydrocephalus appeared to represent products of secretion of the choroid plexus.

238

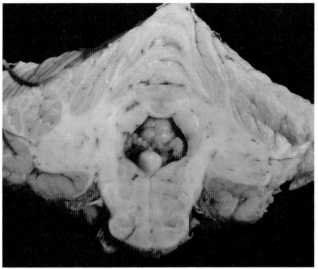

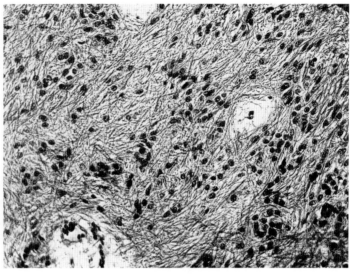

Fig. 117a. Subependymoma of fourth ventricle

Fig. 117b. HE × 200

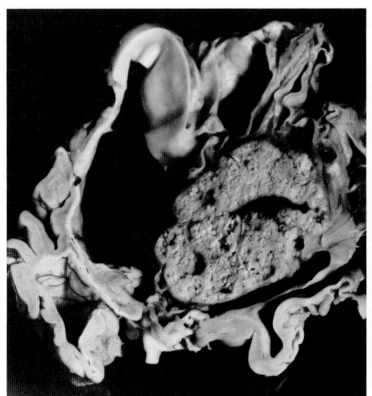

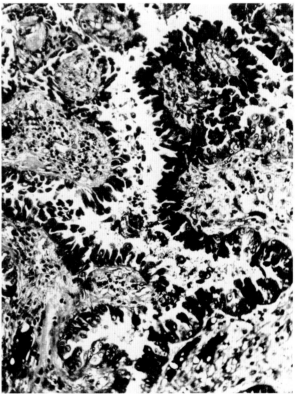

Fig. 117c. Papilloma of choroid plexus of right
lateral ventricle

Fig. 117d. HE × 200

Medulloblastoma is one of the most common tumors of the central nervous system to occur during childhood, although it may also affect young adults; it predominates in males. There is wide acceptance of the view that it is exclusively a cerebellar tumor, especially prone to develop in the posterior vermis, and that it is essentially a neuroblastoma arising from persistent rests of the embryonic external granular layer, particularly in the roof of the fourth ventricle.

The characteristic clinical features are a rapid course of gait ataxia, and early signs of obstructive hydrocephalus, marked tendency to seeding in the cerebrospinal fluid channels manifested by pleocytosis and low sugar, and favorable response to radiotherapy.

Pathologically, it is a circumscribed soft grayish-pink solid tumor, disposed to necrosis but not to hemorrhage or cyst formation, growing down from the vermis into the fourth ventricle, often accompanied by diffuse seeding in meninges and ependyma throughout brain, spinal cord, and nerve roots. Microscopic features are compact sheets of uniform carrot shaped cells with hyperchromatic round nuclei showing abundant mitosis, and sparse cytoplasm that tapers at one end. There is a tendency for the cells to form rosettes around tangles of neurofibrils. The vascular stroma is usually sparse. Mature astrocytes may be present but no indication that glial elements play a role in the neoplastic process.

*Case 1:* A 13-month-old girl was well until ten days prior to admission when following convalescence from a mild upper respiratory infection she developed irritability, nausea, and an unsteady gait. Examination revealed a head circumference of 19.5 inches with the anterior fontanelle patent and bulging. There was complete left and partial right lateral rectus palsy, and bilateral papilledema. Cerebrospinal fluid contained a total protein of 40 mg %. Ventriculography revealed an internal hydrocephalus secondary to a tumor in the posterior fossa, which at craniotomy was found to extend from beneath the vermis into the depths of the fourth ventricle. During attempts to remove the tumor, the patient became apneic and died.

The brain showed a large circumscribed gray tumor that replaced the inferior vermis and an operative tract marked by hemorrhage extending into it; the tumor obstructed the fourth ventricle, resulting in hydrocephalus involving the aqueduct, third and lateral ventricles and in diffuse flattening of the cerebral convolutions (Fig. 118a).

Microscopically, sheets of cells with uniform hyperchromatic nuclei, showing scattered mitotic figures and scant cytoplasm were at times disposed in rosettes around centers containing vague fibrillae (Fig. 118b).

*Case 2:* A 4½ year-old girl developed attacks of occipital headache, vomiting, unsteadiness of gait, irritability, and lethargy over a period of two months. Examination disclosed papilledema, ataxia of gait, and stiffness of neck. A ventriculogram revealed uniformly dilated ventricles. On craniotomy, a soft tumor was partly removed from the vermis. After an initial improvement, death occurred within ten months of the onset of her illness.

The brain contained a circumscribed grayish-red tumor mass in the inferior vermis, associated with local operative trauma and with widespread seeding, as evidenced by the opaque and nodular appearance of the meninges and ependyma (Fig. 118c).

Microscopically, the main tumor mass as well as the seeds of the meninges (Fig. 118d) disclosed the same structure as in Case 1.

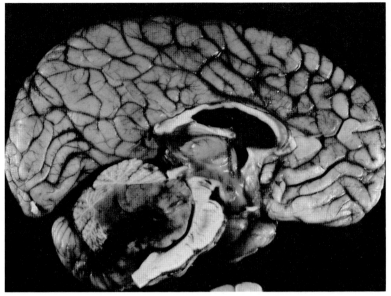

Fig. 118a. Medulloblastoma of inferior vermis

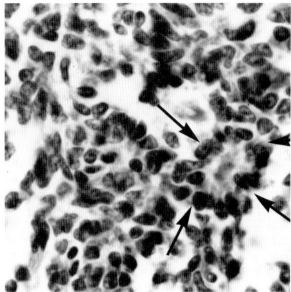

Fig. 118b. HE × 560

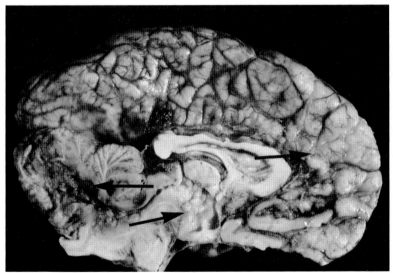

Fig. 118c. Medulloblastoma of inferior vermis accompanied by diffuse
seeding

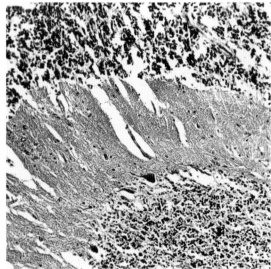

Fig. 118d. HE × 100

In the electron microscope, the tumor cells of medulloblastoma are best characterized by their relative lack of specific differentiation. The cells are closely packed with very little extracellular space (Fig. 119). Occasional, small, adhesive devices are found between adjacent cells. The nucleo-cytoplasmic ratio is high with a relative paucity of cytoplasm. Nevertheless, all the usual organelles, such as Golgi apparatus, mitochondria, microtubules and numerous free ribosomes, are present. Endoplasmic reticulum is usually inconspicuous but is present. Occasional cells may show focal accumulation of fibrils approximately 70–90 Å in diameter. The density of the cytoplasm may vary from cell to cell. This may reflect the presence of two cell types as some believe, or, more likely, is simply a matter of variability of fixation.

The question of the cellular origin of medulloblastoma is unresolved. Virtually all possibilities have been raised. Thus, some believe in a single cell type for the original neoplastic cell and this, according to different authors, may be either glioblastic, neuroblastic, or some cell which normally serves as a precursor to both glia and neurons. Other authors regard the tumor as mixed and deriving from more than one cell type. These speculations are based on the presence or absence of glial-like fibrils and/or microtubules. These criteria are not very specific and it is important to remember that the infiltrating nature of the tumor will result in the entrapment of nonneoplastic cells within the growing mass. It may also be important to point out that, so far, synapses have not been reported within medulloblastomas.

*References*

Kadin, M. E., L. J. Rubinstein, and J. S. Nelson. Neonatal Cerebellar Medulloblastoma Originating from the Fetal External Granular Layer. J. Neuropath. and Expt. Neurol. 29: 583, 1970.

Metakas, F., J. Cervos-Navarro, and F. Gullota. The Ultrastructure of Medulloblastomas. Acta Neuropath. 16: 271, 1970.

Soljima, T. Fine Structure of Medulloblastoma. Gann. 61: 17, 1970.

Waga, S. A Histological and Electron Microscopic Study on Medulloblastomas and Cerebellar Sarcomas. Arch. J. Jap. Chir. 34: 436, 1965.

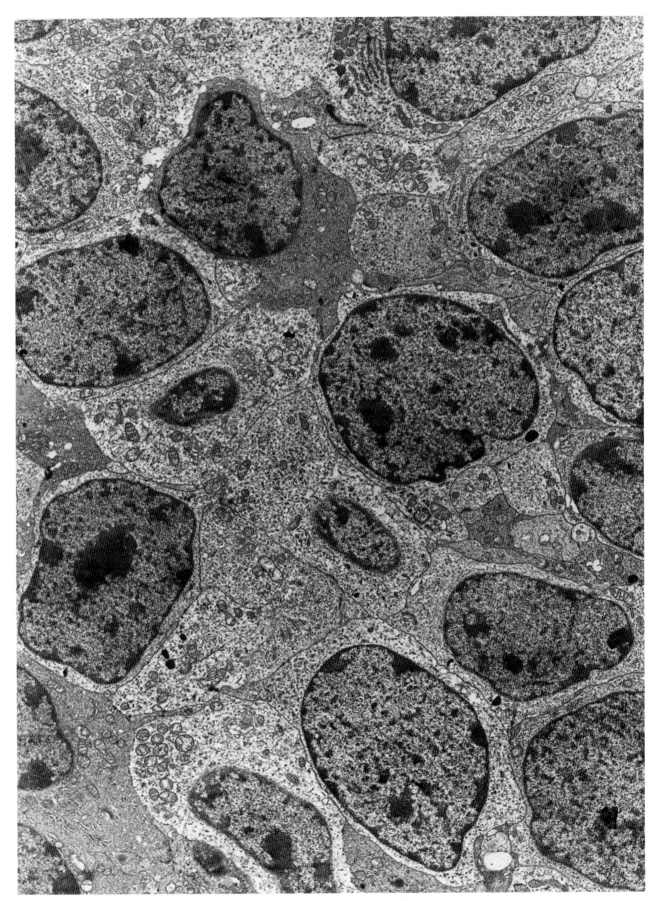

Fig. 119. An electron micrograph of a medulloblastoma × 8,000

Tumors of the pineal body are relatively rare, showing an incidence of less than 1% of intracranial tumors. Since the parenchymal cells of this structure are of neuroepithelial origin, the tumors are usually classified with the gliomas. However, only a small number of them arise from pineal parenchyma, the majority being regarded as teratomas. A classification that has received wide acceptance is that adopted by Russell and Rubinstein: 1) teratoma, 2) pineoblastoma, and 3) pineocytoma.

The teratomas occur predominantly in young males. Their structure bears a close resemblance to testicular seminomas (or dysgerminomas of ovaries). Their midline pineal location and their occurrence in other midline positions, in the form of ectopic pinealoma, also favor such a concept.

The pineoblastomas and pineocytomas are tumors of the parenchymal cells, the former consisting of immature forms, resembling medulloblastoma, while the latter are more mature cells often showing perivascular rosettes. As a group they have no special sex or age predilection.

The clinical course varies, that of the teratomas being more rapid and more prone to seeding. The symptoms are largely those due to compression and infiltration of the tectum, especially upward or downward gaze palsy (Parinaud's syndrome). A syndrome of precocious sexual puberty is common in the younger age group but its interpretation varies from incidental involvement of the hypothalamus to release of a normal inhibiting influence of the pineal body on gonadal development.

## Teratoma of Pineal Body

*Case 1:* A 21-year-old man developed headaches, nausea, vomiting, vertigo, diplopia, tinnitus, ataxia, and visual impairment. Examination revealed bilateral nystagmus, papilledema, paresis of upward gaze, diminished sensation of the face, decreased hearing, dysmetria and ataxia with wide-based gait, and a positive Romberg sign. A ventriculogram revealed a tumor obstructing the aqueduct of Sylvius. The patient died after a Torkildsen procedure.

A partly cystic tumor derived from the pineal body invaded the tectum and tegmentum of the brain stem. (Fig. 120a).

Microscopically, the tumor was composed of nests of large polyhedral epithelioid cells with vesicular nuclei showing occasional mitoses separated by small lymphoid cells (Fig. 120b), closely resembling a seminoma.

## Pineoblastoma

*Case 2:* A 6-year-old girl developed headaches, vomiting, lethargy, and stiffness of the neck and was admitted to a hospital. Examination revealed blurred disc margins and retinal hemorrhages, and by ventriculography, obstruction of the aqueduct due to a mass in the region of the pineal body. A Torkildsen shunt was performed. She was treated with x-rays, receiving a dose of 4,250 r over a period of several months, resulting in remission for the next two years. She then relapsed and an air study demonstrated evidence of tumor in the right hemisphere communicating with the ventricles. At craniotomy, bilateral intraventricular tumor was found. She expired two days postoperatively.

A large grayish tumor that was largely replaced by hemorrhage occupied the region of the pineal body, compressing the tectum and the aqueduct, and had ruptured into the distended lateral ventricles (Fig. 120c).

On microscopic examination, the tumor consisted of a sheet of uniform round cells with hyperchromatic nuclei and scattered mitotic figures surrounded by sparse cytoplasm (Fig. 120d).

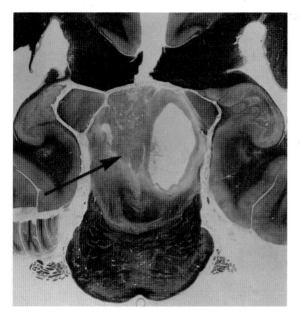

Fig. 120a. Tumor of pineal body

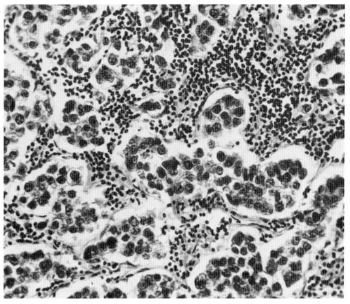

Fig. 120b. HE × 200

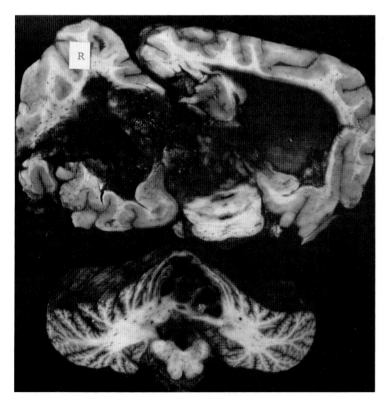

Fig. 120c. Tumor of pineal body with massive hemorrhage,
extending into lateral ventricles

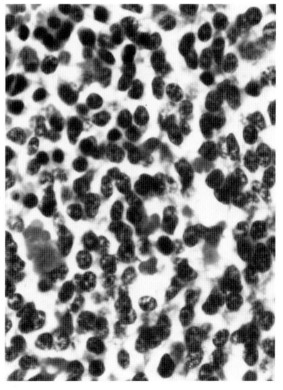

Fig. 120d. HVG × 560

Tumors arising from mature nerve cells are exceedingly rare in the central nervous system, by contrast with their relatively high frequency in the peripheral nervous system. Since they are commonly associated with proliferation of glial elements, to which they owe much of their growth potential, they are better designated as gangliogliomas rather than ganglioneuromas. They have also been classed as hamartomas because of considerations that they represent ectopias of developmental origin.

Pathologically, they are composed of mature ganglion cells associated with well differentiated astrocytes, are slowly growing, lacking signs of rapid division and are often calcified.

Their most common location is in relation to midline structures, such as the floor of the third ventricle, but they may also involve the cerebral and cerebellar hemisphere, particularly in a paramedian location.

## Ganglioglioma of Uncus-Amygdaloid Region

Small tumors, often of a hamartomatous nature, located in anterior or mesial parts of the temporal lobes, have been reported in association with the syndrome of temporal lobe epilepsy.

> *Case:* A 26-year-old man developed at the age of 13 years spells that were manifested by feelings of numbness, hallucinations of smell, taste, hearing, and vision but without apparent loss of consciousness. At the age of fifteen, a neurologic examination, including a pneumoencephalogram, was normal, but several EEGs revealed generalized paroxysmal dysrhythmia with focal activity, initially in the left occipital and subsequently in the left temporal region. He was treated with anticonvulsant medication. In the following ten years he became increasingly withdrawn and expressed paranoid ideas of reference. At the age of eighteen, he had an acute psychotic episode, and on admission to a psychiatric institution a diagnosis of catatonic schizophrenia was made. A course of combined electroshock and insulin therapy led to apparent improvement and he was discharged. Subsequently, he had a number of brief readmissions for similar episodes, during which he received either electroschock or psychotherapy. Psychologic tests revealed a normal intelligence but evidence of a schizophrenic disorder. It was noted, however, that when anticonvulsant medication was stopped, he would either experience grand mal attacks or spells, some of which were characterized by sensations of micropsia or automatic behavior for which he was amnesic. He died from a pulmonary embolism complicating a thrombophlebitis.

The brain showed on section a small ill-defined infiltrating tumor with cystic degeneration, that involved the left uncus-amygdaloid region (Fig. 121a).

On microscopic examination, large ganglion cells with coarse Nissl substance, some of which were binucleated, were scattered through cystic tissue composed of small fibrillary astrocytes (Fig. 121b) and glial fibers (Fig. 121c).

This case is another example of a limbic lesion causing ictal and interictal psychiatric manifestations sufficient to confuse the diagnosis with "functional" mental disorders (see Reference, p. 214).

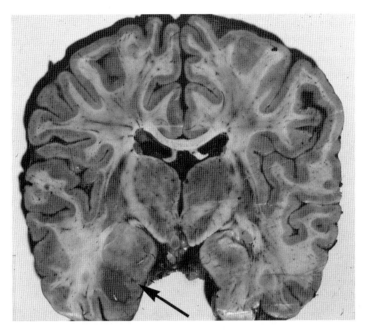

Fig. 121a. Ganglioglioma of left uncus-amygdaloid region

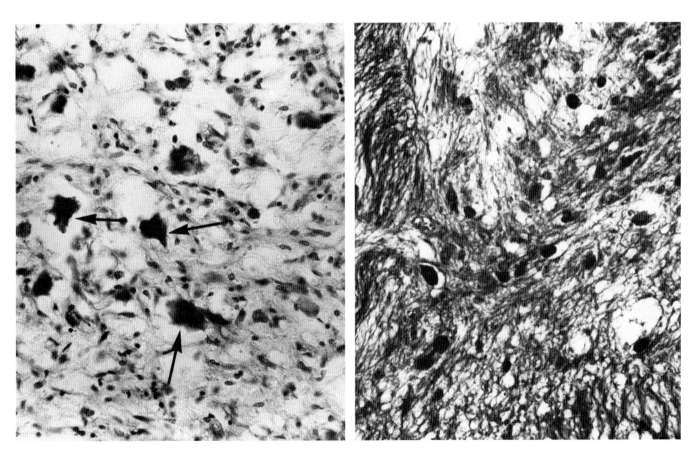

Fig. 121b. Nissel x 200

Fig. 121c. PTAH × 150

## Hamartoma of Tuber Cinereum

A tumor, usually small, attached to the tuber cinereum by a stalk and composed of well differentiated ganglion and glial cells has been reported in a number of cases, with a clinical syndrome of precocious sexual puberty, possibly through a neurosecretory mechanism.

> *Case:* A 37-year-old woman had a history of having contracted syphilis at the age of thirteen years, developed seizures and personality changes and was committed to a mental hospital. The blood Wassermann was positive but there was no evidence of central nervous system lues. (Precocious sexual puberty was implied but not well documented.)

The brain contained a spherical grayish-white tumor of about 1 cm. in diameter, arising from the region of the tuber cinereum, that compressed the third ventricle (Fig. 122a). Microscopically, it was composed of small and medium-sized neurons (A) and fibrillary astrocytes, attached by a stalk of myelinated nerve fibers (B) to the floor of the third ventricle (Fig. 122b).

*Reference*

List, C. F., C. E. Dowman, B. K. Bagchi, and J. Bebin. Posterior Hypothalamic Hamartomas and Gangliogliomas Causing Precocious Puberty. Neurol. 8: 164, 1958.

## Granule Cell Hypertrophy of the Cerebellum

A rare hamartomatous tumor of the cerebellum, known as granule cell hypertrophy of the cerebellum, or Lhermitte-Duclos' disease, is characterized by gross hypertrophy of folia of the cerebellum and microscopically by proliferation largely of the cells of the granule layer, less likely of the Purkinje cells. It is often clinically asymptomatic but may act by increasing intracranial pressure due to obstruction of the fourth ventricle.

> *Case:* A 42-year-old woman complained of severe headaches for about two years, that were considered to be "tension headaches." Since these persisted, she was admitted to a hospital where examination revealed vertigo and nystagmus on sudden changes in position, considered to be due to labyrinthitis. Several months later she underwent surgery for intestinal obstruction, and while recovering from the operation, she suddenly expired, nine hours postoperatively.

The brain was enlarged, weighing 1,880 grams. The most striking change was hypertrophy of the folia of the right cerebellar hemisphere and the adjacent vermis, that compressed and displaced the fourth ventricle to the left (Fig. 122c), causing internal hydrocephalus.

Microscopically, the granule and molecular layers were greatly enlarged, showing replacement of the granule cells by hypertrophied neurons and proliferation of their axons in the molecular layer, amongst which there were scattered Purkinje cells of normal appearance (Fig. 122d).

*Reference*

Ambler, M., S. Pogacar, and R. Sidman. Lhermitte-Duclos Disease (Granule Cell Hypertrophy of the Cerebellum), Pathological Analysis of the First Familial Cases. J. Neuropath. and Expt. Neurol. 28: 622, 1969.

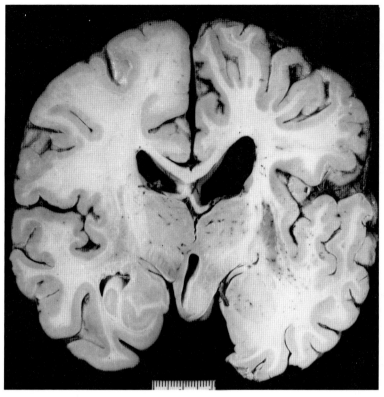

Fig. 122a. Hamartoma of tuber cinereum

Fig. 122b. HE × 100

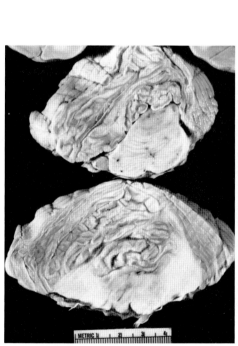

Fig. 122c. Granule cell hypertrophy of cerebellum (sides reversed)

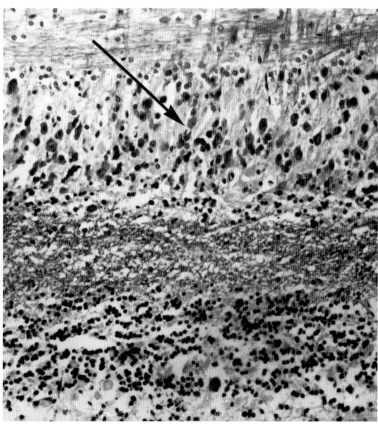

Fig. 122d. Klüver × 175

In a number of conditions, errors in development based on hereditary predisposition tend to produce a complex association of hamartomas and neoplasms in widespread tissues such as skin, nervous system, and internal organs. Because of this they have been designated as phacomatoses and neuroectodermal dysplasias.

One of the prime examples in which the glial and neuronal cells of the central nervous system are so involved, along with those of the skin and viscera, is tuberous sclerosis or Bourneville's disease.

The classic clinical picture of tuberous sclerosis comprises a triad of symptoms, that develop slowly from birth, of mental retardation, convulsions, and adenoma sebaceum of the face, the latter in the form of a maculo-papular rash in butterfly pattern of distribution. Variations are not uncommon such as formes frustes in which, for example, the adenoma sebaceum is absent.

The main pathologic features consist of cortical and subependymal nodules in the brain; retinal phacomas; hyperplasia of sebaceous and sweat glands, vascular and fibrous tissues in the dermis; mixed hamartomas of kidneys, and rhabdomyomas of heart.

> *Case 1:* A 34-year-old man, whose mentally defective and epileptic sister had died at the age of two years, had been developing convulsions and mental retardation since he was seven months old. When finally admitted to a hospital, he had a fine papular eruption on his face, was a low-grade mental defective, could not talk, demonstrated mild spasticity and choreiform movements, and had many grand mal seizures.

The brain which weighed 1,380 grams, presented a normal convolutional pattern but contained slightly raised and umbilicated pearly-white cortical nodules of cartilaginous consistency (arrows) throughout both hemispheres (Fig. 123a).

Sections revealed that the nodules (A) consisted of a white or grayish discolored tissue in which the cortex and white matter could not be distinguished; the enlarged ventricles contained grayish-white, firm nodules (B) that projected into them from the subependymal regions, particularly in the striothalamic areas (Fig. 123b).

Microscopic examination revealed that the cortical nodules underwent a dense hyperplastic gliosis. The cytoarchitecture had disappeared, due to dropout of neurons and hyperplasia of small and large glial elements, in which bizarre giant neurons with abnormally branching dendrites and axons were embedded (Fig. 123c). The subependymal nodules consisted of hyperplasia of glial fibers (lower right) with tendency to calcify (upper left) (Fig. 123d).

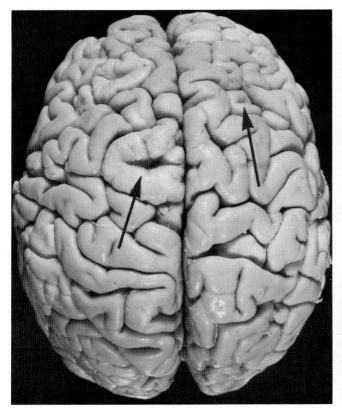

Fig. 123a. Tuberous sclerosis, external
appearance

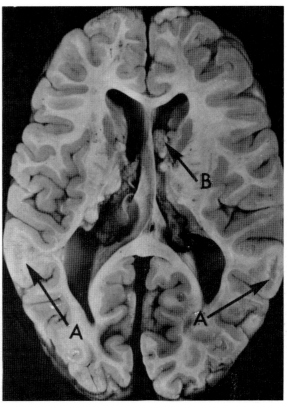

Fig. 123b. Tuberous sclerosis, horizontal
section

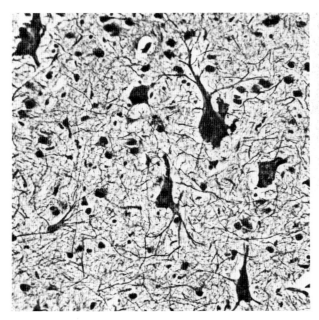

Fig. 123c. von Braunmühl × 250

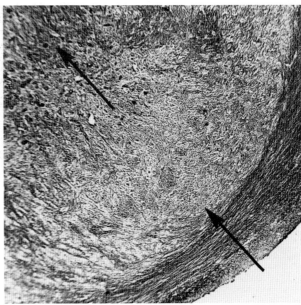

Fig. 123d. Holzer × 24

Other stigmata of developmental disturbances may be present in tuberous sclerosis, such as megalencephaly, hydrocephalus, micropolygyria, and heterotopia.

The retinal phacomas are discrete grayish-white nodules scattered through the fundus (arrows) (Fig. 124a), that microscopically consist of hyperplasia of astrocytes and glial fibers (Fig. 124b).

The renal tumors are pleomorphic and vary from angiomas to myomas, adenomas, and fibrolipomas (A) embedded in the parenchyma of the renal cortex (B) (Fig. 124c).

In a number of instances, the neurologic picture differs from the classic form, being dominated by progressive signs of increased intracranial pressure due to an intraventricular tumor.

> *Case 2:* A 15-year-old girl, whose older sister died of the same disease (confirmed by autopsy) showed signs of arrested development and adenoma sebaceum from early childhood. At the age of nine years, skull x-rays showed evidence of hydrocephalus, and at this time, she became increasingly unable to walk and experienced seizures. Her condition showed progressive deterioration from then on and towards the end she became totally blind, revealing bilateral optic atrophy.

The brain weighed 1,600 grams and, on section through the frontal lobes (Fig. 124d), contained a large partly cystic and hemorrhagic intraventricular tumor mass on the left side that compressed the head of the caudate nucleus and septum pellucidum, blocking the foramen of Monro, and accounting for the hydrocephalus; the right lateral ventricle contained scattered small subependymal firm nodules; there were no visible cortical nodules, possibly masked by signs of generalized pressure.

The microscopic structure of the tumor was that of a gigantocellular astrocytoma (Fig. 124e) that is characteristic of the disorder; it consisted of compactly arranged fascicles of large spindle-shaped astrocytes, containing glial fibers. Scattered foci in the cortex showed the characteristic changes of the disease.

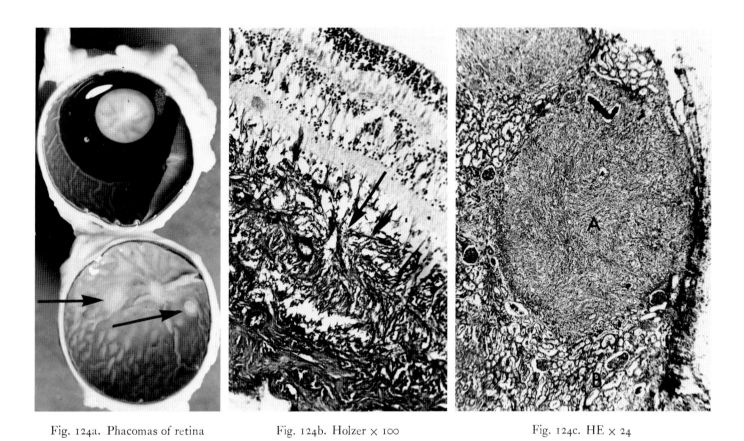

Fig. 124a. Phacomas of retina    Fig. 124b. Holzer × 100    Fig. 124c. HE × 24

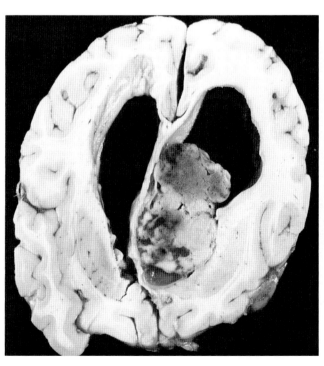

Fig. 124d. Tuberous sclerosis with left sided intraventricular tumor (sides reversed)

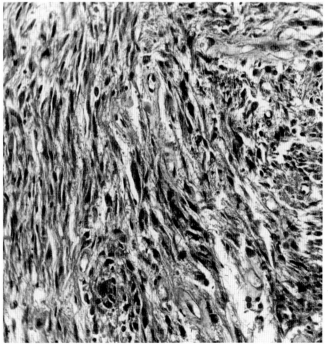

Fig. 124e. HE × 200

This group of tumors comprises miscellaneous forms that take their origin from tissues other than the parenchymal elements of the central nervous system, namely, meninges, peripheral nerve sheaths, blood vessels, the pituitary gland, and from extraneural embryonic cell rests. With some exceptions, they are extrinsic in location, tend to be encapsulated, and have a more favorable prognosis with surgery.

## MENINGIOMAS

Meningiomas are tumors that take their origin largely from the arachnoidal granulations that are derived from the neural crest and that project into the dural sinuses. As a result the most common sites for the development of such tumors are in locations where there is normally a concentration of the arachnoidal cells (Fig. 125a).

The intracranial forms may thus be classified in accordance with location as parasagittal, sphenoid ridge, olfactory groove, parasellar and tuberculum sellar, tentorial, foraminal, and intraventricular. The intraspinal forms may arise from any site, more commonly at the thoracic level, in a subdural location.

Meningiomas are the most common extrinsic intracranial tumors, and in the spinal canal they share a high incidence with the Schwannomas. They prevail in middle age and are more common in females. Their clinical symptomatology depends on location as well as on their slow evolution. Multiple meningiomas are not uncommon.

Grossly, meningiomas are most often globular, homogeneous, firm, and avascular but occasionally they grow en plaque at the base of the brain; some may be relatively vascular. They are encapsulated and are attached to the dura where their surface contains a network of venous channels. Meningiomas invade bone causing hyperostosis and osteolysis but as a rule do not extend beyond the arachnoid membrane to invade the nervous tissue which is only compressed.

> *Case 1:* A 50-year-old woman had a history of headaches for many years. Several months before admission to a hospital, she developed aphasia and disturbance of gait. A few days before admission there was a sudden onset of vomiting, dizziness, right-sided weakness and numbness, and right hemianopsia. Examination revealed euphoria, apraxia, a right homonymous lower-quadrant hemianopsia, right hemiparesis with pyramidal signs, and impairment on the right of sense of position and two-point discrimination, with extinction of all sensory stimuli on bilateral simultaneous stimulation. An electroencephalogram showed evidence of a left fronto-temporal focus. A left carotid arteriogram revealed evidence of a left parietal tumor. Patient died suddenly five hours after angiography.

A large, firm, encapsulated, finely granular, globoid tumor, measuring approximately 7 cm. in maximum diameter, was found attached to the falx in the left frontoparietal region. The tumor caused marked pressure atrophy of the surrounding brain tissue from which it was sharply demarcated, displacing the ventricles downward and to the right (Fig. 125b).

The above case illustrates a parasagittal meningioma that most commonly involves the middle one-third of the convexity of the cerebral hemisphere near the sagittal sinus. The development of localizing signs only at an advanced stage of the tumor precluded an earlier diagnosis and determined the fatal outcome.

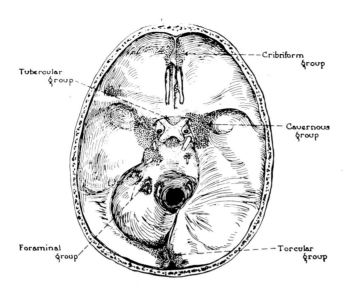

Fig. 125a. Distribution of arachnoidal granulations in
the skull
(*courtesy Percival Bailey*)

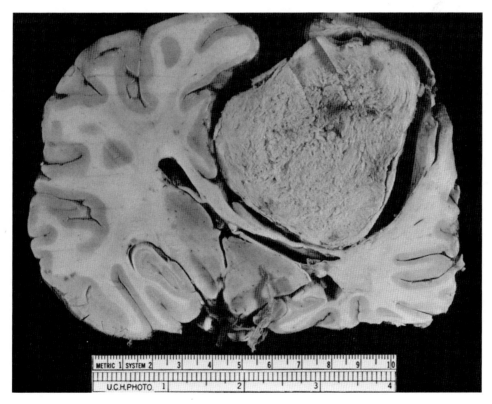

Fig. 125b. Parasagittal meningioma (sides reversed)

*Case 2:* A 61-year-old man developed gradual suppression of vision in both eyes. Four years later examination disclosed bitemporal hemianopsia, which was more marked on the left side. Excretion of 17-ketosteroids was decreased to 5.6 mg per 100 cc in 24 hours. The cerebrospinal fluid was under a pressure of 230 mm of $H_2O$, gave a positive Pandy reaction, contained 178 mg % of total protein, and showed a first-zone rise in the colloidal gold curve. A pneumoencephalogram revealed symmetrical dilatation of the ventricular system. An encapsulated tumor in the suprasellar region was found at operation and partly removed. The further course was one of progressive impairment of vision, personality changes, and mental deterioration. A nodular, encapsulated tumor measuring 3 by 3.5 cm occupied the interpeduncular fossa, obliterating the optic chiasm and other structures in the floor of the third ventricle (Fig. 126a).

The above is an example of a meningioma arising in the region of the tuberculum sellae. Its clinical behavior resembled that of a chromophobe pituitary adenoma.

*Case 3:* A 43-year-old man developed a hearing deficit and tenderness in the right ear over a period of one year, followed by ataxia and blurring of vision. On examination he showed decreased hearing on the right side, diminution of the right corneal and gag reflexes, a tendency to fall to the right, ataxia and nystagmus on lateral gaze. Pneumoencephalography and vertebral angiography led to a diagnosis of a right cerebellopontine angle tumor. On craniotomy, only a part of the tumor could be removed and the biopsy diagnosis was meningioma. He expired two weeks postoperatively of pulmonary complications.

An encapsulated firm and homogeneous globular tumor, measuring 5 cm in maximum diameter compressed the right side of the pons, the middle and inferior cerebellar peduncles, cerebellum, and the roots of cranial nerves 5, 7 and 8, while the fourth ventricle was displaced to the left side (Fig. 126b).

The above case illustrated a cerebellopontine angle location of a meningioma, resembling the clinical symptomatology of an acoustic neuroma.

The histology of meningiomas depends on their origin from closely related mesothelial and stroma cells, and may be one of the following three main types, though often combined:

1. *Meningotheliomatous* or syncitial, consisting of a sheet of uniform cells with only vague cell outlines and with uniformly spherical and vesicular nuclei, showing little tendency to pleomorphism or mitotic activity and separated into lobules by a delicate vascular stroma (Fig. 126c).

2. *Psammomatous* or transitional, in which cells similar to type 1, are disposed in whorls, the centers of which readily undergo hyalinization and calcification resulting in psammoma bodies (Fig. 126d), and

3. *Fibroblastic* or fibrous, characterized by fusiform cells with elongated nuclei that are arranged in intersecting fascicles of parallel streaming forms that produce abundant collagen and reticulin fibers (Fig. 126e).

There are several other histologic varieties that are either rare or controversial as to their inclusion with meningiomas, since they are closely related to tumors of blood vessels. These are angioblastic meningiomas that bear a close resemblance to hemangioblastomas of the cerebellum, and hemangiopericytomas that are believed to arise from pericytes.

A very rare *melanoblastic* variety develops from melanin-bearing cells in the arachnoid, largely around the medulla.

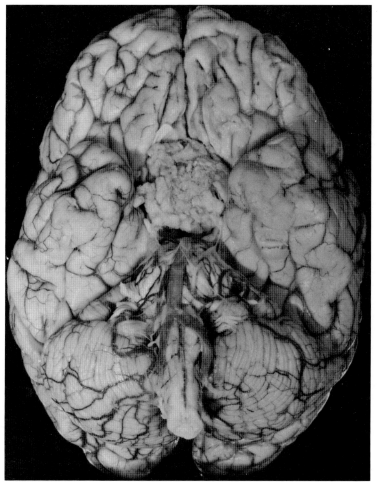

Fig. 126a. Suprasellar meningioma

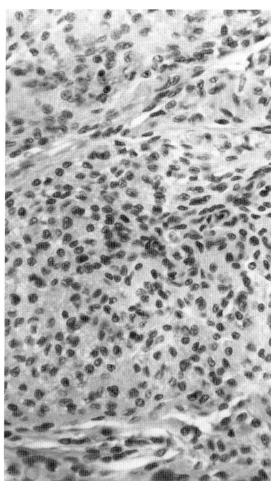

Fig. 126c. HE × 250

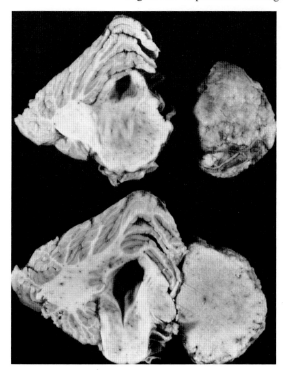

Fig. 126b. Meningioma, right
cerebellopontine angle

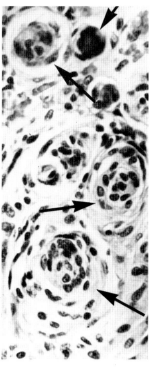

Fig. 126d. HE × 250

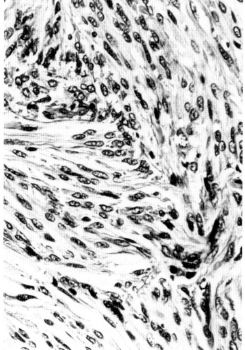

Fig. 126e. HE × 250

One of the most prominent features of meningioma cells is the highly irregular cell surface characterized by the interdigitation of numerous narrow cell processes. Many desmosomes (arrows) are evident along the cell borders so that, for the most part, the extracellular space is quite narrow (Fig. 127). Normal arachnoidal cells also display elongated cell processes which are connected to one another by desmosomes. In contrast to meningiomas, however, the normal leptomeninges are characterized by an ample extracellular space, that is, the subarachnoid space. On the other hand, some areas within meningiomas contain large extracellular spaces which may contain large amounts of collagen, some of which appear much wider than normal. Often, calcium deposits are present in the same areas, around which collagen and tumor cells arrange themselves in a concentric fashion. The tumor cells themselves contain the usual organelles but are often marked by highly irregular nuclei (N) so that, sometimes, extensions of cytoplasm appear within the nucleus. These are the nuclear inclusions described by light microscopy. In addition, some glycogen is occasionally seen but more prominent is the frequent presence of filaments which sometimes accumulate in large numbers.

*References*

Napolitano, L., R. Kyle, and E. R. Fisher. Ultrastructure of Meningiomas and the Derivation and Nature of Their Cellular Components. Cancer. 17: 233, 1963.

Poon, T. P., A. Hirano, and H. M. Zimmerman. Electron Microscopic Atlas of Brain Tumors. Grune and Stratton (New York, 1971).

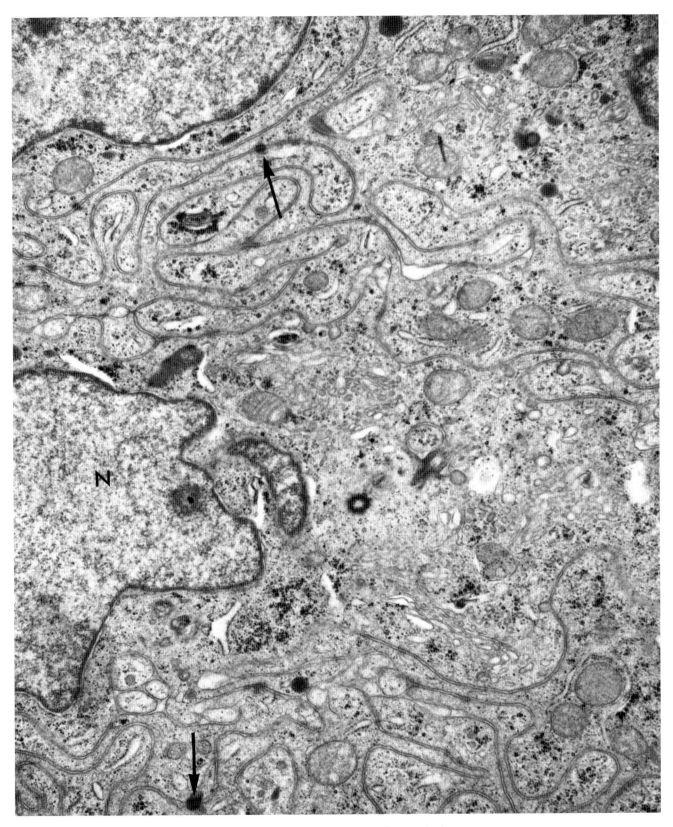

Fig. 127. An electron micrograph of a meningioma ×
30,000 (Hirano, in Progress in Neuropathology, Vol. I.
(H. M. Zimmerman, ed.). Grune and Stratton (New
York, 1971), p. 1.)

An increasing number of primary intracranial sarcomas have been reported in recent years. Their origin is from connective tissue cells located in either the dura or pia-arachnoid and their pial extensions into the substance of the brain. They should not be confused with the occasional sarcomatous changes in a meningioma. As a group they are distinguished by their rapid growth, malignant clinical course, and variable responsiveness to radiation therapy.

They have been classified into a number of different varieties, some of which have been controversial as to their inclusion in this group.

The classification introduced by Kernohan and Uihlein, is probably the most inclusive: 1. Fibrosarcoma, 2. Giant cell sarcoma, 3. Circumscribed sarcoma of the cerebellum, 4. Meningeal sarcomatosis, 5. Hemangiopericytoma, 6. Combined sarcoma and glioma, and 7. Recticulum cell sarcoma or microgliomatosis.

## Fibrosarcoma

Fibrosarcoma may arise from any of the layers of the meninges and from their perivascular pial extensions within the brain, occurring at all ages. It appears as a large local homogeneous mass, that is firm and fleshy, encapsulated but tends to infiltrate the adjacent nervous tissue; it is prone to metastasize through cerebrospinal fluid channels. The microscopic structure is one of spindle shaped cells with variable pleomorphism and mitotic figures and with abundant reticulin fibers.

> *Case:* A 21-year-old man had a recent onset of persistent headaches and blurring of vision. On admission to the hospital he was lethargic and showed papilledema and hyperreflexia. EEG, brain scan, and an arteriogram revealed evidence of a tumor in the right temporoparietal region. At operation, a firm avascular tumor was found located beneath the right temporal lobe attached to the tentorium, diagnosed at biopsy as sarcoma. He had a course of radiation therapy and of cytoxan but there was progressive deterioration and he died three to four months following the onset.

A large tumor that was attached to and infiltrated both the upper surface of the tentorium and the undersurface of the right temporo-occipital region, was partly obscured by postoperative necrosis and hemorrhage (Fig. 128a).

Microscopic examination showed a structure that varied from intersecting bundles of spindle-shaped cells with large hyperchromatic nuclei, and scattered mitoses within the meninges (upper field), to more pleomorphic round and elongated cells in the underlying gray matter (lower field) (Fig. 128b). The entire tumor was pervaded by large amounts of collagen and reticulin fibers, both in the meninges and cortex (Fig. 128c).

Giant cell sarcomas and the circumscribed sarcoma of the cerebellum have each been disputed, the former having been interpreted as a glioblastoma and the latter as an adult form of medulloblastoma.

Combined glioma and sarcoma represents a mixed neoplasm in which the predominant tumor of either type can stimulate reactive neoplasia of the other.

*References*

Kernohan, J. W., and A. Uihlein. Sarcomas of the Brain. Chas. C Thomas (Springfield, Ill., 1962).
Rubinstein, L. J., and D. W. C. Northfield. The Medulloblastoma and the So-called "Arachnoidal Cerebellar Sarcoma." Brain, 87: 379, 1964.

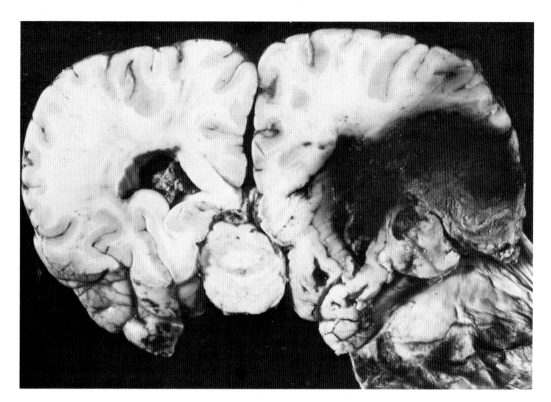

Fig. 128a. Fibrosarcoma, right hemisphere

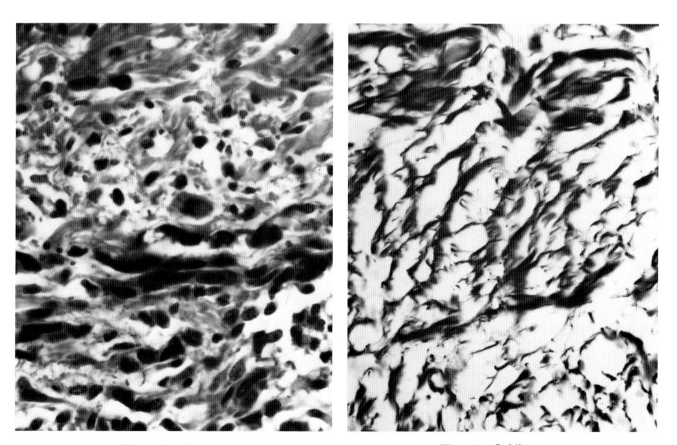

Fig. 128b. HE × 375

Fig. 128c. Laidlaw × 375

## Meningeal Sarcomatosis

These are tumors arising from both reticuloendothelial and fibroblastic cells of the leptomeninges, are of multifocal origin and spread diffusely in the subarachnoid space and in the subependymal tissues. They occur most commonly in infants, follow a rapid clinical course, often resembling a basal meningitis because of predominant location in the posterior fossa, pleocytosis and low sugar in the cerebrospinal fluid, and are prone to result in hydrocephalus.

Pathologically, the meninges show diffuse clouding or milky opacity that may condense into scattered large tumor masses that infiltrate the nervous tissue along the perivascular spaces. The microscopic examination shows a mixture of round anaplastic reticuloendothelial and spindle-shaped fibroblastic cells.

*Case:* A 2-year-old, white boy developed two weeks prior to admission listlessness, anorexia, vomiting, headaches, irritability, weakness of the right side of the face, incoordinated movements of the right eye, dysarthria, and staggering. Examination on admission revealed dilated fixed pupils, nystagmus to the left, absent extraocular movements, proptosis and fifth and seventh nerve palsies on the right side, and a stiff neck. X-rays of the skull and EEGs were normal. Lumbar puncture showed a pressure of 210 mm $H_2O$; a total protein of 108 mg %; sugar of 5 mg % and 7 lymphocytes per cmm. He was treated with antibiotics although there was no cultural evidence of an infectious process. In the further course there was a rising cerebrospinal fluid pressure to 300 mm $H_2O$. Ventriculography was then performed that revealed only dilated ventricles. He followed a rapidly downhill course and expired approximately one month following the onset of his illness.

The brain and spinal cord showed diffuse thickening and opacity of the leptomeninges, that was accentuated around the cerebellum and brain stem, where large grayish-white, firm, and homogenous tumor masses extended from the meninges into the underlying nervous tissue on either side (Fig. 129a).

Microscopically, dense infiltrations of round to spindle-shaped cells, with vesicular nuclei and scattered mitotic figures (Fig. 129b) filled the subarachnoid space and extended through perivascular spaces into the parenchyma where it stimulated a reaction by gemistocytic astrocytes (Fig. 129c). There were large amounts of proliferating reticulin fibers both within the involved meninges and the infiltrated nervous tissue (Fig. 129d).

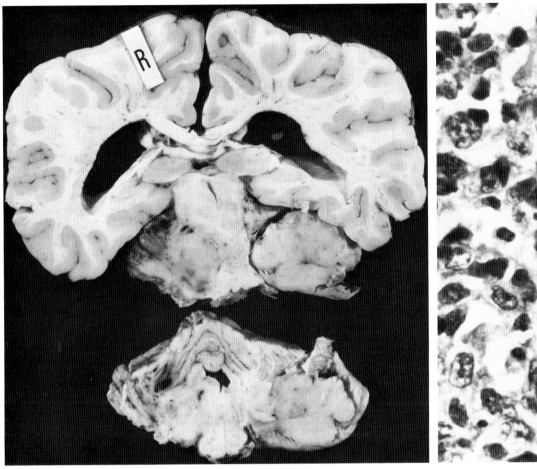

Fig. 129a. Meningeal sarcomatosis

Fig. 129b. HE × 450

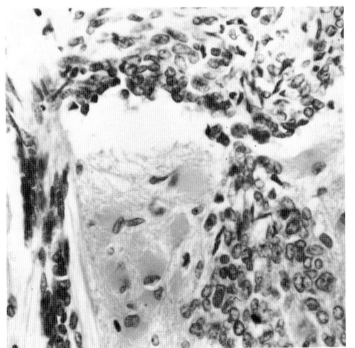

Fig. 129c. HE × 290

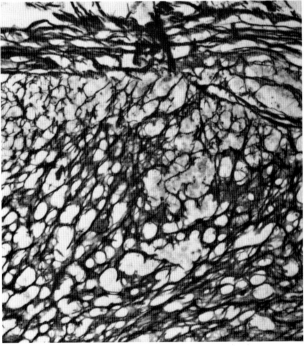

Fig. 129d. Laidlaw × 185

## Reticulum Cell Sarcoma (Microgliomatosis)

Primary tumors of reticuloendothelial cells in the central nervous system are rare but have been receiving increasing attention especially because of their proneness to occur under conditions of an altered immune state. The controversy about their fundamental cell type of origin, as between reticuloendothelial cells or microglia, has been largely resolved as a semantic problem because of the identity of the two cell types, resulting in their designation of either reticulum cell sarcoma or microgliomatosis.

Clinically, these tumors occur predominantly in middle or advanced age and follow a rapid and malignant clinical course that may be amenable to some extent to radiation therapy. Their tendency to multifocal dissemination presents diagnostic difficulties.

Pathologically, they vary greatly from large tumor masses to miliary infiltrates, resembling encephalitis. The cell types vary from reticulum cells to microglia in shape and staining reactions, associated with some lymphocytes, and condense around blood vessels where they induce concentric rings of reticulin fibers, as well as infiltrate the local meninges.

*Case 1:* A 45-year-old woman developed progressive weakness of the right side one week before admission. Examination showed a mild right-sided impairment of vibratory and position sense and in two-point discrimination, and hyperactive reflexes with an extensor plantar response on the right side. A lumbar puncture disclosed pressure of 140 mm $H_2O$, a total protein of 60 mg %, the gamma globulin being 12.3 mg (twice normal). On the assumption of a demyelinating disorder, she was started on intravenous ACTH, and showed improvement. Two months later she was readmitted with numbness and weakness of the left side, blurring of vision, intellectual impairment, left homonymous hemianopsia and sensory deficit to position and vibratory sense and stereognosis on the left. A brain scan revealed foci in the midbrain and in the right inferior parietal region. Pneumoencephalography showed displacement of the ventricles to the left. A right temporoparietal craniotomy was performed and a biopsy disclosed perivascular cuffing with mononuclear cells of undetermined type. A month postoperatively she became comatose, with a dilated right pupil and expired five months after the onset of symptoms.

The brain contained a large fleshy, gray, and partly hemorrhagic tumor, that appeared to be made up of several confluent masses, occupying the region of the basal ganglia on the right side, obliterating the right lateral and third ventricles, and displacing the ventricles to the left; an operative tract led into its superior surface (Fig. 130a). A small tumor nodule was also found in the cortex of the left inferior central region (at another level).

Microscopically, the tumor consisted of a patternless sheet of closely packed mononuclear cells of large and medium size with hyperchromatic nuclei, frequently showing mitosis, and with sparse cytoplasm, along with rare lymphocytes (Fig. 130b). In less compact areas, the tumor cells showed a distinct perivascular arrangement, the intervening nervous tissue containing numerous microglial cells along with scattered astrocytes (Fig. 130c).

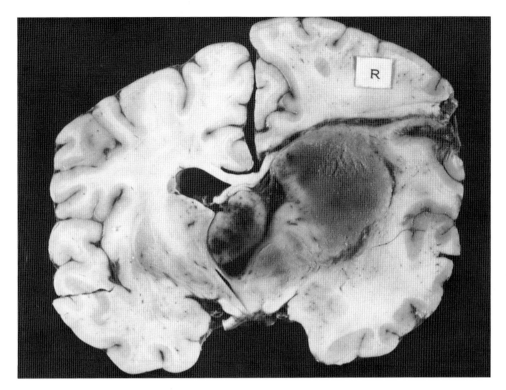

Fig. 130a. Reticulum cell sarcoma (microgliomatosis)

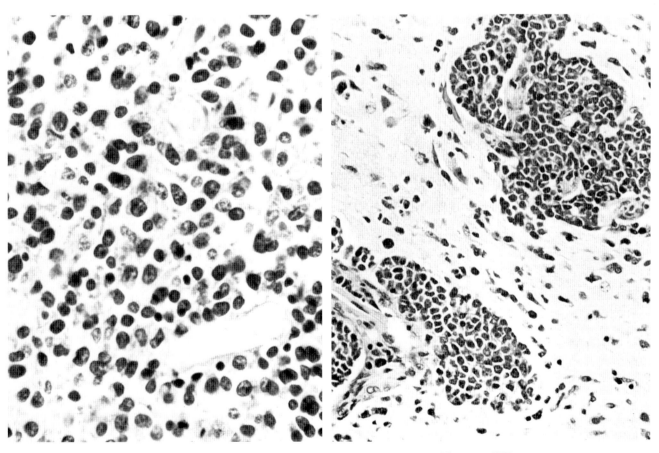

Fig. 130b. HE × 375

Fig. 130c. HE × 180

## Reticulum Cell Sarcoma (Microgliomatosis) (Continued)

In a few instances, *Waldenström's* syndrome with macroglobulinemia and disseminated reticuloendotheliosis, has been associated with a reticulum cell sarcoma of the brain, giving rise to speculation about the presence of abnormal immunoglobulins in this type of tumor, as illustrated in the following case:

*Case 2:* A 73-year-old man became mentally confused four months prior to admission to a hospital. Examination showed fever, petechial hemorrhages in mucosa of mouth, productive cough, hiccoughs, enophthalmos with partial ptosis and marked photophobia on the right, flat optic discs, mental confusion, and positive snout reflex. Hematologic evaluation, including immuno-electrophoresis and bone marrow aspiration, led to a diagnosis of Waldenström's macroglobulinemia; because of the prominent neurologic symptoms, the condition was designated as the Bing-Neel syndrome. An echo-encephalogram and skull films showed a pineal shift of 6 mm to the left and an EEG a decreased alpha activity over the right hemisphere. Later, the patient developed a left homonymous hemianopsia, a mild left hemiparesis with hyperactive reflexes, bilateral plantar extensor signs, and absent abdominal and cremasteric reflexes. A bilateral carotid arteriogram showed displacement of the anterior and middle cerebral complex to the left, indicative of a mass in the right temporal lobe. Patient underwent a craniotomy, biopsy being inconclusive. Postoperatively, patient continued to be lethargic, although the tumor decreased in size by angiography. He then received three plasmaphoreses with improvement after each one; however, he developed pneumonitis and expired five months after the onset of the neurologic symptoms.

General autopsy findings revealed infiltrates of lymphocytes, lymphoblasts, and plasma cells in lymph nodes, bone marrow, and spleen.

The brain showed a poorly outlined area of demyelination in the central white matter of the right occipital lobe that merged with subacute necrosis of the surrounding cortex, and an operative hematoma in the right parietal region (Fig. 131a).

On microscopic examination, large mononuclear cells with hyperchromatic nuclei and occasional mitoses (Fig. 131b), intermingled with lymphocytes, were found infiltrating the leptomeninges and perivascular spaces of the gray and white matter (Fig. 131c). In the diffusely demyelinated white matter, confluent infiltrates by the same mononuclear cells were intimately associated with, and largely replaced by, gitter cells and astrocytes while microglia predominated in the involved cortex.

### References

Adams, J. H., and J. M. Jackson. Intracranial Tumors of Reticular Tissue. J. Path. Bact. 91: 369, 1966.

Dutcher, T. F., and J. L. Fahey. The Histopathology of the Macroglobulinemia of Waldenström. J. Nat. Cancer Inst. 22: 887, 1959.

Gunderson, C. H., J. Henry, and N. Malamud. Plasma Globulin Determinations in Patients with Microglioma. J. Neurosurg. 35: 406, 1971.

Schneck, S. A., and I. Penn. Cerebral Neoplasms Associated with Renal Transplantation. Arch. Neurol. 13: 77, 1965.

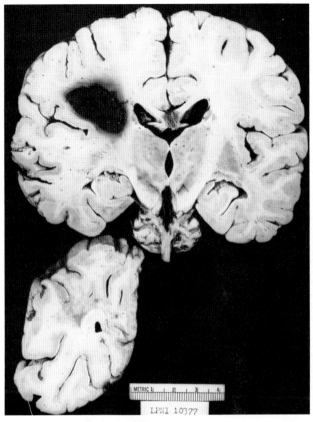

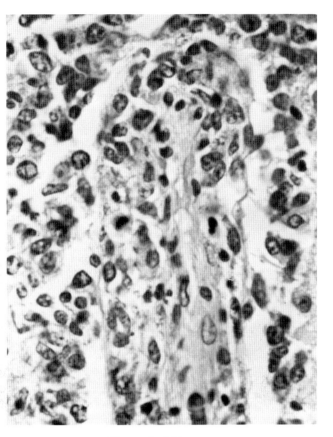

Fig. 131a. Reticulum cell sarcoma with Waldenström's syndrome (sides reversed)

Fig. 131b. HE × 375

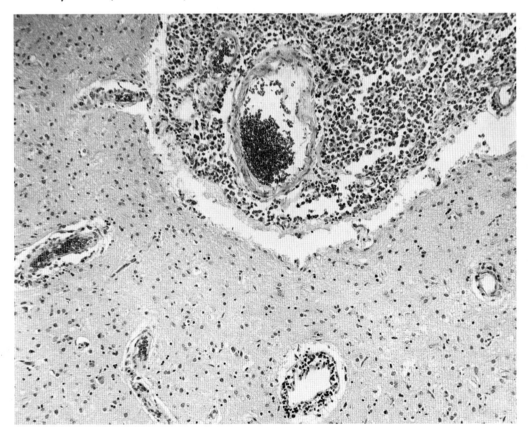

Fig. 131c. HE × 120

Tumors arising from the sheaths of nerve roots have been variously designated as schwannoma or perineurial fibroblastoma, depending upon whether they are believed to orginate from the sheath of Schwann or from the endoperineurium, the former view receiving wider acceptance. Neurofibroma on the other hand is believed to represent a diffuse proliferation of similar cells in peripheral nerves and occurs most often in von Recklinghausen's disease. Although the two types differ in their biologic growth, their close cytologic kinship often makes their separation difficult.

## Schwannoma

Schwannomas are solitary intracranial or intraspinal tumors that are more common in middle age and are slow growing. Intracranially, their incidence is about 8% of intracranial tumors, their most common location being in the sheath of the acoustic nerve where they induce a characteristic cerebellopontine angle clinical syndrome. Intraspinal Schwannomas are as common as intraspinal meningiomas, where they tend to develop from the sheaths of predominantly dorsal nerve roots, either as extra- and/or intradural growths (Fig. 132a).

Pathologically, the tumors are encapsulated, spherical growths, varying from a few millimeters to several centimeters. They are attached to the nerve root which is only included in the capsule, arising distally to the leptomeningeal attachment and expanding centripetally. They may be firm and of homogeneous appearance but more frequently tend to cystic changes, deposition of fat and hemorrhage. The microscopic picture shows a structure of either a solid fibrillary form characterized by interlacing bundles of elongated spindle cells, interrupted by palisading of nuclei and Verocay bodies, rich in reticulin fibers (type A of Antoni) and/or a loose textured form given to microcysts and fatty metamorphosis (type B of Antoni).

> *Case:* A 33-year-old woman complained of vertigo and right-sided headaches for an indeterminate period of time that led to partial removal of a right-sided acoustic tumor. On re-examination six months later she still complained of headaches and was markedly ataxic; there were bilateral papilledema, nystagmus to all directions of gaze, bilateral deafness that was more marked on the right side, and bilateral pyramidal tract signs. The cerebrospinal fluid pressure was 300 mm of $H_2O$. Following a shunt from the lumbar subarachnoid space to the left Fallopian tube, she ran a high fever and expired.

The brain contained a large encapsulated tumor with variegated appearance of firm, fatty, and hemorrhagic areas, attached to the right side of the pons throughout its extent which it compressed but did not infiltrate; there was narrowing and displacement of the fourth ventricle, resulting in hydrocephalus; the shunting tube was in place in the right lateral ventricle (Fig. 132b).

Microscopically, (Fig. 132c) areas showing palisading of nuclei (A) were associated with small spindle-shaped cells disposed in fascicles (B). Other areas contained a loose tissue with alternating fibers and foam cells (Fig. 132d) in which large amounts of sudanophilic fat were deposited while the fibers stained for reticulin (Fig. 132e).

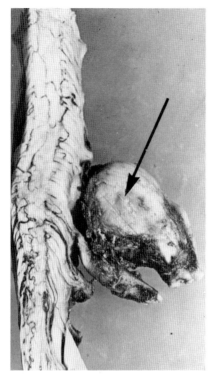

Fig. 132a. Schwannoma of spinal cord

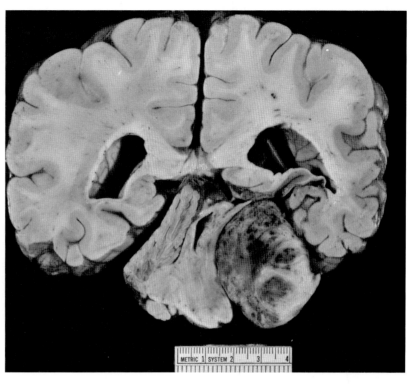

Fig. 132b. Acoustic schwannoma, right side

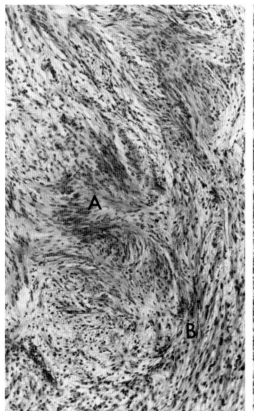

Fig. 132c. HE × 100

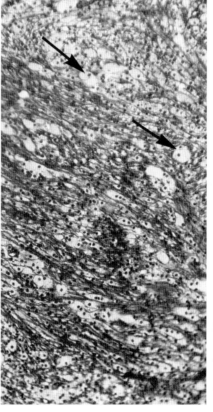

Fig. 132d. Heidenhain's aniline blue × 200

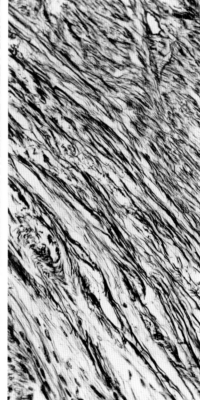

Fig. 132e. Laidlaw × 200

## Peripheral Nerve Sheath Tumor in Electron Microscopy

The cells comprising these tumors are usually arranged in palisade fashion with abundant extracellular space. The cells are elongated and essentially spindle-shaped. The widest part contains the nucleus and usual perinuclear organelles. The cytoplasmic processes extend into a wide extracellular space but often approach other processes quite closely. Basement membrane (BM) surrounds many of the processes (Fig. 133) but when several processes approach one another very closely, they form a small bundle with no basement membrane between adjacent processes. Instead, the entire bundle is surrounded by a basement membrane. Collagen is present in varying amounts in the wider extracellular spaces (E). In addition, spindle-shaped structures, Luse bodies, which display a periodicity of 1,000–1,200 Å, are occasionally present in the extracellular space. Luse bodies, while not confined to peripheral nerve sheath tumors, are, nevertheless, a characteristic feature of this tumor. The blood vessels of these tumors are often lined by fenestrated endothelium.

The cellular origin of the tumors is unknown. Some authors, on the basis of cell shape and the presence of large amounts of collagen, regard these tumors as fibroblastic in nature; others emphasize the presence of basement membrane and the location of the tumor and consider the tumor of Schwann cell origin. On the other hand, one should not totally disregard the perineurial cells which normally display both basement membrane and abundant collagen in the nearby extracellular spaces. Furthermore, it is interesting that perineurial cell processes often form small, basement membrane-covered bundles with no basement membrane between adjacent processes.

*References*

Cravioto, H. The Ultrastructure of Acoustic Nerve Tumors. Acta. Neuropath. 12: 116, 1969.
Hirano, A., H. M. Dembitzer, and H. M. Zimmerman. Fenestrated Blood Vessels in Neurilemmoma. Lab. Invest. 27: 305, 1972.

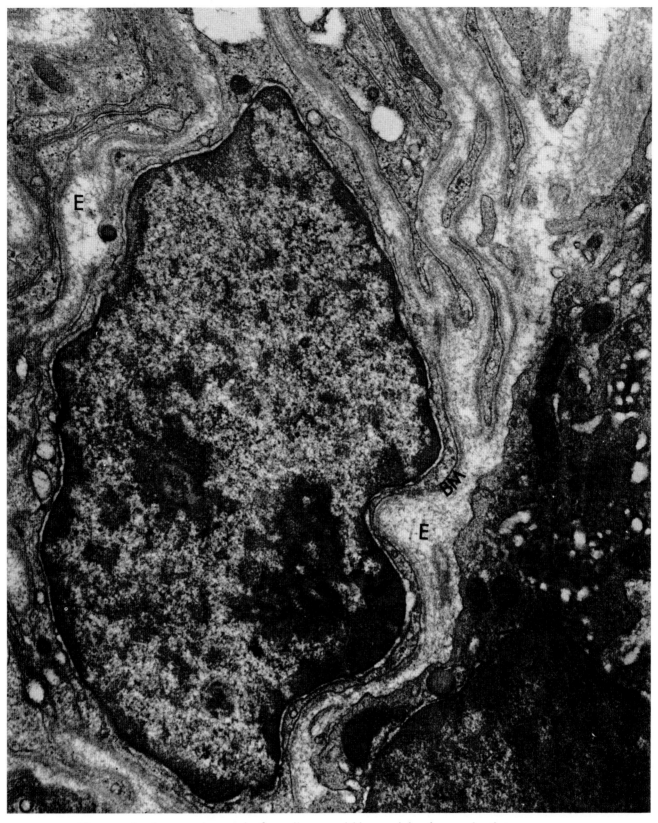

Fig. 133. An electron micrograph of a perikaryon within a peripheral nerve sheath tumor × 30,000

## Von Recklinghausen's Neurofibromatosis

Von Recklinghausen's disease, like tuberous sclerosis, is based upon a dominant heredo-familial tendency to hyperplasia and neoplasia of neuroectodermal and mesodermal tissues. Neurofibromatosis refers to its predominant manifestation, however, there are diverse other features, such as various cutaneous lesions including cafe-au-lait spots, bony changes, multiple meningiomas, gliomas, such as astrocytomas of optic nerves, intramedullary astrocytomas and ependymomas of the spinal cord, and disseminated hamartomatous hyperplasia of Schwann, meningeal and glial cells.

The multiple tumors of nerve fibers involve various cranial and spinal nerve roots, especially acoustic tumors that are frequently bilateral, and of peripheral nerves and ganglia including those of the sympathetic system. Histologically, the characteristic features of neurofibroma, namely, diffuse proliferation of collagen and reticulin fibers embedded in a matrix of mucopolysaccharides with inclusions of axis cylinders, are often combined with manifestations characteristic of solitary Schwannomas.

Clinically, the disorder follows a chronic course. However, it is prone to undergo malignant changes, giving rise to neurofibrosarcomas that are apt to metastasize.

*Case:* A 23-year-old man with negative family history was well until the age of seven when he had the gradual onset of right facial weakness and numbness. At age nine numerous subcutaneous firm nodules were discovered and a mass diagnosed neurofibroma was excised from the right upper forearm. At age seventeen, he developed tinnitus and deafness on the right side, staggering gait, slurred speech, dysphagia, and thickness of the tongue. Six months before his death, examination revealed bilateral nystagmus on lateral gaze, depressed corneal reflexes and decreased sensibility on the right, a complete right peripheral facial palsy with diminished taste, decreased hearing on the right, absent gag reflex with movement of the uvula up and to the left, deviation of the tongue to the right on protrusion, a wide-based gait with tendency to fall to the right, and left-sided papilledema. Angiography and pneumo-encephalography disclosed evidence of a mass in the brain stem in the region of the foramen magnum. Craniotomy revealed an intramedullary glioma in the upper cervical cord, and patient received radiotherapy. However, he showed progressive deterioration with increasing ataxia and bilateral deafness and expired despite chemotherapy with BCNU, vincristine, and CCNU.

The brain showed multiple large encapsulated tumors involving the roots of both eighth nerves, the right fifth and the left ninth and tenth nerves, that compressed the brain stem and the fourth ventricle (Fig. 134a). Countless small nodules involved the nerve roots of the spinal cord and extended down along the nerve fibers of the cauda equina (Fig. 134b).

Microscopically, the disseminated growths along the course of the nerve fibers (Fig. 134c), showed proliferation of Schwann and perineurial cells with scattered axis cylinders (Fig. 134d) and abundant collagen and reticulin fibers.

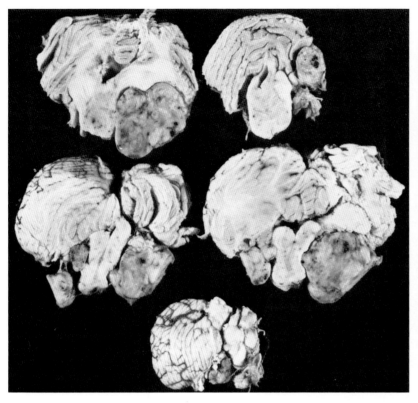

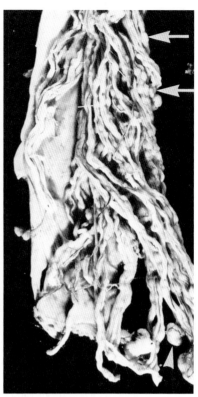

Fig. 134a. Bilateral tumors of cranial nerves in von Recklinghausen's disease

Fig. 134b. Neurofibromatosis of cauda equina, in von Recklinghausen's disease

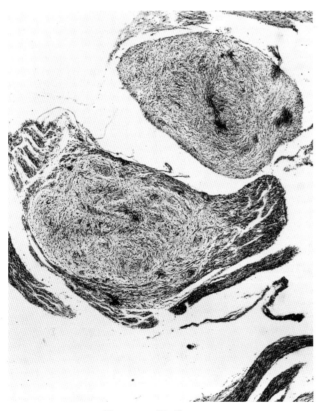

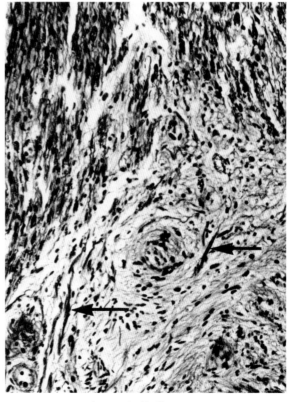

Fig. 134c. Bodian × 34

Fig. 134d. Bodian × 150

Tumors arising from blood vessels are classified into hemangiomas, which are essentially malformations or hamartomas, and hemangioblastomas, which are true neoplasms.

## Hemangiomas

Hemangiomas represent persistent embryonic vascular channels with anomalous structure of their walls causing changes in the surrounding tissues through alteration in hemodynamics incidental to shunts in the circulation. They may be classified into capillary telangiectasias and arteriovenous malformations.

The capillary *telangiectasias* are frequently asymptomatic but may become clinically evident through repeated hemorrhages or large size. They are commonly located in the pons and cerebral and cerebellar white matter. Grossly, they are unencapsulated reddish to brownish, at times calcified lesions. Microscopically, they consist of dilated vascular channels lined by a thin layer of connective tissue associated with gliosis and hemosiderin-containing macrophages in the intervascular tissue (Fig. 135a and b).

### Arterio-venous Malformations

A-V malformations are also known as serpentine or cirsoid angiomas. The arteries and veins composing them are abnormally developed in calibre and length resulting in tortuous vascular masses. They are most common on the lateral aspect of the cerebral hemispheres where they tend to be wedge-shaped with the base in the leptomeninges and apex directed towards the ventricles. The afferent arteries in such location are the middle cerebral branches and the efferent veins are drained either through the enlarged cortical veins to the superior sagittal sinus or via the internal cerebral veins to the vein of Galen. Other cerebral vascular territories may be involved. Less common sites are the midbrain, cerebellum, and spinal cord. Microscopically, the enlarged blood vessels show intimal sclerosis, mural fibrosis, defects in elastica and media, nodular thickening, calcification, and thrombosis. The adjacent meninges and nervous tissue show pigmentation from recurrent hemorrhage and degeneration due to compression and impaired circulation.

> Case: A 36-year-old man was admitted to a hospital with a history that in the past one and one-half years he experienced recurring episodes of unconsciousness and generalized seizures. On admission, examination revealed evidence of deterioration in attention, recent memory, and abstract reasoning. In the hospital he had a number of ictal episodes, characterized by outbursts of violence. An angiogram demonstrated a large A-V malformation involving an extensive area in both frontal lobes, that was considered inoperable. He was treated with dilantin. About a month after admission he died following a seizure associated with coma.

Coronal sections through the frontal lobes at a level behind the genu of the corpus callosum revealed large numbers of dilated vascular channels involving branches of the anterior cerebral arteries and tributaries of the septal and subependymal veins, with chronic hemorrhagic necrosis of the adjacent nervous tissue and terminal intraventricular massive hemorrhage (Fig. 135c).

Microscopically, there were greatly dilated arteries and veins with either thin or irregularly thickened walls, at times associated with chronic organized thrombi and with gliosis, cystic degeneration, and calcification of the intervascular cerebral tissue (Fig. 135d).

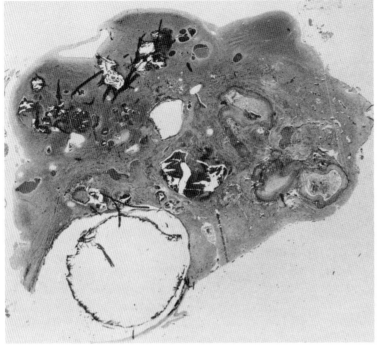

Fig. 135a. Hemangioma of pons

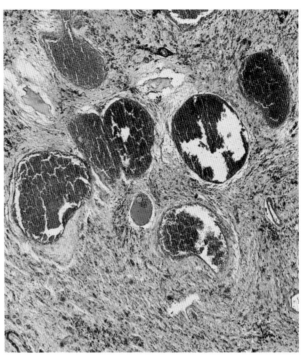

Fig. 135b. HVG × 32

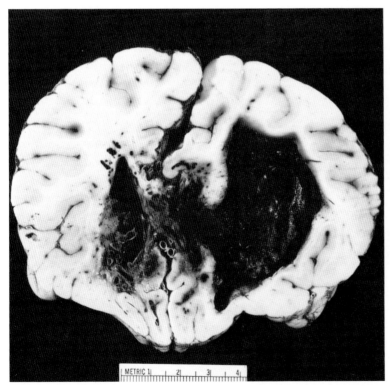

Fig. 135c. Arteriovenous malformation

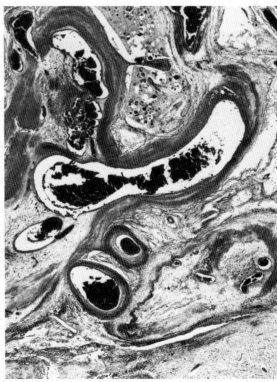

Fig. 135d. HVG × 15

This is a condition of angiomatosis that involves the skin of the face and the leptomeninges and is thus included among the neurocutaneous syndromes, although, unlike other forms, there is no definite evidence of hereditary transmissions. A port-wine nevus, confined to the distribution of the various branches of the trigeminal nerve is present on one side of the face, that may be associated with affection of the eye in the form of buphthalmos or congenital glaucoma. It is usually but not always associated with angiomatosis of the leptomeninges in the parieto-occipito-temporal regions on the same side as the nevus; the meningeal changes may however be bilateral.

Pathologically, the meninges, both grossly and microscopically, contain an excessive number of malformed and thin-walled veins. These may extend into the underlying cortex and/or involve the deep veins. A characteristic cortical calcification ensues as a result of stasis that causes scalloped opacities that are visible in x-rays of the skull. The condition ultimately leads to some degree of cortical atrophy and gliosis with a corresponding syndrome of hemiplegia, mental retardation, and seizures.

> *Case:* A 17-year-old boy with negative family history was born with a port-wine nevus in the right temporal region. His early development appeared normal, however, from the age of four years he began to regress mentally, had uncontrolled seizures and developed at first a left hemiplegia followed by spastic quadriplegia. An EEG disclosed slow waves and spikes in the right temporoparietal region, followed later by similar changes on the left side. A pneumoencephalogram disclosed localized calcification on the right; an angiogram was negative. The patient died in status epilepticus.

The brain showed excessive vascularity and congestion of the meninges, primarily in the right temporo-parieto-occipital region (Fig. 136a) that also involved a limited area in the left temporal region.

Microscopic examination disclosed an increased number of thin-walled vascular channels in the leptomeninges and large amounts of calcium deposits in the superficial layers of the cortex, outlining the configuration of the gyri (Fig. 136b).

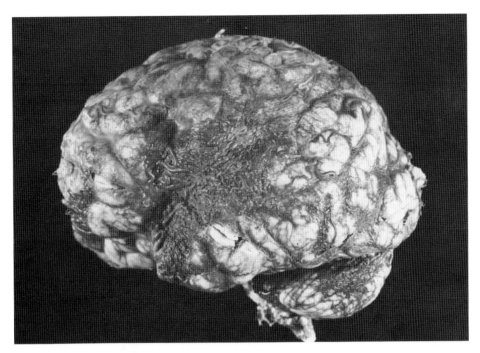

Fig. 136a. Sturge-Weber-Dimitri's
disease (sides reversed)

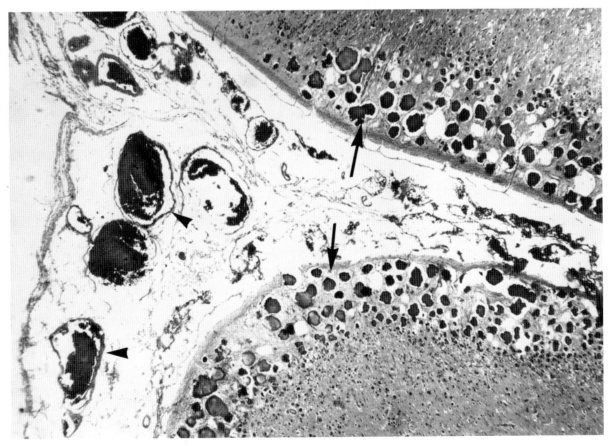

Fig. 136b. HE × 28

## Hemangioblastoma of Cerebellum

Hemangioblastomas involve the cerebellum, as a solitary tumor, with relatively high frequency amongst the posterior fossa tumors of adults. Any part of the cerebellum may be affected, especially the paramedian region. A rare site is the area postrema. A common clinical sign is polycythemia, presumably due to erythropoietic activity by the tumor.

The gross pathologic feature is that of a cyst with a relatively small mural nodule, while its content may vary from clear yellow fluid to frank hemorrhage.

Microscopically, the tumor nodule is composed of dilated capillaries lined by endothelial cells, and of stromal cells that frequently possess a foamy cytoplasm laden with granules of sudanophilic lipid. The entire lesion is pervaded by reticulin fibers outlining the basement membranes of the blood vessels. The adjacent pia is occupied by tumor but the wall of the cyst is devoid of tumor tissue.

*Case:* A 57-year-old man was admitted to a hospital with the chief complaints of progressive weakness of his legs, infrequent headaches, and double vision. On examinaton he was lethargic; unable to converge his eyes; had weakness of upward and right lateral gaze with nystagmus on left lateral gaze. There was marked hypotonia and weakness of all extremities, especially the lower, and trunkal ataxia. Deep tendon reflexes were absent to hypoactive. Patient had a sudden cardiorespiratory arrest and expired before any studies could be done.

Grossly, a large cyst of about 3 cm. occupied the paramedian region of the left cerebellar hemisphere and contained a solid spherical hemorrhagic nodule of less than 1 cm. in its posterior part, while the cyst extended forward compressing the roof of the fourth ventricle (Fig. 137a).

Microscopically, dilated vascular channels, lined by endothelial cells, were associated with closely packed cells containing pleomorphic nuclei and partly vacuolated cytoplasm (Fig. 137b) that were separated by a diffuse network of reticulin fibers.

### von Hippel-Lindau's Disease

In a small percentage of cases, hemangioblastoma of the cerebellum is associated with multiple hemangioblastomas in the central nervous system and in one or both retinae, along with lesions in viscera such as cysts in the pancreas, hypernephroid tumors of kidneys, etc. Known as von Hippel-Lindau's disease, it has a kinship with the phacomatoses and like them has a heredofamilial basis.

*Case:* A 53-year-old man, with a family history of cerebellar hemangioblastoma, diagnosed in 50% of his siblings, was admitted to the hospital because of right-sided occipital headaches of five months' duration. Examination revealed obtundation, ataxia with tendency to fall to the right, and borderline papilledema. The cerebrospinal fluid had an opening pressure of 160 mm of $H_2O$ and 69 mg % of total protein. A PEG showed filling only of the basal cisterns. An IVP revealed the presence of a right kidney tumor. A posterior fossa exploration disclosed a left cerebellar cystic tumor which was subtotally removed. He expired postoperatively of a perforated acute duodenal ulcer.

The general autopsy findings consisted of cysts in the pancreas, hemangiomas of spleen, and bilateral adenocarcinoma of kidneys.

The brain showed a partly cystic and partly solid yellowish tumor involving the superior portion of the left cerebellar hemisphere near the midline, obscured by operative trauma (Fig. 137c). Histologically, it was a hemangioblastoma, with vacuolated stromal cells (Fig. 137d) and diffuse reticulin fibers (Fig. 137e).

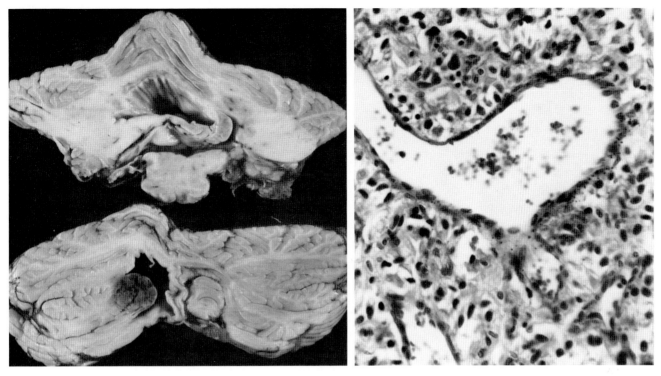

Fig. 137a. Hemangioblastoma of left cerebellar hemisphere

Fig. 137b. HVG × 250

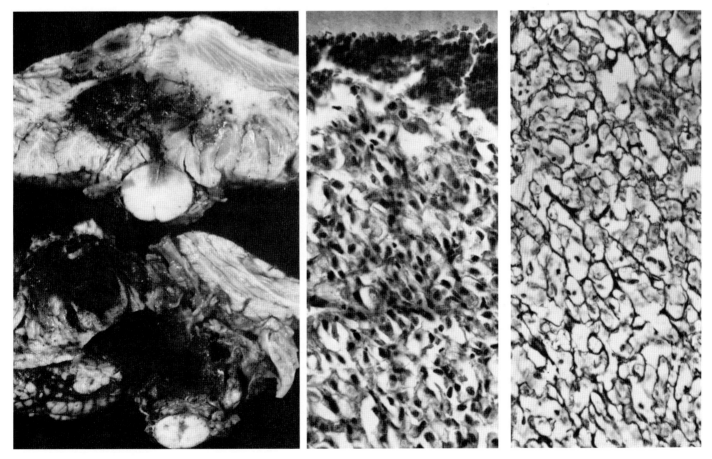

Fig. 137c. Hemangioblastoma of cerebellum in von
Hippel-Lindau's disease

Fig. 137d. HVG × 250

Fig. 137e. Laidlaw × 250

Tumors arising from the anterior lobe of the pituitary gland are classified in accordance with their origin from either chromophobe, eosinophil (alpha) or basophil (beta) cells of the gland. Of these, only the chromophobe and eosinophilic adenomas are of clinical significance.

## Chromophobe Adenoma

Chromophobe adenomas are three times as common as the eosinophilic form, have their maximum growth on the periphery of the gland and thus often tend to extend beyond their initial position in the enlarged sella into adjacent structures. They predominate at middle age. Their earliest clinical manifestations, in addition to signs of hypopituitarism, are due to compression of the optic chiasm, producing the classic bitemporal hemianopsia; on occasion they may break through the diaphragm of the sella early, compressing one or other optic tract, to produce hemianopsias. Compression of the third ventricle, base of frontal or temporal lobes result in a variety of additional symptoms including personality changes. Pathologically, the tumors are usually characterized by an encapsulated globular homogeneous mass. Microscopically, the pattern is either sinusoidal or diffuse.

*Case:* A 42-year-old man had a history of progressive visual loss in the left eye for approximately one year. Three weeks prior to admission he noted restriction of vision in both temporal fields, left greater than right, as well as bifrontal headaches, increasing fatiguability and irritability, and decreasing libido. Examination revealed a bitemporal hemianopsia; visual acuity was 20/30 in the right eye and 20/100 in the left eye; pupils were small and reacted well to light, and there was no papilledema. Skull x-rays showed an enlarged sella. Bilateral carotid arteriograms revealed that the intracranial portion of both internal carotid and anterior cerebral arteries were displaced upwards, suggestive of a neoplasm in the region of the pituitary gland. Endocrine examination revealed mild signs of hypothyroidism and hypogonadism. Patient underwent a left frontal craniotomy, revealing a prefixed optic chiasm. A very brisk hemorrhage ensued after puncture of the mass of the tumor. The bleeding was finally controlled, however, precluding any further attempt to remove the tumor. Postoperatively, patient remained in a semi-comatose state, developed hypotension, Cheyne-Stokes respiration, and diabetes insipidus. His left pupil was dilated and he became completely unresponsive and expired.

The brain contained a large encapsulated extrinsic midline tumor that compressed the optic chiasm. It was partly replaced by operative hemorrhage; there was compression of the left middle cerebral artery, causing acute infarction of the cortex and basal ganglia in the vascular territory (Fig. 138a).

Microscopic examination showed the tumor to consist of a diffuse sheet of uniform round cells with hyperchromatic nuclei, without mitoses, and sparse cytoplasm, lacking eosinophilic or basophilic staining granules (A) surrounded by a capsule of connective tissue (B) around which there were remains of the normal gland (C) (Fig. 138b).

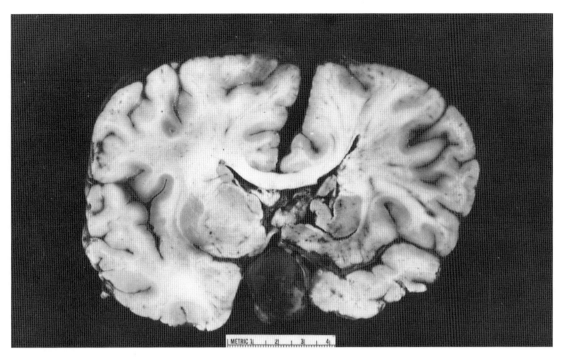

Fig. 138a. Chromophobe adenoma (with P. O.
hemorrhage)

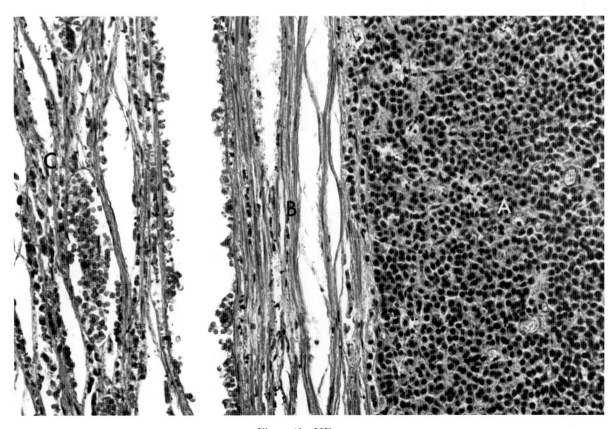

Fig. 138b. HE × 225

## Chromophobe Adenoma in Electron Microscopy

As in most neoplasms, two elements comprise the tumor mass of chromophobe adenomas. The first are the parenchymal epithelial cells (Fig. 139). These are cuboidal in shape and are characterized by the presence of scattered membrane-bound dense-core secretory granules approximately 1,000–1,500 Å in diameter (arrows). In addition, lipofuscin deposits and/or multilamellated dense bodies may sometimes be seen. At the surface of blood vessels, which comprise the second element of the tumor mass, the epithelial cells are covered by a common basement membrane which abuts on a relatively wide collagen-containing extra-cellular space. The endothelium of the blood vessels is, itself, covered by a basement membrane, and, unlike the cerebral vasculature, is fenestrated in many areas.

*References*

Hirano, A., U. Tomiyasu, and H. M. Zimmerman. The Fine Structure of Blood Vessels in Chromophobe Adenoma. Acta Neuropathol. 22: 200, 1972.

Zanbrano, D., L. Amezua, G. Dickmann, and E. Franke. Ultrastructure of Human Pituitary Adenomas. Acta Neurochir. 18: 78, 1968.

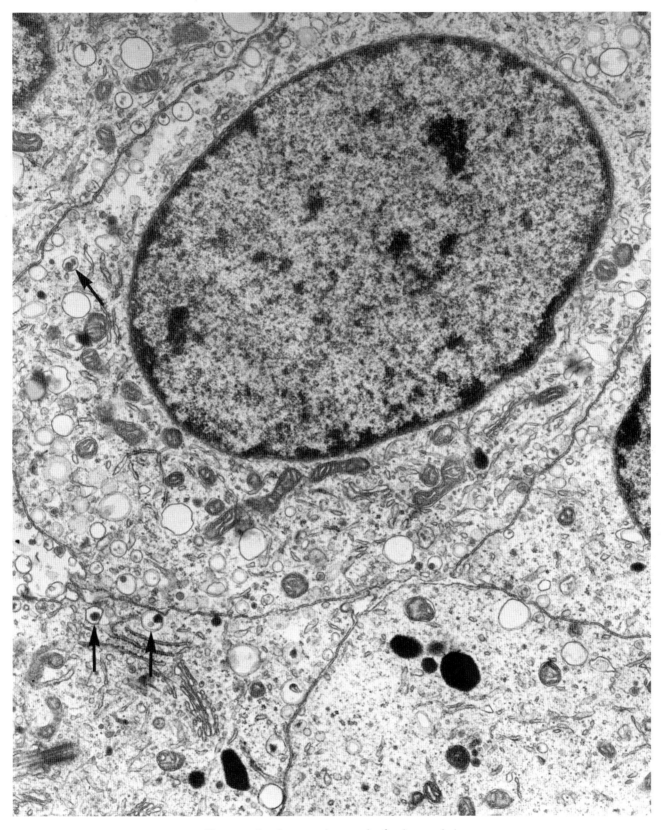

Fig. 139. An electron micrograph of a chromophobe
adenoma × 19,000

## Eosinophilic Adenoma

Eosinophilic adenomas are generally smaller tumors and are more centrally located in the pituitary gland than the chromophobe type. They give rise to a characteristic clinical picture of eosinophilic hyperpituitarism—namely, acromegaly or giantism. Such a syndrome may also result from diffuse hyperplasia of the specific cells without adenoma formation.

*Case:* A 40-year-old man developed, in the course of four years, symptoms of acromegaly, enlargement of the testes, and gynecomastia. The circulating growth hormone was estimated to be four times the normal value. In spite of x-ray therapy he followed a downhill course.

The pituitary gland was enlarged, and showed a diffuse hyperplasia of round cells with eccentric nuclei and eosinophilic granules separated by a scant stroma (Fig. 140a).

## Eosinophilic Adenoma in Electron Microscopy

In all essential features, the fine structure of eosinophilic adenomas is closely similar to that of chromophobe adenoma. They differ substantially, however, in that various organelles are much more prominent in parenchymal cells of the eosinophilic adenoma. The secretory granules are more numerous and much larger (Fig. 140b). They usually measure between 3,000 and 5,000 Å. Furthermore, as might be expected, the Golgi apparatus and the rough endoplasmic reticulum are highly developed.

*Reference*

Schelin, U. Chromophobe and Acidophil Adenomas of the Human Pituitary Gland. A Light and Electron Microscopic Study. Acta Path. Microbiol. Scand. (Suppl.) 158: 1, 1962.

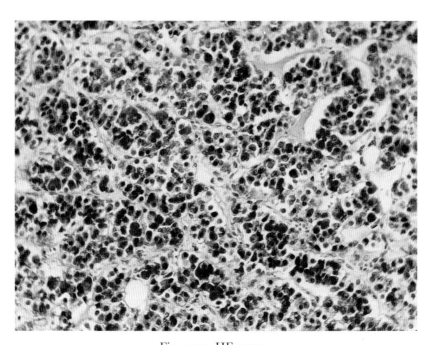

Fig. 140a. HE × 200

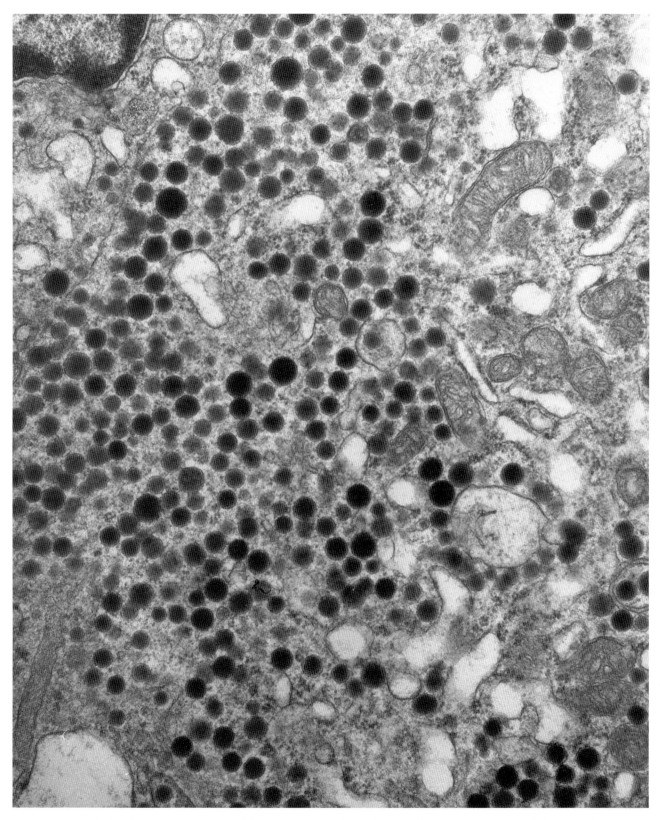

Fig. 140b. An electron micrograph of the secretory granule in the cytoplasm of a tumor cell within an eosinophilic adenoma × 40,000

The central nervous system is one of the most common sites for the development of congenital tumors based on embryonic cell rests, although they are relatively rare among the intracranial tumors. They include craniopharyngiomas; epidermoids, dermoids, and teratomas; paraphysial cysts; lipomas and chordomas. With few exceptions, they are slowly growing, some predominating in childhood but many occurring in later years of life. They are usually situated in median or paramedian locations.

## Craniopharyngiomas

Of the congenital tumors, craniopharyngiomas or Rathke-pouch cysts are the most common, with an incidence of 3% of all intracranial tumors. They arise from the region of the hypophysial stalk, presumably on the basis of epithelial cell rests. However, their exact pathogenesis is not clear, as they may represent either a form of epidermoid cyst or metaplasia of the cells of the pars tuberalis of the hypophysis. Their common location is suprasellar. About one half occur in childhood and the remaining have a predilection for adults of middle age. Their symptomatology is dominated by signs of pituitary and hypothalamic dysfunction, depending on the age of occurrence, and by signs of compression of the optic chiasm, as well as of increased intracranial pressure. They are usually cystic (Fig. 141a), although some may be solid, the cysts containing a fluid rich in cholesterin crystals and varying amounts of calcium; although circumscribed, they tend to invade the third ventricle to the walls of which they become adherent.

Microscopically (Fig. 141b), the usual pattern is that of a single layer of columnar epithelium surrounding a loose collection of stellate cells within which cystic degeneration tends to occur associated with cholesterin and calcium deposits.

*Case:* A 25-year-old man was well until the age of 14 years when he had the onset of headaches, nausea, and vomiting and impairment of visual acuity. Examination at that time led to a diagnosis of a calcified suprasellar mass and a subtotal resection of a craniopharyngioma was accomplished. One year later he had a recurrence of his tumor and at this time he was found to be retarded, 17-ketosteroid output in the urine was below normal, and there was underdevelopment of his secondary sex characteristics. Skull films showed perisellar calcification on the right for which he was reoperated. He was maintained on cortisone and thyroid extract. Later examinations revealed bilateral optic atrophy and bitemporal upper quadrant defect. He began having spells with a blacking-out sensation. Hypoglycemia developed with a sugar level of 60 mg %. On his last admission, skull x-rays showed a greatly enlarged sella, erosion of the anterior portion of the dorsum sellae and suprasellar calcification. Pneumoencephalogram revealed the tumor to extend anteriorly, indenting the floor of the anterior horns, and posteriorly around the pons, causing marked backward displacement of the aqueduct and fourth ventricle. He underwent a right frontotemporal craniotomy with subtotal removal of tumor but developed severe diabetes insipidus, and expired of cardiac arrest.

The brain showed an extensive encapsulated cystic lesion in both interpeduncular and prepontine locations, the cysts containing a yellowish mass of congealed fluid, interspersed with flakes of calcium and cholesterin crystals (Fig. 141c).

Microscopically, only remnants of cuboidal squamous epithelial cells were found (A), surrounding cysts filled with eosinophilic hyaline and basophilic calcified material (B), scattered foreign-body giant cells and large amounts of cholesterin crystals (C) (Fig. 141d).

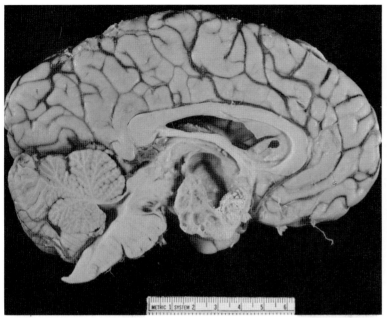

Fig. 141a. Craniopharyngioma

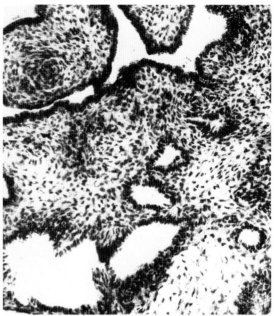

Fig. 141b. HE × 100

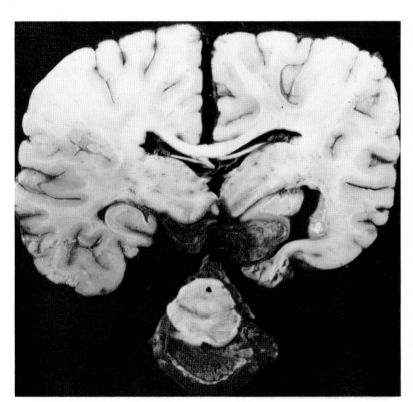

Fig. 141c. Craniopharyngioma spreading into a prepontine location

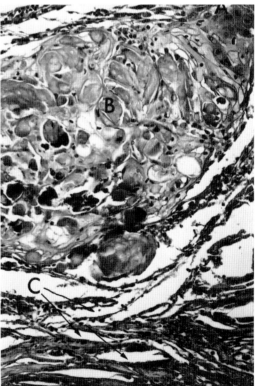

Fig. 141d. HE × 100

## Craniopharyngiomas in Electron Microscopy

As revealed by the electron microscope, craniopharyngiomas consist of nests of cells often arranged around a central keratin-containing space (K). The parenchymal cells of the tumor are essentially the same as the epidermis but differ in some details of shape and arrangement (Fig. 142). The cells abutting the keratin-containing region are sometimes closely fitting squamous cells but more often they tend to have small, irregular separations at the borders of which the cells are connected by well developed and abundant desmosomes (arrows). Within these cells, prominent tonofibrils may be seen. The irregular spaces between these cells are the small reticulated cysts (C) visible in the light microscope. As one moves radially from the kertain-containing area towards the basal region of the cell nest, the cells become more compactly arranged until, at the basal layer, the cells are cuboidal and quite closely packed. These cells are covered by a basement membrane which separates the epithelial mass from a large connective tissue space which constitutes the large cysts seen in the light microscope. These spaces frequently contain a network of reactive glial processes.

*Reference*

Ghatak, N. R., A. Hirano, and H. M. Zimmerman. Ultrastructure of a Craniopharyngioma. Cancer. 27: 1465, 1971.

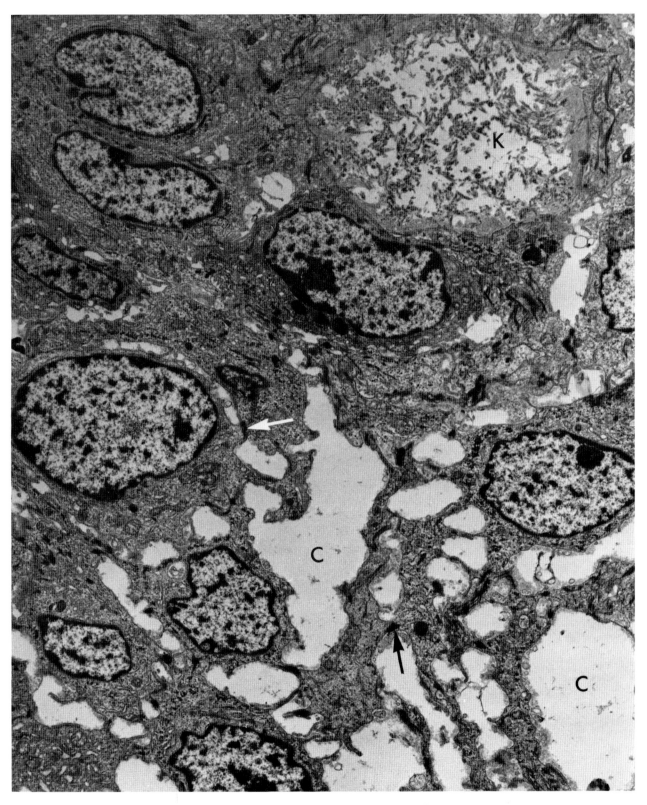

Fig. 142. An electron micrograph of a craniopharyngioma × 8,000

## Epidermoid and Dermoid Cysts

Epidermoid cysts are rare intracranial and intraspinal lesions that arise from epidermal rests in diploe of skull, meninges, brain, and spinal column and occur in adults of all ages. Their most common intracranial location is in the cerebellopontine angle, sella turcica and temporal lobes, while the intraspinal forms occur most frequently in the region of the conus.

They consist of encapsulated masses with grumous flaky content that has a characteristic pearly sheen. Microscopically, the thin cyst wall is composed of an outer layer of connective tissue adjacent to the compressed nervous tissue and an inner layer of squamous epithelium with granules of keratohyalin, while the contents are made up of layers of desquamated cornified epithelial cells.

The dermoid cysts differ from the epidermoids in that they contain elements of the entire skin.

*Case:* A 17-year-old boy developed symptoms at the age of five years that led to a diagnosis of a tumor in the pineal region. He was treated with a ventriculocisternal shunt and radiation and was well until six months prior to demise. At this time he developed signs of increased intracranial pressure and was admitted to the hospital. Examination revealed right exotropia and reduced visual acuity, nystagmus that was most marked on upward gaze, sluggish reaction of pupils, action tremor and cogwheel rigidity on the left side. Ventriculography disclosed a tumor mass in the third ventricle. He was treated with a ventriculovenous shunt but expired postoperatively.

The brain contained an extensive encapsulated mass, consisting of shiny and flaky tissue, in the parapineal region (Fig. 143a) that extended from the aqueduct to the third ventricle.

Microscopically, there were variations in thickness and structure of the wall composed of squamous epithelium (A) undergoing cornification and desquamation and of dermal structures such as sweat glands (B) with secondary inflammation and foreign-body giant cells (C) (Fig. 143b).

## Teratomas

Teratomas are tumors composed of derivatives of two or three germinal layers. They are exceedingly rare in the central nervous system, are more apt to occur in young children and follow a malignant clinical course.

*Case:* A four-year-old girl developed, over a period of eight months, the following symptoms in sequence: left ophthalmoplegia, a bruit over the left eye, headaches, personality changes, signs of diabetes insipidus, anorexia, cachexia, bilateral pyramidal signs, exophthalmos, and optic atrophy of the left side. Angiography outlined a tumor containing anomalous vessels at the base of the brain, which was confirmed at operation.

Autopsy disclosed erosion of the base of the skull by two large encapsulated vascular tumor masses lying at the base of the brain. These greatly compressed and displaced the temporal lobes, the basal ganglia, and optic tracts, filled the third ventricle and compressed the lateral ventricles (Fig. 143c). The tumor also invaded the pituitary gland and the third, fifth, and sixth cranial nerve roots on the left side.

Microscopically, squamous epithelium (A), undifferentiated mesenchyme (B), and glandular epithelium arranged in acini (C) represented structures derived from the three germinal layers (Fig. 143d). There were many mitoses in the cells, suggesting a malignant change.

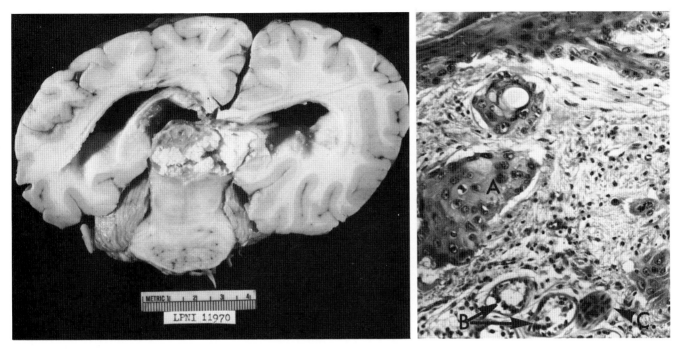

Fig. 143a. Dermoid cyst, parapineal region

Fig. 143b. HE × 135

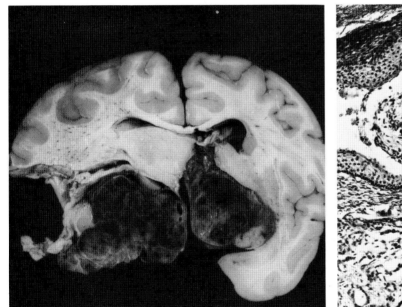

Fig. 143c. Teratoma at base of brain

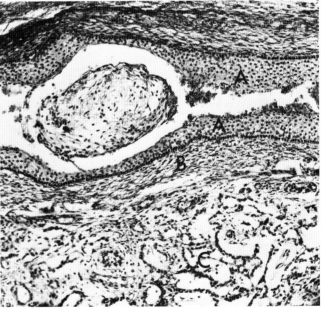

Fig. 143d. HE × 85

## Colloid Cysts of Third Ventricle

A small group of tumors, known as colloid or paraphysial cysts, develop in the region of the junction between the third ventricle and foramen of Monro, conducive to intermittent obstruction of the circulation of the cerebrospinal fluid. As a result, intermittent symptoms of hydrocephalus, relieved by changing the position of the head, aid in diagnosis that can be confirmed by pneumoencephalography. The pathogenesis is controversial as between its origin from an embryonic structure known as the paraphysis, from ependyma, or choroid plexus.

The cysts vary greatly in size. They consist of a thin capsule composed of single, epithelial, and connective tissue layers and a content of colloid material.

*Case:* A 27-year-old man was admitted to a hospital with a history of severe headaches of about one month's duration, followed by vomiting, convulsions, and semicoma. On admission, changes in posture either precipitated or relieved the symptoms of headaches and alterations in consciousness. A PEG disclosed evidence of a mass in the third ventricle that was confirmed by craniotomy. Because of adhesions it was not possible to remove it. He expired of complicating meningitis.

The brain showed an encapsulated mass containing a gelatinous yellowish semisolid material that protruded forwards from the third ventricle near the foramina of Monro and was adherent to the undersurface of the body of the fornix (Fig. 144a).

Microscopically, the cyst wall consisted of an inner layer of cuboidal epithelium (A) and an outer layer of connective tissue (B) surrounding amorphous colloid material (C) that showed a positive staining reaction with PAS, equally noted in small cysts within the capsule (Fig. 144b).

## Chordomas

Chordomas are rare tumors derived from primitive notochordal tissue, that arise intracranially from various sites at the base of the skull, especially the region of the clivus, and intraspinally most commonly in the sacrococcygeal area. They occur largely in the third to fifth decades of life.

In structure they resemble the tissue of the notochord, the cells either possessing a granular cytoplasm, some of which is glycogen and fat, or are vacuolated forms filled with a mucinous material, referred to as physaliferous cells.

*Case:* A 31-year-old man had a two months' history of increasing neck pain and muscle spasm. Just prior to admission to a hospital he became nauseated, vomited, and developed diplopia. Examination revealed palsies of cranial nerves VI, IX, X, and XII, on the right side. X-ray of the skull suggested pressure erosion of the right lateral margin of the foramen magnum. Angiography showed lateral and dorsal displacement of the basilar artery from right to left and a right vertebral angiogram disclosed a large avascular mass anterior and to the right of the basilar artery. A right suboccipital craniectomy was then performed, disclosing an encapsulated soft tumor, anterior and lateral to the medulla, diagnosed chordoma. Postoperatively, he expired of respiratory difficulty.

The base of the medulla and lower part of the pons were unequally compressed by a solid grayish-white mass that was partly obscured by operative hemorrhage (Fig. 144c).

Microscopic examination revealed large uniform round cells with eccentric nuclei and with variations from granular to vacuolated cytoplasm (A) surrounded by a capsule of connective tissue (B) that adhered to but did not infiltrate the brain stem (C) (Fig. 144d).

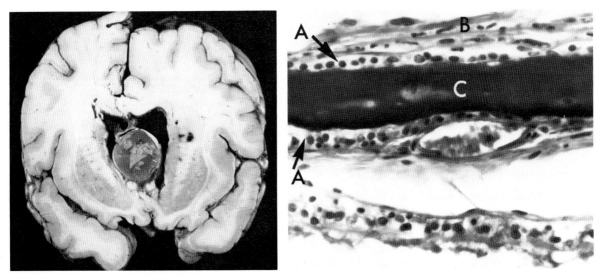

Fig. 144a. Colloid cyst of third ventricle

Fig. 144b. Periodic acid Schiff × 300

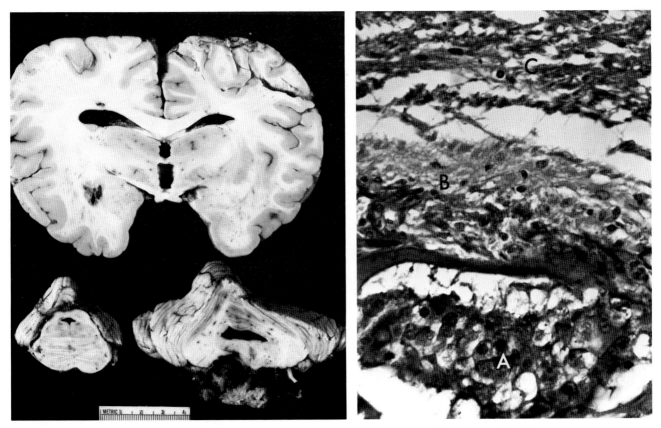

Fig. 144c. Chordoma, base of lower pons

Fig. 144d. LFB-PAS × 300

## Metastatic Tumors

Metastatic tumors in the central and peripheral nervous system are common but their precise incidence has varied in different statistics. Probably 5% of malignant systemic tumors metastasize to the brain. The largest number are carcinomas, less frequently sarcomas and melanomas. They usually originate from tumor emboli in arterial blood stream, gaining entrance into the nervous tissue by permeation of Virchow-Robin spaces, less commonly by direct penetration. The most common sources are lung and breast carcinomas, followed by renal and alimentary carcinoma, melanoma, and chorioepithelioma.

Pathologically, they are more often multiple than single in a ratio of approximately 70–30%. They are more apt to involve the cerebral and cerebellar gray matter, especially in borders with white matter, than the brain stem, spinal cord, or peripheral nerves. On occasion they disseminate widely in the cerebrospinal fluid channels by seeding. Variations in size are common, from miliary to large tumors. The characteristic gross features are discrete borders surrounded by edema, the latter often massive, even in the presence of small tumors.

The clinical manifestations are more often characterized by generalized than localized signs and by abrupt onset.

### METASTATIC CARCINOMA

*Bronchogenic* carcinoma is probably the single, most common site for cerebral metastases, often leading to misdiagnosis because of predominant cerebral symptoms in the presence of an occult primary lesion.

> *Case:* A 51-year-old man had a history of an abrupt onset of vertigo, intermittent headaches, and ringing in his ears one month before admission to a hospital. On admission he was mentally confused, showed papilledema and multiple retinal hemorrhages, ataxia of gait, and nystagmus on left lateral gaze. Brain scan revealed an abnormal increase in the posterior fossa. Chest tomograms demonstrated a mass lesion in the right hilar region, diagnosed by biopsy as a bronchogenic carcinoma. A ventriculogram revealed one tumor bulging into the left lateral ventricle and another into the fourth ventricle. He underwent a ventriculo-auricular shunt with a Pudenz valve. Postoperatively, his condition deteriorated and he died on the thirteenth postoperative day.

The brain contained multiple discrete partly hemorrhagic and necrotic tumor nodules of variable size, involving principally the gray matter of the cerebral cortex, caudate nucleus and cerebellum bilaterally, accompanied by diffuse edema, resulting in narrowing of the ventricles (Fig. 145a).

Microscopically, the tumor nodules were composed of closely packed small cells with round to oval hyperchromatic nuclei showing many mitotic figures, that compressed the adjacent nervous tissue, as in the cerebellum (Fig. 145b).

### METASTATIC MELANOMA

Malignant melanomas of the skin and other less common or unknown sources, are very prone to produce cerebral metastases.

The accompanying illustration is from a case in which generalized cerebral symptoms developed rapidly following excision of a malignant melanoma of the skin of the neck.

The brain showed diffuse dissemination of black to brownish pigmented tumor tissue throughout the leptomeninges (Fig. 145c) that extended into the underlying nervous tissue (Fig. 145d) from the pia-arachnoid (A) along the perivascular spaces (B).

294

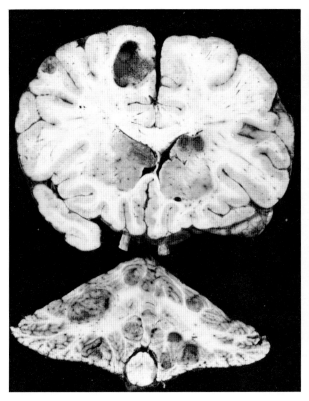

Fig. 145a. Multiple cerebral metastases of bronchogenic carcinoma

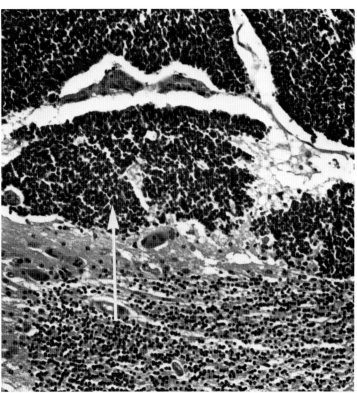

Fig. 145b. HE × 170

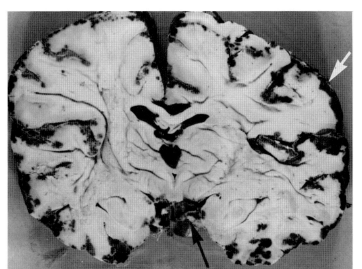

Fig. 145c. Multiple metastatic melanoma

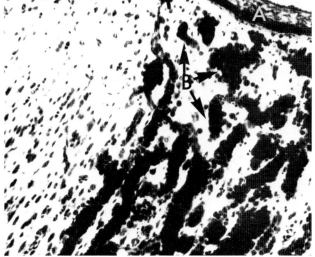

Fig. 145d. Nissl × 100

## Metastatic Tumors in Electron Microscopy

From light microscopic observation, we know that metastatic tumors retain the cytological features of their original sites and are clearly different from neuronal or glial cells. This characteristic is even more distinct when metastatic tumors are examined in the electron microscope. For example, plasmacytomas display the elaborately developed rough endoplasmic reticulum which practically fills the cytoplasm of the tumor cells. Similarly, the large accumulations of glycogen found in renal carcinoma are also seen in cerebral metastases. In addition, the highly developed desmosomes (arrows) found in various well differentiated carcinomas are found in metastatic tumors and they are quite different from the desmosomes seen in ependymal cells or astrocytes, either neoplastic or normal (Fig. 146). A further example of this characteristic, namely the retention of the original cytological features, concerns the morphology of the small vessels supplying the tumor. In some parts of the body, such as endocrine glands and kidney, among others, the capillary endothelium contains many pores known as fenestrae. This is unlike most of the brain where the endothelium is nonfenestrated. Not surprisingly, the blood vessels in renal carcinoma are fenestrated as in the normal kidney. Interestingly, when such tumors metastasize to the brain, the vasculature retains this feature. Thus, we may conclude that the growing metastatic neoplasm in the brain induces the formation of these specialized blood vessels which presumably arise from nonfenestrated cerebral vessels.

*Reference*

Hirano, A., and H. M. Zimmerman. Fenestrated Blood Vessels in a Metastic Renal Carcinoma in the Brain. Lab. Invest. 26: 465, 1972.

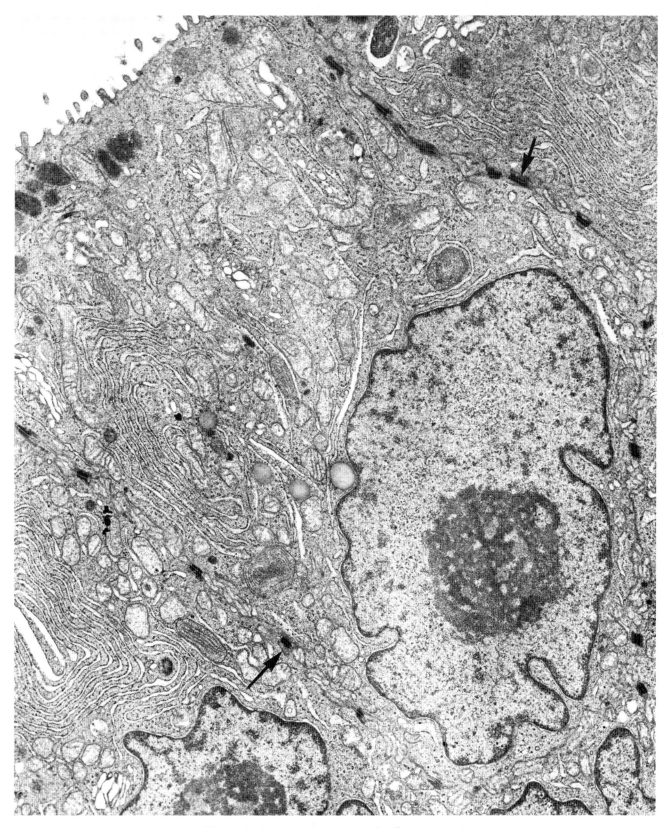

Fig. 146. An electron micrograph of a metastatic
carcinoma to the brain × 17,000

Different varieties of systemic sarcoma may metastasize to the brain and spinal cord though less commonly than the carcinomas. Of these, malignant lymphomas, either lymphosarcoma or Hodgkin's disease, are noteworthy.

The most common mode of metastasis is by extension through cranial and vertebral bones into the underlying dura, leptomeninges, and nervous tissue. Both the granuloma and sarcoma varieties of *Hodgkin's disease* may act in this manner.

> *Case 1:* A 42-year-old man had a diagnosis of Hodgkin's disease for which he received many courses of nitrogen mustard, chlorambucil, and x-ray therapy. Four years later, he developed episodes of twitching of the right side of the face, followed by right facial weakness, slurring of speech, and weakness of the right leg. The total protein of the cerebrospinal fluid was elevated. X-rays of the pelvis and the fifth lumbar vertebral body showed evidence of infiltration; on skull x-ray, there was displacement of the calcified pineal gland inferiorly and posteriorly. He received x-ray therapy to both lateral regions of the skull and lumbar spine but after a period of improvement, developed weakness of the left as well as the right leg, and frequent episodes of unconsciousness. He expired of respiratory failure after five months of hospitalization.

The brain showed a large nodular grayish-white firm tumor mass that extended from the dura into the underlying meninges and cerebral tissue in the region of the left middle and inferior frontal gyri, associated with edema and displacement of the ventricles to the right side (Fig. 147a).

Microscopically, the tumor showed the characteristic structure of Hodgkin's granuloma with infiltration by lymphocytes, plasma cells, eosinophils, reticulum and Reed-Sternberg cells, interspersed with collagen and reticulin fibers (Fig. 147b).

Metastatic *rhabdomyosarcomas* are tumors that rarely metastasize to brain or spinal cord.

> *Case 2:* A 39-year-old woman developed a lump on the right side of the neck, associated with paralysis of the recurrent laryngeal nerve. A tumor nodule was removed from this region. About eight months later she began to notice blurring of vision, inability to close her right eye, difficulty in swallowing, and loss of sensation in the right half of her face. Examination revealed signs of paralysis of cranial nerves V, VI, VII, VIII, IX, X, XI, and XII on the right side. A ventriculogram disclosed generalized hydrocephalus.

Autopsy revealed a firm, fleshy tumor adherent to the brain stem and cerebellum in the region of the right cerebellopontine angle, greatly compressing, displacing, and partly infiltrating these structures (Fig. 147c).

The histologic appearance of the tumor was one of parallel bundles of spindle-shaped cells with large hyperchromatic nuclei and with striated muscle fibers in the cytoplasm (Fig. 147d).

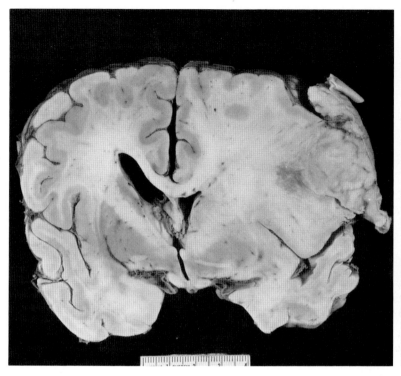

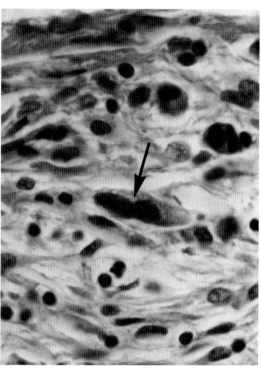

Fig. 147a. Metastatic granuloma in Hodgkin's disease, left hemisphere (sides reversed)

Fig. 147b. HE × 560

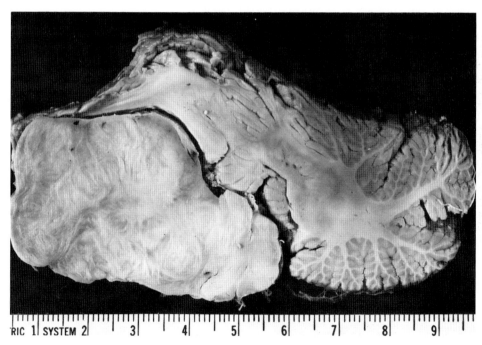

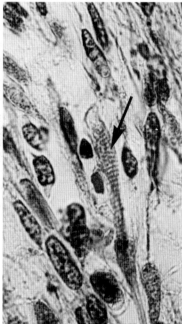

Fig. 147c. Rhabdomyosarcoma, right side of brain stem (sides reversed)

Fig. 147d. HVG × 900

The central nervous system manifestations of the acute and chronic forms of leukemia are usually due to hemorrhages, either subdural or intracerebral, that develop in the terminal stages of the disorder. These result from either leukostasis, related to intravascular leukemic infiltrations or accompanying thrombocytopenia.

*Case 1:* A 5-year-old boy had symptoms of lymphocytic leukemia for about five months. Terminally, he developed coma, associated with right hemiplegia.

Multiple petechial hemorrhages were disseminated through the gray and white matter of the brain; these coalesced into massive hemorrhages in the thalamus and pons on the left, where they involved the pyramidal fibers (Fig. 148a). The hemorrhages occurred in association with metastatic nodules of leukemic cells (Fig. 148b).

Less commonly leukemic infiltrates may involve diffusely the leptomeninges, causing hydrocephalus, or penetrate the roots of cranial and spinal nerves resulting in cranial nerve palsies, radicular pains, and manifestations of polyneuropathy.

*Case 2:* A 35-year-old cyclotron engineer developed radicular pain and paresthesias in the lower extremities, followed by headaches, impaired vision, epileptiform attacks, ocular and facial palsies, and episodes of delirium. Examination in the hospital revealed also bilateral papilledema, flaccid paralysis of the lower extremities, and paralysis of bladder and rectal sphincters. The cerebrospinal fluid contained from 2,000 to 5,000 mononuclear cells per cmm and a total protein varying between 104–172 mg %. Examination of the blood revealed evidence of monocytic leukemia. The clinical course was progressively downhill over a period of six months.

Autopsy findings confirmed the diagnosis of leukemia with widespread involvement of many of the body tissues. The leukemic infiltrations in the central nervous system were most abundant in the leptomeninges, and in and about the roots of various cranial and spinal nerves (Fig. 148c).

The cells were mononuclear forms with large hyperchromatic and lobulated nuclei (A) and many mitotic figures (B) (Fig. 148d).

*Reference*

Litteral, E. B., and N. Malamud. Leukemia with Predominant Neurologic Manifestations. Neurol. 5: 740, 1955.

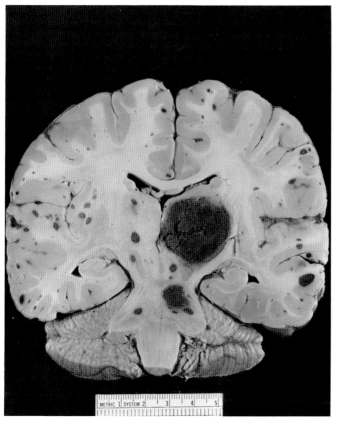

Fig. 148a. Multiple hemorrhages in leukemia (sides reversed)

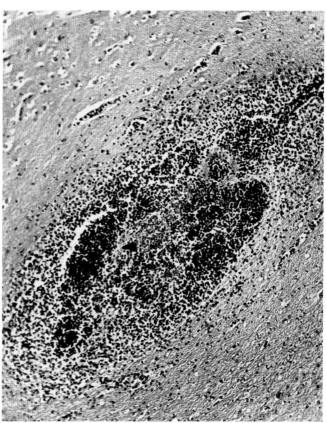

Fig. 148b. HE × 100

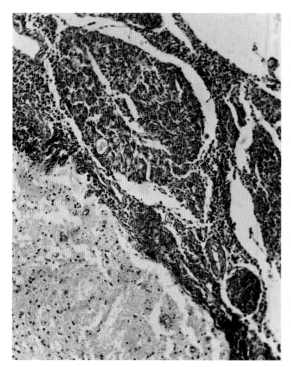

Fig. 148c. HVG × 50

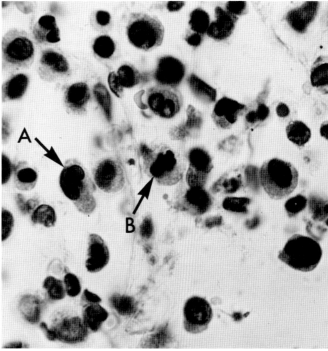

Fig. 148d. HVG × 900

In recent years an increasing number of cases have been reported in which nonmetastatic neurologic complications occur in association with malignant systemic tumors.

The underlying lesions appear to be of a degenerative and/or inflammatory type and tend to involve specific parts of the central and/or peripheral nervous system.

The following syndromes have been described, primarily in cases of carcinoma: 1) subacute cortical cerebellar degeneration; 2) sensorimotor polyneuropathy; 3) motor neuron disorder, and 4) mixed forms of encephalomyelitis in combination with any of the above syndromes.

The pathogenesis has remained obscure as to whether toxic, metabolic, nutritional, hyperergic, or viral causes are responsible.

### Subacute Cortical Cerebellar Degeneration

*Case 1:* A 66-year-old man complained of nausea, vomiting, diplopia, vertigo, and disturbance of gait for one month before admission to a hospital. On examination he exhibited an ataxic wide-based gait, a positive Romberg sign, marked dysarthria, unsustained horizontal and rotatory nystagmus, and incoordination on heel-to-knee test. All laboratory studies, including x-rays of the chest, ventriculograms, and cerebrospinal fluid tests, were negative. Death occurred four months after the onset of his illness.

The autopsy revealed a bronchogenic carcinoma of the "oat cell" type.

The cerebellum showed depletion and degeneration of the neurons of the dentate nucleus (Fig. 149a) accompanied by reactive proliferation of microglia, fat-laden gitter cells, and astrocytes. There was also diffuse dropout of Purkinje cells, although less marked.

A similar syndrome may develop in the course of malignant lymphomas, as illustrated by the following case of Hodgkin's disease:

*Case 2:* A 35-year-old man gradually developed headaches, vertigo, nausea and vomiting, ataxia, and nystagmus. Examination revealed a tumor of the right inguinal region, which was diagnosed by biopsy as Hodgkin's disease. Neurologically, he showed dysarthria, coarse tremor, past-pointing and rebound phenomena in the upper extremities, and ataxia of the lower extremities. The condition was one of progressive decline during the next year and a half in spite of x-ray therapy.

Autopsy revealed Hodgkin's disease involving the spleen, lymph nodes, and bone marrow.

The essential findings in the central nervous system were diffuse degenerative changes in the cerebellum, affecting primarily the Purkinje layer, where most of the neurons disappeared and were replaced by gliosis in the Bergmann and molecular layers (Figs. 149b and c).

In neither of the previous cases was there any evidence of an inflammatory reaction.

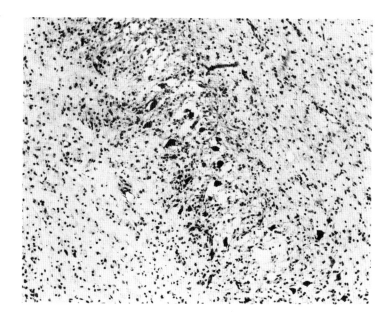

Fig. 149a. Nissl × 100

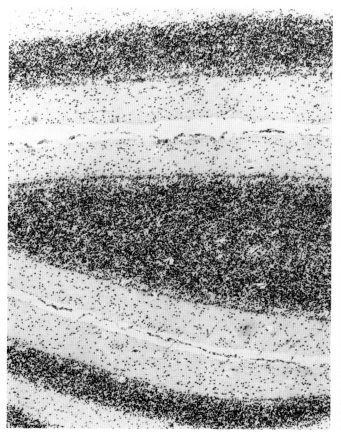

Fig. 149b. Nissl × 50

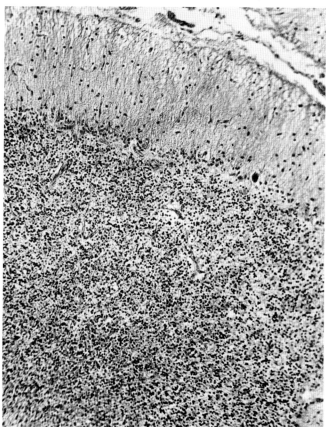

Fig. 149c. HE × 100

## Mixed Form with Polyneuropathy and Encephalomyelitis

*Case:* A 64-year-old man was admitted to a hospital several months after he developed progressive numbness and weakness of his hands and feet. Examination revealed hypesthesia, decrease in vibratory and position sense and of 2-point discrimination, and hypoactive to absent tendon reflexes. The cerebrospinal fluid protein was elevated to 88 mg %. He lost 20 lb in weight over an eight-week period. There were no findings to indicate the presence of a systemic malignant tumor, including a negative chest x-ray, G. I. series, and urinalysis. In his further course, his neurologic condition continued to deteriorate to a point of complete deafferentation so that he no longer had any sensory perception. There was also generalized weakness and muscle wasting. In the last few weeks of his life, he developed signs of mental deterioration, finally lapsing into a state of coma and died one and one-half years following the onset of his illness.

The general autopsy revealed a small undifferentiated ("oat cell") bronchogenic carcinoma with metastases to hilar lymph nodes and terminal bronchopneumonia.

The brain and spinal cord showed no gross changes.

Microscopic examination revealed complete demyelination of the dorsal columns of white matter throughout the spinal cord (Fig. 150a) as well as of the dorsal roots in which fat-laden foam cells (A) replaced the destroyed myelin associated with infiltration of the adjacent meninges by lymphocytes (B) (Fig. 150b). There was depletion and axonal reaction of anterior horn cells associated with moderate perivascular cuffing with lymphocytes and diffuse proliferation of microglia (Fig. 150c). The peripheral nerves were diffusely demyelinated. The cerebral cortex, especially of the temporal lobes, revealed marked inflammatory reaction, characterized by perivascular cuffing, microglial nodules (arrow) and diffuse microglial and astroglial proliferation associated with neuronal depletion (Fig. 150d).

In this case, the outstanding feature was the presence of widespread inflammatory reaction, both chronic and acute, in association with a degenerative polyneuropathy, suggestive of possible viral etiology.

*Reference*

The Remote Effects of Cancer on the Nervous System, ed. by Brain, W. R , and F. Norris. Grune and Stratton (New York, 1965).

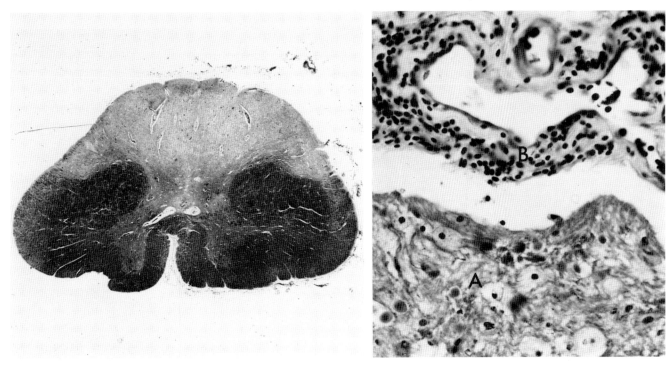

Fig. 150a. Weil stain of spinal cord

Fig. 150b. Weil × 250

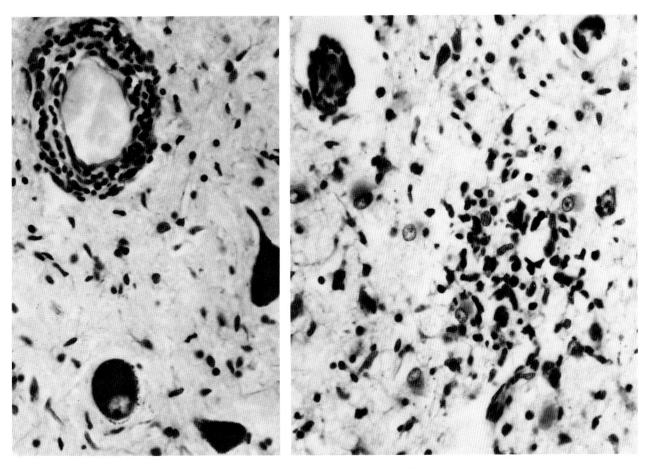

Fig. 150c. Nissl × 310

Fig. 150d. Nissl × 310

## Progressive Multifocal Leukoencephalopathy (PML)

In malignant lymphomas a multifocal demyelinating disorder has been reported with rapidly progressive generalized or focal neurologic signs having their onset in the late stages of the systemic disease. The demyelinating process is characterized by unique changes in oligodendroglia in the form of either enlarged basophilic nuclei and/or eosinophilic inclusions, and by reactive astrocytes with bizarre nuclei, in the presence of mild inflammatory reaction.

*Case 1:* A 43-year-old man was admitted to a hospital with a history of having developed a lymphosarcoma, approximately one year previously for which he was treated with nitrogen mustard. Two months prior to admission, he developed seizures, and on admission he was noted to be lethargic. There were large matted lymph nodes in the cervical, axillary, and inguinal areas, but the neurologic and spinal fluid examinations were unremarkable. A course of methotrexate therapy was begun, but his condition continued to deteriorate with increasing lethargy. Pneumonia developed that responded to antibiotics. By this time he was stuporous, developed a positive Babinski sign on the right side, and several days later, a flaccid hemiplegia on the left side. He expired approximately three months following the onset of his neurologic disorder.

The general autopsy findings confirmed widespread sarcoma of lymph nodes and splenomegaly.

The brain showed on section extensive demyelination of the white matter in both frontal lobes, more on the right side, that appeared to represent confluence of countless discrete pinpointed or linear foci (Fig. 151a). This was confirmed in myelin stains, the demyelinative foci having their predilection in the white matter although involving also the lower layers of the cortex. The lesions contained large numbers of fat-laden macrophages (A) and many enlarged amphophilic nuclei of oligodendroglia (B) (Fig. 151b). There were scattered giant astrocytes with large lobulated nuclei (Fig. 151c).

The condition of PML, however, is not confined to complications of lymphomas but has been reported in association with carcinomatosis, sarcoidosis, and chronic systemic infections as illustrated in the fllowing case:

*Case 2:* A 38-year-old woman, with a long history of many obscure infectious illnesses, had in the last six years of her life attacks of pyelonephritis that were often accompanied by signs of uremia. During her last attack she developed for the first time blurring of vision, weakness of the left arm, bilateral pyramidal signs in the lower extremities, an ataxic gait, and signs of pseudobulbar paralysis. The cerebrospinal fluid was free of cells, but contained 218 mg of protein per 100 cc; there was a first-zone rise in the colloidal gold curve. She died in coma five months after the last attack.

Countless demyelinative foci were disseminated throughout the white matter of the brain, including the richly myelinated areas of thalamus, subthalamus, and cerebral peduncles (Fig. 151d). In higher magnifications the reactive cells were both altered oligodendroglia (as in the previous case) and hypertrophied bizarre astrocytes with multinucleation and eosinophilic inclusions (Fig. 151e).

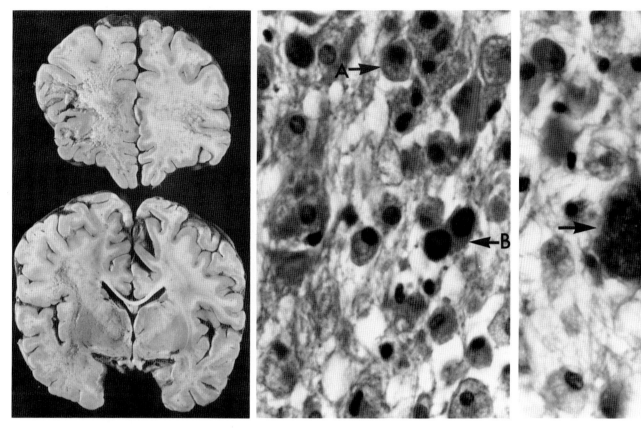

Fig. 151a. Demyelinative lesions in progressive multifocal leukoencephalopathy

Fig. 151b. HE × 560

Fig. 151c. HE × 560

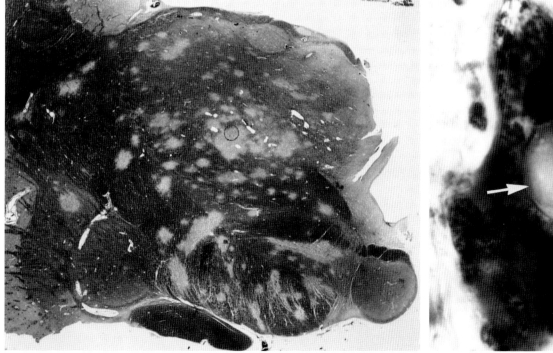

Fig. 151d. Weil stain

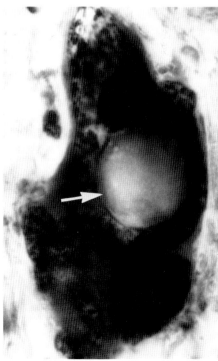

Fig. 151e. HE × 1125

## Progressive Multifocal Leukoencephalopathy (PML) in Electron Microscopy

In the electron microscope, some of the nuclei of glial cells associated with demyelinating foci are seen to contain both spherical and filamentous inclusions (Fig. 152). Sometimes these particles are arranged in a crystalloid mass. The spherical particles measure approximately 400 Å in diameter. From a morphological point of view, the spherical particles are indistinguishable from papova virions. The immunological nature of the particles is currently a matter of extensive study.

*References*

Padgett, B. L., G. M. ZuRhein, D. L. Walker, R. J. Eckroada, and B. H. Dessel. Cultivation of Papova-like Virus from Human Brain with Progressive Multifocal Leucoencephalopathy. The Lancet. 1257–60, 1971.

Silverman, L., and L. J. Rubinstein. Electron Microscopic Observations on a Case of Progressive Multifocal Leucoencephalopathy. Acta Neuropath. 5: 215, 1965.

Weiner, L. P., R. M. Herndon, and O. Narayan. Cyopathic, Immunofluorescent and Electron Microscopic Characteristics of Agents Isolated from Progressive Multifocal Leukoencephalopathy in Cell Cultures. Am. J. Path. 63: 5a, 1972.

ZuRhein, G. M. Association of Papova-virions with a Human Demyelinating Disease (Progressive Multifocal Leukoencephalopathy). Progr. med. Virol. 11: 185, 1969.

ZuRhein, G. M., and S. M. Chou. Particles Resembling Papova-viruses in Human Cerebral Demyelinating Disease. Science. 148: 1477, 1965.

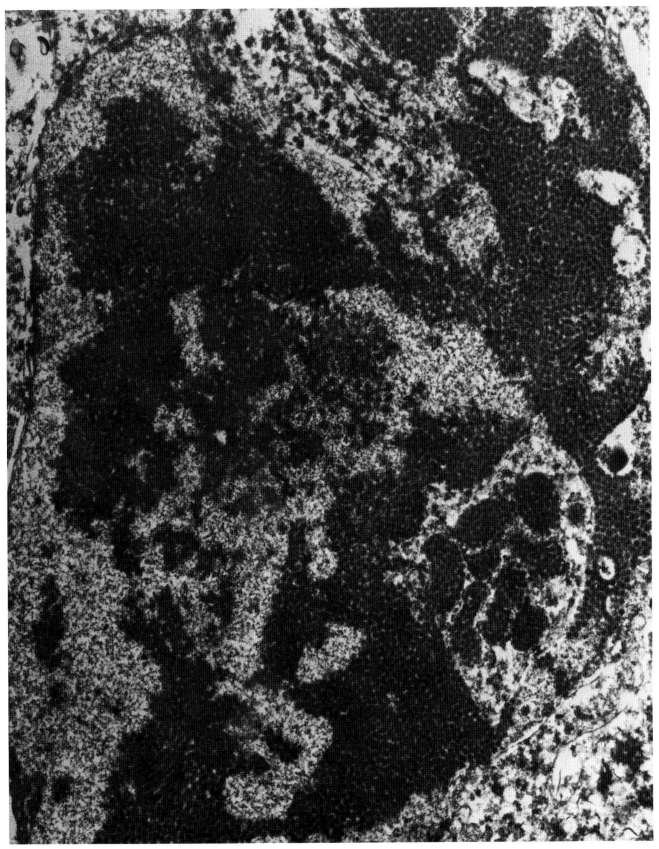

Fig. 152. An electron micrograph of a nucleus in an altered glial cell of a case of progressive multifocal leukoen-cephalopathy. Masses of dense spherical or filamentous structures are present within the nucleus, × 25,000.

In the course of treatment with ionizing radiation of either intra- or extra-craniospinal tumors, neurologic complications due to radionecrosis of the normal nervous tissue may develop. It has been generally accepted that this depends on the tolerance dose, calculated to be 3,300–4,300 r administered in twenty-eight to forty-two days for spinal cord and 4,500–5,000 r in thirty days for brain tissue. The duration of the latent period has varied from three months to seven or more years.

The pathology of radionecrosis is characterized by predilection for white matter and by a combination of parenchymal and vascular changes, often of disproportionate degree. The parenchymal changes are characterized by edema, liquefaction and coagulation necrosis, plasmatic infiltration by proteins, fibrin and pseudocalcium, reduction in oligodendroglia, sparse reaction by microglia and gitter cells, and hypertrophy of astrocytes, sometimes with formation of multinucleated giant cells. The vascular changes consist of fibrinoid necrosis, hyalinosis and fibrosis of vessel walls, and formation of telangiectasias.

The pathogenesis of radionecrosis remains speculative as between interdependence or independence of the parenchymal and vascular changes.

## Postirradiation Necrosis

*Case 1:* A 22-year-old man received, over a period of twenty days, a calculated dose of approximately 5,000 r to the cervical region for a nasopharyngeal carcinoma, which responded favorably. Ten months later he developed signs of an ascending myelitis with a level at C6. He died of respiratory difficulties four months after the onset of the neurologic complication.

The autopsy revealed no recurrence of the carcinoma.

Throughout the swollen cervical spinal cord there was an acute necrotizing myelopathy involving the white matter and sparing the gray matter (Fig. 153a). It was characterized by diffuse disintegration of myelin and axons, accompanied by scattered macrophages, and by fibrinoid necrosis of the walls of blood vessels surrounded by fibrin, red blood cells and polymorphonuclear leucocytes in the perivascular zones (Fig. 153b).

*Case 2:* A 33-year-old woman was admitted to a hospital with a history that one and one-half years previously she was operated on for a low grade astrocytoma of the left frontal lobe, followed by 6,000 r of x-ray therapy, with remission of symptoms. She was readmitted because of recent onset of increasing mental confusion and convulsive episodes. Examination revealed disorientation, lethargy, a facetious attitude, and hyperactive deep reflexes on the right side. A carotid angiogram disclosed bowing of the right anterior cerebral artery to the left and a tumor blush in the right frontal lobe. Her condition progressively worsened and she died approximately eight months after her last hospital admission.

The brain showed remains of a cystic glioma confined to a limited area in the inferior frontal gyrus on the left side (A) and extensive necrosis of the white matter of the right frontal lobe (B) and adjacent part of the corpus callosum, with normal appearance of the intervening tissue (Fig. 153c).

Microscopically, the tumor was a well differentiated fibrillary astrocytoma. The necrotic white matter was largely liquefied, showing only minimal glial reaction and contained scattered congested blood vessels with necrotic walls (Fig. 153d), while the adjacent cortex contained only reactive astrocytes.

*References*

Malamud, N., E. B. Boldrey, W. K. Welch, and E. J. Fadell. Necrosis of Brain and Spinal Cord Following X-ray Therapy. J. Neurosurg. 11: 353, 1954.

Van Cleave, C. D. Irradiation of the Nervous System, Rowman and Littlefield (New York, 1963).

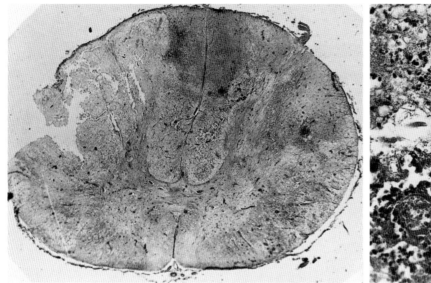

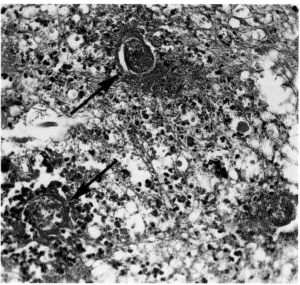

Fig. 153a. Radionecrosis of spinal cord

Fig. 153b. Hematoxylin van Gieson × 100

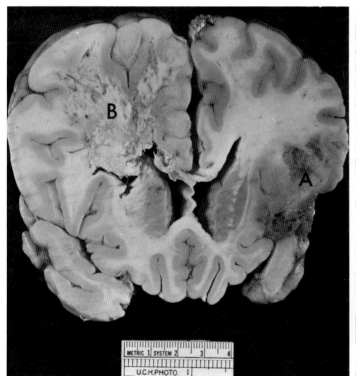

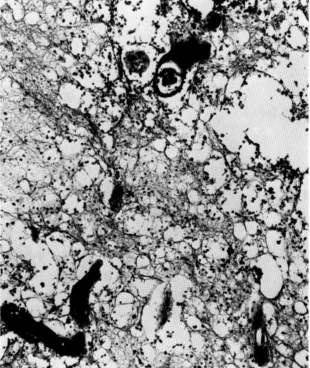

Fig. 153c. Radionecrosis of right frontal lobe and glioma of
left frontal lobe (sides reversed)

Fig. 153d. Weil × 70

## Postirradiation Fibrosarcoma

A rare complication of radiation therapy is the development of malignant fibrosarcoma as a result of irradiation of the connective tissue of meninges and blood vessels. Such a change appears to occur after an unusually long latent interval that is apt to induce neoplastic proliferation of vascular tissue and hypertrophic astroglia with bizarre nuclear division.

*Case:* A 17-year-old girl had an occipital craniotomy at the age of nine years for a tumor of the vermis, diagnosed medulloblastoma. It was followed by x-ray therapy, consisting of 4,500 r to the posterior fossa and lateral ventricles, 465 r to the cervicothoracic cord and 325 r to the lumbar cord, over a period of forty-five days. For the next eight years she remained virtually symptom free. After that she began to develop signs of increasing intracranial pressure and bilateral homonymous hemianopsia, more marked on the right. A ventriculogram now revealed a large tumor in the left parieto-occipital region, considered to be recurrence of the original tumor. A course of radiation therapy was again administered, consisting of 3,300 r over a period of seventy-seven days. But, although she improved slightly, her right-sided hemianopsia persisted and her general condition deteriorated; she expired nine months following the relapse.

The biopsy of the original vermis tumor showed the typical structure of a medulloblastoma, being composed of closely packed oval cells with hyperchromatic nuclei infiltrating the cerebellar tissue (Fig. 154a).

The brain at autopsy revealed a large grayish-white firm, homogeneous and fairly well circumscribed tumor mass that replaced the mesial parts of the left parieto-occipital region (A), obliterating the posterior horn and causing terminal brain stem hemorrhages through transtentorial herniation, while cystic scar tissue marked the site of the old operation in the vermis (B) (Fig. 154b).

Microscopically, there was no trace of the original tumor in the vermis, and only gliosis remained, associated with proliferation of numerous small blood vessels (Fig. 154c) and scattered multi-nucleated giant cells.

The tumor in the left hemisphere showed the structure of a fibrosarcoma (Fig. 154d), with interlacing bundles of spindle cells that appeared to arise from the walls of proliferated blood vessels (as well as from adjacent meninges). The cells contained pleomorphic nuclei with scattered mitoses, and reticulin and collagen fibers, interspersed with bizarre multi-nucleated giant cells (Fig. 154e).

*Reference*

Noetzli, M., and N. Malamud. Postirradiation Fibrosarcoma of the Brain. Cancer. 15:617, 1962.

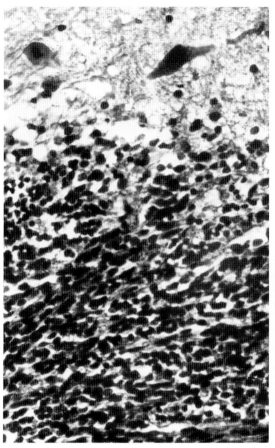

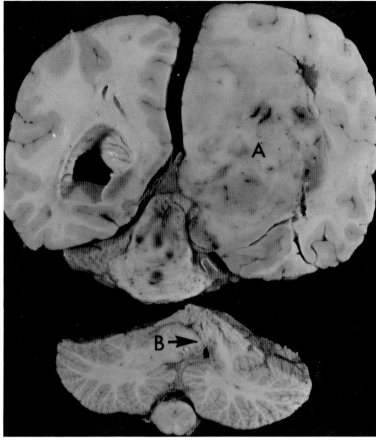

Fig. 154a. HE × 375

Fig. 154b. Sarcoma in left occipital lobe (sides reversed); operative scar in vermis of cerebellum

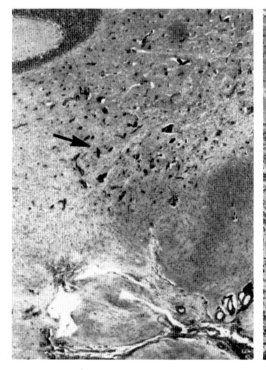

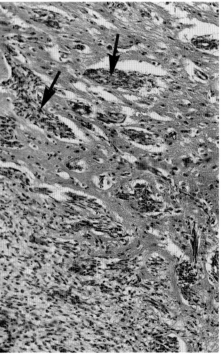

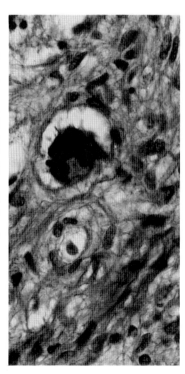

Fig. 154c. Hematoxylin van Gieson × 20

Fig. 154d. Hematoxylin van Gieson × 70

Fig. 154e. Hematoxylin van Gieson × 375

# VIII
## *Degenerative Disorders*

Degenerative diseases comprise a great variety of primary degenerative conditions of obscure etiology. They have been variously interpreted as abiotrophic disorders on the assumption of a constitutional predisposition to involution, as system disorders because of selective involvement of one or other neuroanatomic system, and as heredodegenerative diseases caused by hereditary transmission. However, each of these interpretations has been criticized as inadequate. Abiotrophy is an obscure concept. A predilection for distinct neuroanatomic systems applies to some but not to other forms in this group. An hereditary background has been established in only some conditions, whereas in others, showing similar clinical and pathoanatomic features, such evidence is lacking. Exogenous or endogenous metabolic disturbances cannot be ruled out as etiologic factors.

### SENILE-PRESENILE DEMENTIAS

In the group of dementias associated with advanced age there has been a tendency to include a variety of degenerative and vascular disorders that have little in common with the exception of the clinically prominent organic brain syndrome (C.B.S.).

The accompanying Table lists the neuropathologic diagnoses in a large series of cases with clinical diagnosis of C.B.S.

Several inferences may be drawn from the table:

1. A distinction often made between senile and presenile dementia of Alzheimer has no justification except for the arbitrary separation in accordance with the age of onset. It would be preferable to include both under a diagnosis of Alzheimer's disease, regardless of age, as is evident from their pathologic similarity. Furthermore, the terms "senile-presenile" imply that these conditions are in some way related to normal aging, which is a controversial point. 2. Pick's and Creutzfeldt-Jacob's diseases, often included with the presenile dementias, are entirely separate conditions; and, 3. The degenerative and vascular disorders, though they may coexist, are independent entities.

### ALZHEIMER'S DISEASE

The clinical picture of Alzheimer's disease is dominated by progressive impairment of cognitive functions, especially of recent and retentive memory, accompanied by secondary emotional and personality changes. Aphasia, apraxia, and agnosia may be present but are ill defined. Other neurologic signs are relatively mild except terminally, when convulsions often occur.

Pathologically, the distinctive features are: diffuse atrophy of the brain (Fig. 155) involving primarily the cerebral cortex, and specific microscopic changes in the form of senile plaques, neurofibrillary tangles, and granulovacuolar bodies.

*Reference*

Malamud, N. Neuropathology of Organic Brain Syndromes Associated with Aging. Aging and the Brain. Plenum Publishing Corp. (New York, 1972), pp. 63–87.

TABLE. NEUROPATHOLOGIC DIAGNOSIS IN 1,225 CASES OF CHRONIC BRAIN SYNDROME

| Neuropathologic Diagnosis | | Age Range | Number of Cases |
|---|---|---|---|
| Senile Brain Disease ) | Alzheimer's Disease | 65-98 | 416 (34%) |
| Presenile Brain Disease ) | | 40-64 | 103 (8.4%) |
| Pick's Disease | | 35-72 | 35 (2.8%) |
| Creutzfeldt-Jakob's Disease | | 43-86 | 32 (2.7%) |
| Arteriosclerotic Brain Disease | | 42-100 | 356 (29%) |
| Mixed Senile-Arteriosclerotic Brain Disease | | 62-94 | 283 (23%) |

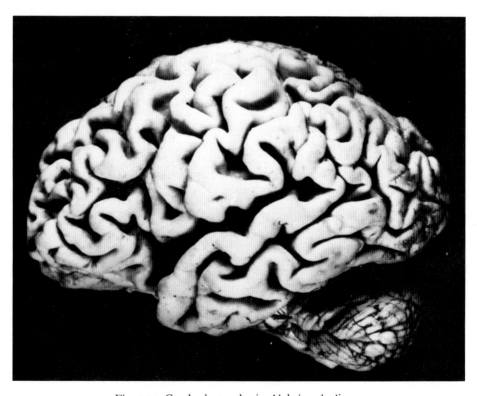

Fig. 155. Cerebral atrophy in Alzheimer's disease

*Case 1: Alzheimer's Disease (form of senile dementia)* A 79-year-old man developed increasing depression and paranoid ideation following the death of his wife five years before hospitalization. On admission to a hospital he showed marked confusion, memory defects, especially for recent events, and nominal aphasia. There were senile changes in the skin, cornea, and lens, and peripheral arteriosclerosis. An electroencephalogram was interpreted as a diffusely slow record. Because of his agitated depression, he was treated with electroshock. He succumbed to a pulmonary embolus from a thrombophlebitis of the leg.

The weight of the brain was 1,220 grams. The leptomeninges were moderately fibrotic; the cortex was diffusely atrophied, but the basal arteries showed only mild atherosclerosis. The atrophy was characterized by uniform narrowing of gyri and widening of sulci throughout all the lobes. Coronal sections disclosed diffuse thinning of the cerebral cortex, including that of the hippocampal formation, associated with dilatation of the subarachnoid spaces Sylvian fissures and lateral ventricles, and relative preservation of all subcortical structures (Fig. 156a).

*Case 2: Alzheimer's Disease (form of presenile dementia)* A 67-year-old woman was well until the age of 53 when she became forgetful, unable to carry out complex tasks, and was depressed. Her condition progressively deteriorated, necessitating commitment to a state hospital five years following the onset. Examination at this time showed a breakdown in speech and mental associations with tendency to perseveration, washing and dressing apraxia, impairment of memory, and disorientation. Physical, neurologic, and laboratory examinations were negative except for a diffusely abnormal electroencephalogram that indicated a convulsive susceptibility. The further course was one of progressive decline and she expired of bronchopneumonia.

The brain showed generalized atrophy of the gyri and on section widespread cortical atrophy, including the hippocampal formation with compensatory dilatation of the subarachnoid spaces and lateral ventricles (Fig. 156b).

The microscopic findings, in keeping with the gross changes, were identical in the two cases, irrespective of the age of occurrence and the differing clinical diagnoses of senile dementia and Alzheimer's disease.

In Nissl preparations there was a diffuse loss of neurons and nonspecific changes in those surviving, accompanied by increase in reactive fibrillary astrocytes (Fig. 156c).

With the PAS method, a positive reaction was noted in the walls of some of the arterioles (congophilic angiopathy) (Fig. 156d) and, in particular, in so-called senile plaques, some of which contained central cores (Fig. 156e). These structures also gave a positive reaction with Congo red for amyloid and have been referred to in the literature as congophilic changes.

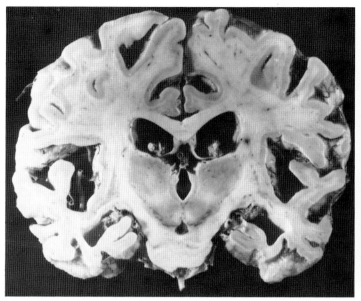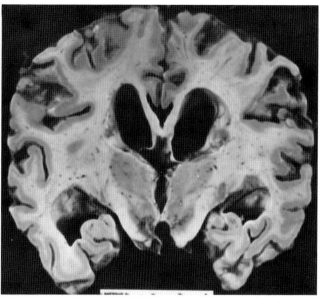

Fig. 156a. Cerebral atrophy in "senile" dementia    Fig. 156b. Cerebral atrophy in "presenile" dementia

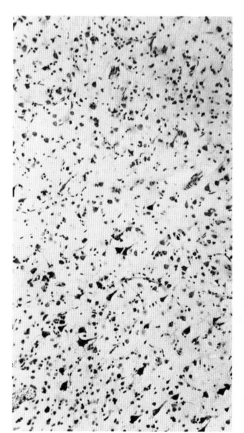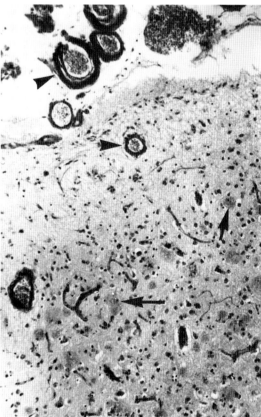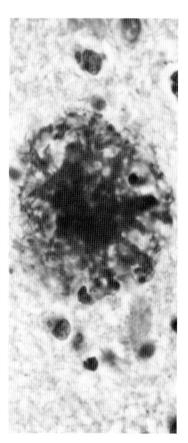

Fig. 156c. Nissl × 100    Fig. 156d. PAS × 100    Fig. 156e. PAS × 450

ALZHEIMER'S DISEASE (continued)

In silver nitrate preparations (methods of Bielschowsky and other modifications), the following specific changes became especially prominent:

1) *Senile plaques* (Fig. 157a) in large numbers, distributed in all layers of the cortex throughout all lobes, though varying in intensity. The plaques appeared as spherical aggregates, from 5–150 μ in diameter, of a diffuse filamentous or granular argyrophilic structure, with or without a dense central core (Fig. 157b).

2) *Neurofibrillary tangles* (Fig. 157c), characterized by proliferation, agglutination, and alteration of strongly argyrophilic neuronal fibrils that extended into dendrites but not axons. They were most numerous in the hippocampal formation, very common in the cerebral cortex, infrequent in basal ganglia and brain stem, and absent in the cerebellum. They showed many variations in shape, from flame-like to globose.

3) *Granulovacuolar bodies* (Fig. 157c and d) consisting of intracytoplasmic argyrophilic granules of about 1.5 μ in diameter within clear halos. These were virtually confined to the pyramidal layer of the hippocampus.

The interdependence of the three types of changes may be assumed from their constant association in Alzheimer's disease, although they differ in relative numbers and regional predilection. It is noteworthy, however, that the neurofibrillary tangles (and in some instances the granulovacuolar bodies) occur in the absence of senile plaques in a number of unrelated disorders such as in the parkinsonism-dementia-ALS syndrome of the island of Guam and in chronic encephalitis.

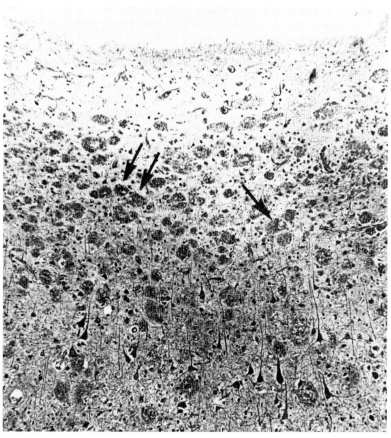

Fig. 157a. von Braunmühl × 75

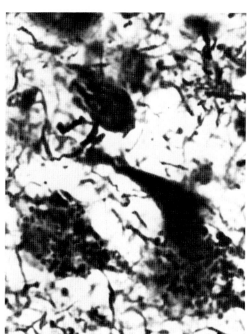

Fig. 157b. von Braunmühl × 450

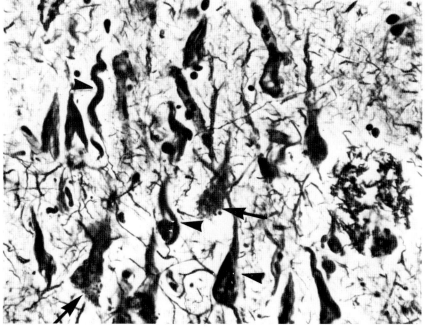

Fig. 157c. von Braunmühl × 280

Fig. 157d. von Braunmühl × 720

## Senile Plaques in Electron Microscopy

In the electron microscope, the senile plaque is seen to be composed primarily of neuronal and glial processes surrounding an amyloid core (Fig. 158). The amyloid, which is indistinguishable from that found in any part of the body, is composed of radially arranged hollow filaments, 60–90 Å in diameter. Interspersed among the filaments are occasional, randomly arranged dense bodies.

The glial processes derive from either astrocytes or reactive microglia. The astrocytes often form a sheet-like investment around the amyloid core and appear similar to reactive astrocytes seen in various conditions. Specifically, they may contain lipid inclusions and large accumulations of glial filaments.

In addition to glial processes, a large part of the plaque is composed of altered, often distended, neuronal processes. The most common alterations are usually high numbers of mitochondria and dense bodies. These changes are responsible for the elevated activities of both oxidative enzymes and hydrolases, respectively, which are associated with senile plaques. Frequently, the mitochondria themselves show deviations in appearance from those seen in normal neuronal processes. In addition, various fibrillary alterations are seen within the neuronal processes. The best known among these are the Alzheimer-type neurofibrillary tangles, that consist of "twisted tubules." In addition, tubulo-vesicular material of unknown derivation is frequently found within the neuronal processes. Furthermore, other, normal components are often present in unusually high numbers. These include the 100 Å neurofilaments, the 240 Å microtubules, and synaptic vesicles, both with and without dense cores.

The origin of the senile plaques and the relationships among the various constituents is unknown. The electron microscope, however, has clearly delineated the Alzheimer-type neurofibrillary tangle from the amyloid core.

*References*

Gonatas, N. K., and P. Gambetti. The Pathology of the Synapse in Alzheimer's Disease. Ciba Foundation Symposium on Alzheimer's Disease and Related Conditions. (G.E.W. Wolstenholme and M. O'Connor, eds.). Churchill (London, 1970), p. 169.

Lampert, P. Fine Structural Changes of Neurites in Alzheimer's Disease. Acta Neuropath. Suppl. V, 49, 1971.

Nikaido, T., J. Austin, R. Rinehart, L. Trueb, J. Hutchinson, H. Stukenbrok, and B. Miles. Studies in Aging of the Brain. I. Isolation and Preliminary Characterization of Alzheimer Plaques and Cores. Arch. Neurol. 25: 198, 1971.

Terry, R. D., N. K. Gonatas, and M. Weiss. Ultrastructural Studies in Alzheimer's Presenile Dementia. Amer. J. Path. 44: 269, 1964.

Wisniewski, H. M., and R. D. Terry. Reexamination of the Pathogenesis of the Senile Plaque. Progress in Neuropathology, Vol. II (H. M. Zimmerman, ed.). Grune and Stratton (New York, 1973), p. 1.

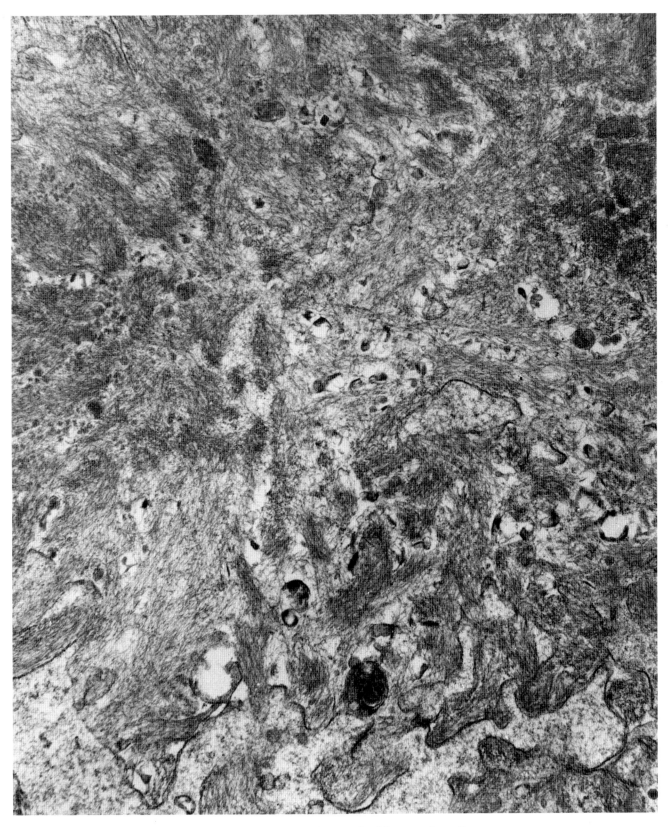

Fig. 158. An electron micrograph of the core of a senile
plaque × 20,000

## Alzheimer's Neurofibrillary Tangles in Electron Microscopy

The electron microscopic elucidation of neurofibrillary tangles (NF) was originally achieved by Terry. Since then, it has been established that the components of the neurofibrillary tangle are unlike any normally occurring cellular constituents. They consist of bundles of parallel fibrils (Fig. 159a), which show characteristic periodic constrictions about 800 Å apart in longitudinal sections (Fig. 159b). The thickness of the fiber varies from approximately 300 Å midway between constrictions to approximately 100 Å at the constriction itself.

Cross sections of the fibrils may appear either annular or arciform (Fig. 159c). On the basis of the longitudinal and cross-sectional profiles, some authors have suggested that the fibrils may be "twisted tubules." The fine structure of the tangles is the same regardless of the involved neuron or underlying disease condition.

The origin of the tangles is still unknown but they apparently are not simply structural distortions of either the 240 Å microtubules or the 100 Å neurofilaments which are normal parts of the neuron. On the other hand, the molecular components of the tangles may eventually prove to be derived from some normally occurring organelle. The depth of our ignorance concerning these structures is, in part, owing to the lack of adequate experimental models. While various fibrillary alterations have been experimentally induced in different laboratory animals, it should be noted that the characteristic "twisted tubule" of Alzheimer-type neurofibrillary tangles has not been reported in animals.

*References*

Hirano, A. Neurofibrillary Changes in Conditions Related to Alzheimer's Disease. Ciba Foundation Symposium. Alzheimer's Disease and Related Conditions. (G.E.W. Wolstenholme and M. O'Connor, eds.). Churchill (London, 1970), p. 185.

Terry, R. D. The Fine Structure of Neurofibrillary Tangles in Alzheimer's Disease. J. Neuropath. & Exper. Neurol. 32: 629, 1963.

Wisniewski, H., R. D. Terry, and A. Hirano. Neurofibrillary Pathology. J. Neuropath. & Exper. Neurol. 29: 163, 1970.

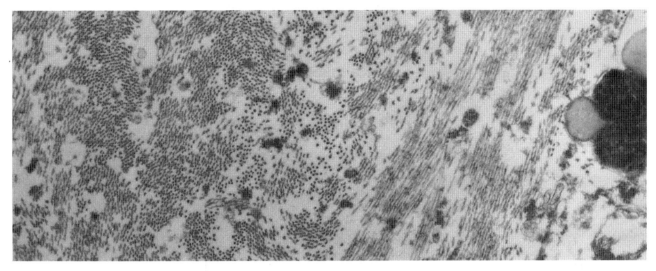

Fig. 159a. Electronmicrograph of a NF tangle and a melanin deposit in the perikaryon of a neuron in locus caeruleus of a case of postencephalitic parkinsonism × 24,000 (Hirano, in Progress in Neuropathology, Vol. I. (H. M. Zimmerman, ed.). Grune and Stratton (New York, 1971), p. 1.)

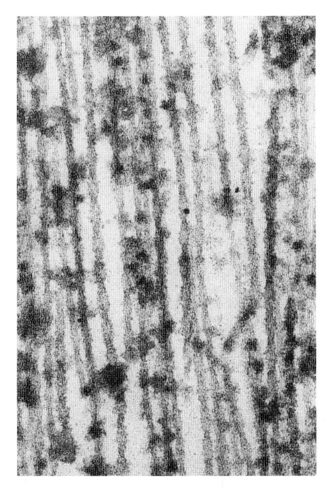

Fig. 159b. Electronmicrograph of longitudinal sections through the twisted tubule of NF tangle × 112,000

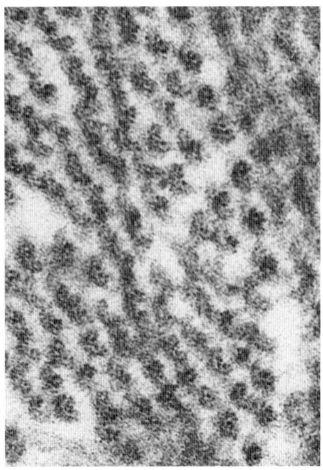

Fig. 159c. Electronmicrograph of cross and oblique sections through the twisted tubule of a NF tangle × 320,000

## Granulovacuolar Bodies in Electron Microscopy

Electron microscopic study has revealed that the granulovacuolar bodies (GV) consist of a membrane-bounded vacuole containing a highly osmiophilic granular core (Fig. 160). Except for the core, the vacuole appears empty.

The nature and origin of these bodies as well as their role in the disease process is still obscure but their morphology suggests a lysosomal nature.

*Reference*

Hirano, A., H. M. Dembitzer, L. T. Kurland, and H. M. Zimmerman. The Fine Structure of Some Intra-ganglionic Alterations. J. Neuropath. and Exper. Neurol. 27: 167, 1968.

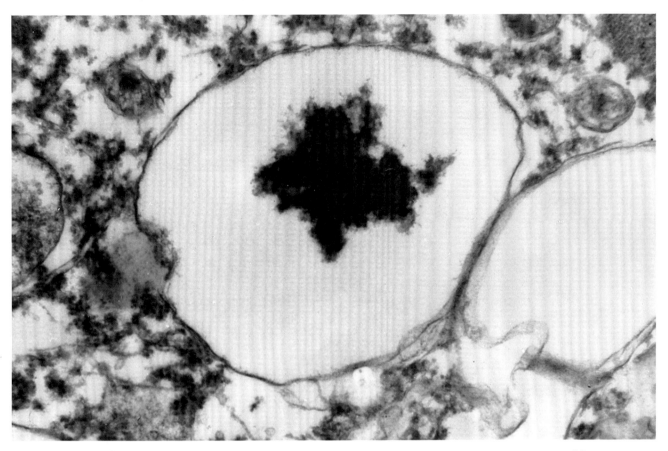

Fig. 160. Electronmicrograph of a GV body in a pyramidal cell of Sommer's sector × 45,000 (Hirano, J. Neuropathol. Exper. Neurol. 27: 167, 1968)

## The Eosinophilic Rod-Like Inclusion in Light and Electron Microscopy
## (Hirano Body)

Eosinophilic rod-like inclusions may be found in both the normal aged brain and in a variety of degenerative diseases, such as Alzheimer's disease, Pick's disease, parkinsonism-dementia complex on Guam, etc. For the most part, this alteration is confined to Sommer's sector and immediately adjacent areas but on rare occasions has been seen in other areas as well.

In the optical microscope, it is rod-like in shape and of indeterminate length (Fig. 161a), appearing strongly eosinophilic and refractile. As revealed by the electron microscope, the structure is intracytoplasmic and consists of a layered arrangement of electron dense lines about 100–150 Å thick, interspersed with layers of regularly arranged circular densities about 60–100 Å in diameter (Fig. 161b). In some sections, the structures display a herringbone-like pattern or a lattice-like structure. The origin and precise nature of this structure remains to be clarified.

### References

Hirano, A. Pathology of Amyotrophic Lateral Sclerosis, in Slow, Latent, and Temperate Virus Infections. (D. C. Gajdusek, and C. J. Gibbs, Jr., eds.) NINDB Monograph No. 2, National Institutes of Health (Washington, 1965), p. 23.

Hirano, A. Progress in the Pathology of Motor Neuron Disease. Progress in Neuropathology, Vol. II. (H. M. Zimmerman, ed.) Grune and Stratton (New York, 1973), p. 181.

Schochet, S. S., Jr., P. O. Lampert, and R. Lindenberg. Fine Structure of the Pick and Hirano Bodies in a Case of Pick's Disease. Acta. Neuropath. 11: 330, 1968.

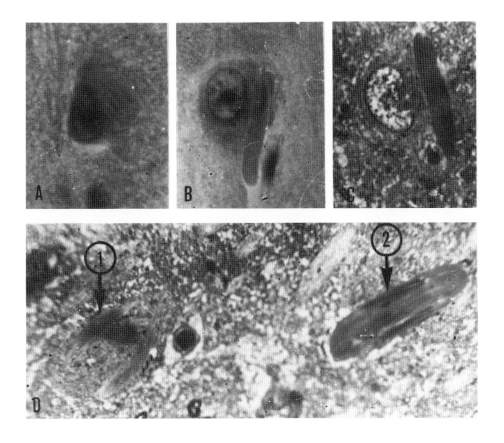

Fig. 161a. Eosinophilic rod-like structures in Sommer's sector; rods may be found
either in the perikaryon (A, D1) or in the processes (B, C, D2) × 1,000 A and B:
paraffin embedded H and E; C and D: epon embedded; toluidine blue
(Hirano et al., J. Neuropathol. Exper. Neurol. 27: 167, 1968)

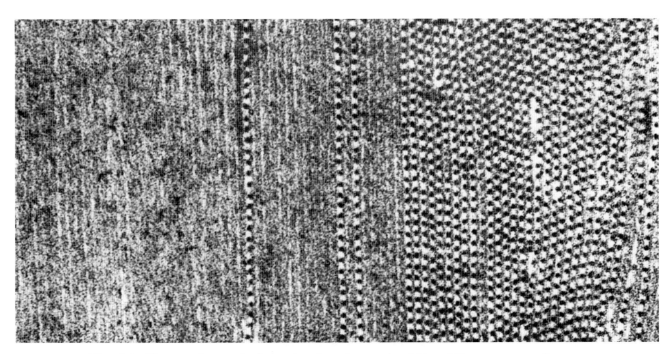

Fig. 161b. Electronmicrograph of a section through an eosinophilic rod-like structure × 165,000

## Alzheimer's Disease and Down's Syndrome

Although the etiology of Alzheimer's disease remains unknown, recently reported findings of an association with Down's syndrome suggest the possible role of a fundamental alteration of the chromosomal state in Alzheimer's disease.

In the accompanying Table, a survey of the incidence of the neuropathologic changes characteristic of Alzheimer's disease in a series of cases of Down's syndrome is compared with that in a miscellaneous group of mental retardation without Down's syndrome. It can be seen that in all patients with Down's syndrome who have survived past age forty, there were changes of Alzheimer's disease, usually of severe degree. By contrast, the group without Down's syndrome showed only occasionally, and at that mild changes, that were limited to a small number of patients of very advanced age. It suggests that the chromosomal abnormalities in Down's syndrome might predispose to development of the neuropathologic changes characteristic of Alzheimer's disease.

The following case serves as an illustration:

*Case:* A 51-year-old man had been an inmate of an institution for the feeble-minded since childhood. He showed the typical features of Down's syndrome. One year before his death there was a noticeable clinical change: he developed epileptic seizures, aged prematurely, and deteriorated rapidly.

The brain showed malformation of the convolutional pattern of the type commonly seen in cases of Down's syndrome that was partly obscured by superimposed signs of diffuse severe cortical atrophy (Fig. 162a).

Microscopically, countless senile plaques and neurofibrillary tangles were present throughout the cortex (Fig. 162b), while granulovacuolar bodies were noted only in the hippocampus.

*Reference*

Jervis, G. A. Early Senile Dementia in Mongoloid Idiocy. Am. J. Psychiat. 105: 102, 1948.
Malamud, N. Neuropathology of Organic Brain Syndromes Associated with Aging. Aging and the Brain. Plenum Publishing Corp. (New York, 1972), pp. 63–87.

| Type | Total No. Cases | Below Age 40 | No. Cases with AD | Above Age 40 | No. Cases with AD |
|------|-----------------|--------------|-------------------|--------------|-------------------|
| MR with Down's Syndrome | 347 | 312 | 5 (1.6%) * | 35 | 35 (100%) ** |
| MR without Down's Syndrome | 813 | 588 | 0 | 225 | 31 (14%) *** |

\* Age range 20-38: all with mild changes of AD.

\*\* Age range 42-69: 60% with severe, 40% with moderate changes of AD.

\*\*\* Age range 54-86: all with mild changes of AD.

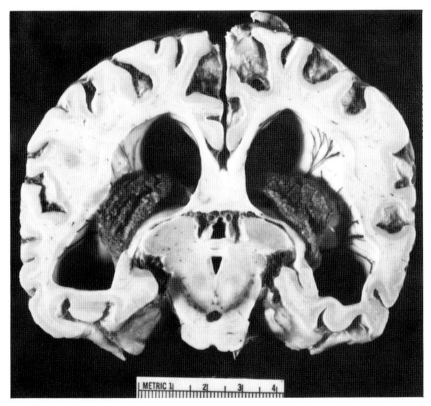

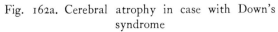

Fig. 162a. Cerebral atrophy in case with Down's syndrome

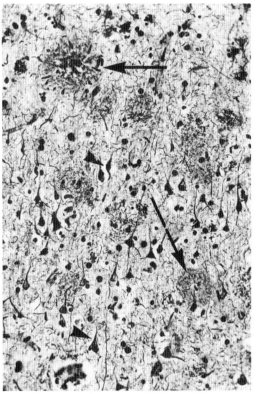

Fig. 162b. von Braunmühl × 200

Pick's disease, also known as lobar atrophy, is a relatively rare disorder, usually occurring at a middle age range of forty to sixty years and therefore often classified as a form of pre-senile dementia. It is clinically manifested by progressive dementia, in which however memory impairment is not a feature, and well-defined symptoms of aphasia, apraxia, or agnosia. There is strong evidence of a Mendelian dominant autosomal mode of inheritance.

Pathologically, the consistent finding is sharply circumscribed atrophy involving symmetrical parts of the frontal, temporal, and parietal lobes, singly or in various combinations. The selection of areas of atrophy is in the phylogenetically recently acquired, while sparing the older sensori-motor, regions. The virtual sparing of the hippocampal formation might be correlated with the preservation of recent and retentive memory.

Microscopically, nonspecific degeneration of the cortex is associated with argyrophilic inclusions in inflated neurons (Pick cells). There is absence of senile plaques, neurofibrillary tangles, or granulovacuolar changes.

*Case:* A 24-year-old man developed over a period of about a year increasing signs of emotional apathy and reduction in spontaneous speech and activity. On initial examination general orientation and memory were intact, but impairment of abstract thinking was evident from the psychologic tests. A pneumoencephalogram showed evidence of atrophy of the frontal lobes. In the next two years there was rapidly progressive deterioration. Toward the end, examination disclosed aphasia, apraxia, agnosia, echolalia, festinating gait, and cogwheel rigidity. The family history revealed the same disease in an older brother and in the mother.

The brain showed circumscribed atrophy of parts of the frontal, temporal, and parietal lobes, sparing the major parts of the superior temporal, pre- and postcentral gyri, and the occipital lobes (Fig. 163a).

Microscopically, Nissl preparations showed reduction in neurons, associated with increase in reactive glia, most marked in the supragranular layers of the cortex (Fig. 163b). In higher magnifications, there were scattered large swollen neurons showing chromatolysis and eccentricity of nuclei (Fig. 163c) that in silver nitrate preparations demonstrated argentophilic inclusions in the absence of senile plaques or neurofibrillary tangles (Fig. 163d).

Electron microscopic studies of the argyrophilic inclusions in biopsied material have revealed the presence of ribosomes, vesicles, lipochrome and microtubules in addition to the 100 Å neurofilaments but not "twisted tubules." Some authors consider the inclusions similar to the alterations observed in chromatolysis.

*References*

Brion, S., J. Mikol., and Psimaras. Recent Findings in Pick's Disease. Progress in Neuropathology, Vol. 2 (H. M. Zimmerman, ed.). Grune and Stratton (New York, 1973), p. 421.

Malamud, N., and R. W. Waggoner. Generalogic and Clinicopathologic Study of Pick's Disease. Arch. Neurol. and Psychiat. 50: 288–303, 1943.

Wisniewski, H. M., J. M. Coblentz, and R. D. Terry. Pick's Disease. A Clinical and Ultrastructural Study. Arch. Neurol. 26: 97, 1972.

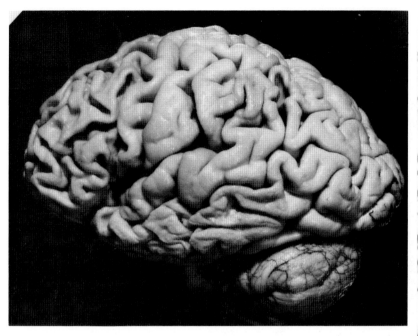

Fig. 163a. Cerebral atrophy in Pick's disease

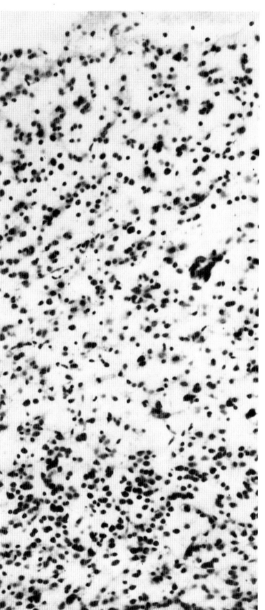

Fig. 163b. Nissl × 140

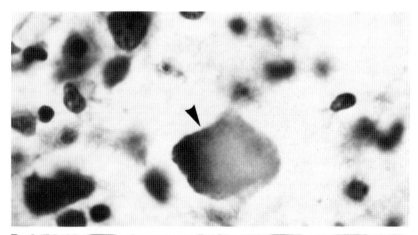

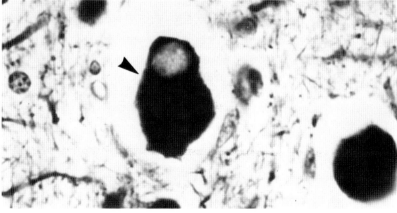

Fig. 163c. Nissl × 720 (above)
Fig. 163d. von Braunmühl × 720 (below)

First reported by Creutzfeldt in 1920 and later more completely described by Jakob in 1921–1923, this is a relatively uncommon disorder. It has been included with the presenile dementias because of predominant occurrence of dementia in an age range of forty to sixty years. There has been some controversy with respect to its nosologic position, yet there is ground for accepting it as a clinicopathologic entity.

The clinical course is comparatively rapid, varying from several months to a few years. It is characterized by progressive dementia in combination with various sensorimotor disturbances involving pyramidal, extrapyramidal, lower motor neuron, cerebellar, and visual systems. A characteristic change in the electroencephalogram has been reported in the form of synchronous bursts of slow waves with repetitive spike and wave activity.

Corresponding pathologic changes occur that have a predilection for either motor or sensory cortex, basal ganglia, cerebellum, brain stem and/or spinal cord. The histologic picture is dominated by a spongy type of degeneration, with or without astroglial reaction, depending on its degree, that at times is accompanied by inflated neurons, yet lacking the specific argyrophilic changes characterizing Alzheimer's and Pick's diseases.

The etiology has remained unknown, the majority of cases being sporadic while a few are familial. Whatever biochemical changes found have been considered to be secondary. Recent experimental work has directed attention to a transmissible agent, possibly in the nature of a slow acting virus.

The accompanying Table lists the clinicopathologic variants that may be included under the term of Creutzfeldt-Jakob's disease. These are illustrated by the following four cases:

### Corticostriatocerebellar form:

*Case:* A 62-year-old man was well until July 1968 when, following a minor head injury, he developed rapidly increasing mental confusion, impairment of recent memory, ataxia, vertigo, and involuntary tremors. Examination in September of 1968 revealed difficulty with mentation; hyperactive deep tendon reflexes; unsustained clonus in the right foot; diminished superficial abdominal reflexes; past pointing of the upper extremities and dysmetria in the lower extremities; a positive Romberg's sign; and bilateral horizontal and vertical nystagmus on lateral gaze. Cerebrospinal fluid examination was normal. An angiogram and pneumoencephalogram were negative; an electroencephalogram was "abnormal." Three months later he became mute, unable to swallow foods, showed marked spasticity, a palmomental reflex, and a right homonymous hemianopsia. He died in April of 1969, approximately nine months following the onset.

The brain showed diffuse atrophy of the cerebral cortex, with accentuation in frontal lobes, corpus striatum and cerebellar cortex, associated with corresponding dilatation of the ventricular system (Fig. 164a).

Microscopically, a diffuse spongy state was present in the cortex and striatum, with innumerable vacuoles occurring both around and between neurons (Fig. 164b). In higher magnifications, inflated neurons with central chromatolysis and eccentric nuclei were scattered amongst others showing nonspecific changes, accompanied by few reacting micro- and astroglia (Fig. 164c). The cerebellar folia showed severe degeneration that was especially pronounced in the granular layer, where a similar spongy state could be demonstrated (Fig. 164d).

TABLE. 32 CASES OF CREUTZFELDT-JAKOB'S DISEASE

| Predominant Clinical Signs and Symptoms | Predominant Pathology | Number of Cases |
|---|---|---|
| 1. Dementia | Cortex - diffuse | 9 |
| 2. Dementia with amaurosis & with myoclonus | Cortex - parieto-occipital | 4 |
| 3. Dementia with motor neuron disease | Cortex - diffuse; upper or lower motor neuron | 7 |
| 4. Dementia with Parkinsonism or chorea | Cortex - diffuse; (basal ganglia - striatum, thalamus, substantia nigra) | 4 |
| 5. Dementia with ataxia | Cortex - diffuse; cerebellum | 8 |

Sex: M 22, F 10    Duration: range 4 mos. - 5 yrs.
                               average 20 mos.

Age: range 43 - 86 yrs.
     average 58 yrs.

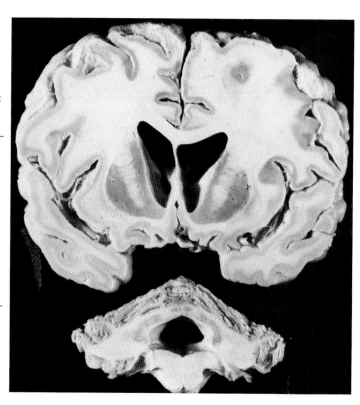

Fig. 164a. Corticostriatocerebellar form of Creutzfeldt-Jakob's disease

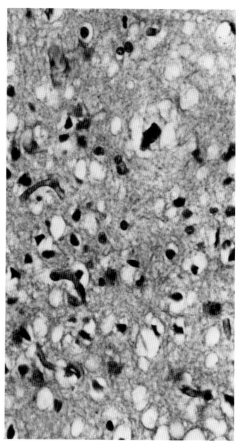

Fig. 164b. LFB-PAS × 310

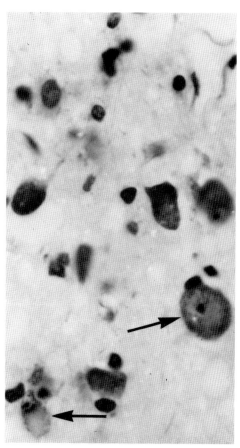

Fig. 164c. Nissl × 560

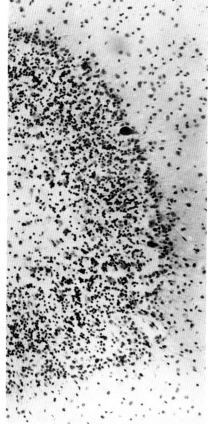

Fig. 164d. Nissl × 100

## Corticoparieto-occipital (Heidenhain's) form:

*Case:* An 86-year-old man was admitted to a hospital on February 15, 1962 because of rapid development of aphasia and mental confusion in the course of one month. There was evidence of gross visual impairment and bilateral positive Hoffmann's signs. Cerebrospinal fluid contained 87 mg % of total protein and showed a gold curve of 1122110000. A pneumoencephalogram revealed evidence of diffuse cerebral atrophy. An electroencephalogram showed dysrhythmic spike and slow wave discharges which were nonfocal. He later developed involuntary rhythmic myoclonic movements. His further course was one of progressive decline and he expired on June 2, 1962, approximately four months following the onset.

The most significant gross changes were severe atrophy of the cortex in posterior parietal and occipital regions, including the calcarine areas (Fig. 165a). The microscopic changes were spongy degeneration throughout all layers of the atrophic cortex with astroglial response only in the less vacuolated areas (Fig. 165b).

## Corticospinal form:

*Case:* A 53-year-old man had a six months' history of personality changes followed by generalized weakness, especially of the left leg. On admission to a hospital, examination revealed hyperactive deep tendon reflexes in the left lower extremity, associated with a Babinski sign, and with diminished abdominal reflexes on that side. A lumbar puncture disclosed a total protein of 60 mg %, and a colloidal gold curve of 1122111000. An electromyogram showed scattered denervation fibrillations as evidence of lower motor neuron disease, in recordings from various muscles of both upper and lower extremities. One year later the patient began experiencing episodes of mental confusion. The weakness had now progressed to involve all limbs, and fasciculations were present in many muscle groups. Subsequently, bulbar signs of dysarthria, dysphagia, and drooling developed. He became intermittently incontinent. In a repeat spinal fluid, total protein determination was 75 mg %. The patient died following an illness of three years.

The brain was grossly unremarkable.

Microscopically, a spongy state was noted in many areas of the cerebral cortex, often characterized by pseudolaminar distribution in layers II and III (Fig. 165c). A striking change involved the entire upper and lower motor neuron system, including the Betz cell region of the motor cortex, the pyramidal tracts in the medulla (Fig. 165d) and throughout the spinal cord, the motor cranial nuclei of VII, X and XII, and the anterior horn cells of the spinal cord.

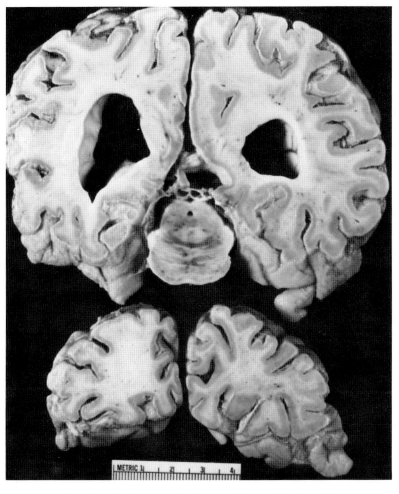

Fig. 165a. Parietooccipital form of Creutzfeldt-Jakob's
disease

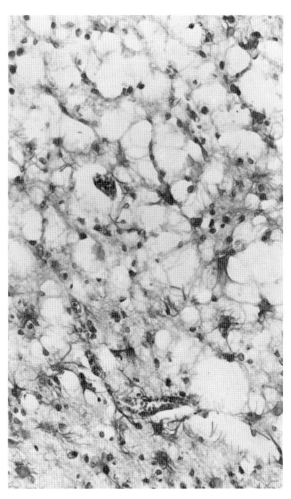

Fig. 165b. Holzer × 100

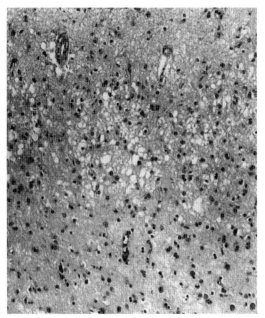

Fig. 165c. HE × 80

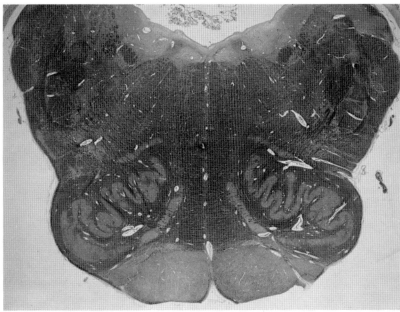

Fig. 165d. Weil stain of medulla

## Corticonigral form:

*Case:* A 55-year-old man developed over a period of six months increasing tremor of the left hand, difficulty with position sense of the left leg and hand. On examination he tended to drag his left leg; there was a positive Romberg sign and reflexes of the left lower extremity were increased. Carotid arteriograms were negative; a pneumoencephalogram showed evidence of cortical atrophy, but a biopsy from the right frontal lobe was inconclusive. Later, he showed signs of dementia, marked rigidity in all extremities, more on the left side, with cogwheel rigidity of the left hand and forced grasping of the right hand. He became bedridden, incontinent, and expired approximately two and one-half years following onset of his symptoms.

The brain showed mild to moderate diffuse atrophy of the cortex, that was most marked in the parasagittal parietal regions, along with bilateral atrophy and loss of pigment in the substantia nigra (Fig. 166a).

Microscopically, the atrophic cortex showed a pseudolaminar spongy state, predominantly in the upper layers (Fig. 166b) that under higher magnification contained inflated pale neurons, undergoing chromatolysis, along with others showing nonspecific changes, associated with moderate astro- and microglial reaction (Fig. 166c). The substantia nigra was depleted of neurons, some of the melanin pigment being taken up by reactive phagocytes, while the remaining neurons showed the same tendency to swelling and chromatolysis as in the cortex (Fig. 166d).

It appeared that the same criteria of spongy degeneration with inflated neurons, previously outlined, applied equally to this case, although it closely resembled the syndrome recently reported by Rebeiz, et al., as a separate entity.

*References*

Brownell, B., and D. R. Oppenheimer. An Ataxic Form of Subacute Presenile Polioencephalopathy (Creutzfeldt-Jakob's Disease). J. Neurol. Neurosurg. Psychiat. 28: 350, 1965.
Kirschbaum, W. R. Jakob-Creutzfeldt Disease. New York, American Elsevier Pub. Co. 1968.
Nevin, S., W. H. McMenemey, S. Behrman, and D. P. Jones. A Subacute Form of Encephalopathy Attributable to Vascular Dysfunction. Brain. 83: 519, 1960.
Rebeiz, J. J., E. H. Kolodny, and E. P. Richardson. Corticodentatonigral Degeneration with Neuronal Achromasia. Arch. Neurol. 18: 20, 1968.
Siedler, H., and N. Malamud. Creutzfeldt-Jakob's Disease. J. Neuropath. and Expt. Neurol. 22: 381–402, 1963.

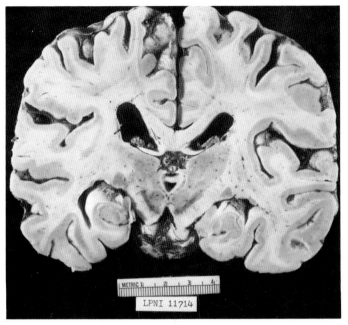

Fig. 166a. Corticonigral form of Creutzfeldt-Jakob's disease

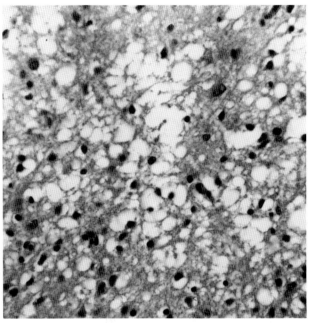

Fig. 166b. HE × 250

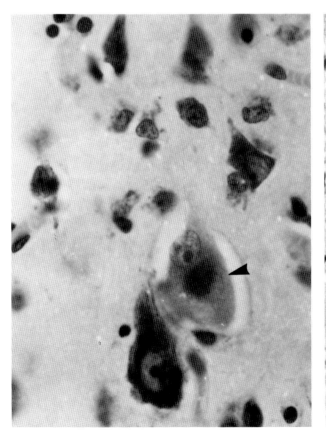

Fig. 166c. Nissl × 560

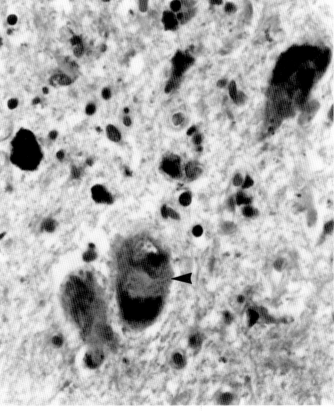

Fig. 166d. HE × 560

## Creutzfeldt-Jakob's Disease in Electron Microscopy

In the electron microscope, the spongy change of Creutzfeldt-Jakob's disease is seen to be a vacuolation within neurons and astrocytes. The vacuoles are electronlucent and often membrane-bounded (Fig. 167). In neurons, many of the vacuoles comprise an entire, distended synaptic terminal and the limiting membrane is actually the plasma membrane itself. Reactive astrocytes are swollen and similar to those found in other conditions as well. They contain excessive accumulations of glial fibrils, lipid granules, glycogen granules, etc. Occasionally, distended neuronal processes contain accumulations of mitochondria, some of which appear altered; dense bodies, fibrillary material; and synaptic vesicles either with, or without, dense cores.

Both neurological and histological abnormalities have been induced after prolonged incubation in chimpanzees following inoculation with brain tissue of patients with Creutzfeldt-Jakob's disease. On this basis, a "slow acting" viral etiology has been postulated for this disease. Subsequently, Lampert found "curled membranous fragments" within the cortical vacuoles similar to those which had previously been found in chimpanzees inoculated with material from patients with Kuru's disease, also attributed to infection by a so-called "slow" virus. In addition, some authors have reported the presence of small particles which they interpreted as viral-like in nature.

*References*

Bignami, A., and L. S. Forno. Status Spongiosus in Jakob-Creutzfeldt Disease. Electron Microscopic Study of a Cortical Biopsy. Brain. 93: 89, 1970.

Bots, G. Th. A.M. Virus-like Particles in Creutzfeldt-Jakob Disease. Acta Neuropath. 18: 267, 1971.

Chou, S. M., and J. D. Martin. Kuru-plaques in a Case of Creutzfeldt-Jakob Disease. Acta Neuropath. 17: 150, 1971.

Gonatas, N. K., R. D. Terry, and M. Weiss. Electron Microscopy Study in Two Cases of Jakob-Creutzfeldt Disease. J. Neuropath and Exper. Neurol. 24: 575, 1965.

Hirano, A., N. R. Ghatck, A. B. Johnson, M. J. Partnow, and A. J. Gomori. Argentophilic Plaques in Creutzfeldt-Jakob Disease. Arch. Neurol. 26: 530, 1972.

Lampert, P. W., D. C. Gajdusek, and C. J. Gibbs, Jr. Experimental Spongiform Encephalopathy (Creutzfeldt-Jakob Disease) in Chimpanzees. J. Neuropath. and Exper. Neurol. 30: 20, 1971.

Vernon, M. L., L. Horta-Barbos, D. A. Fuccillo, J. L. Sever, J. R. Baringer, and G. Birnbaum. Virus-like Particles and Neucleo-Protein-type Filaments in Brain Tissue from Two Patients with Creutzfeldt-Jakob Disease. Lancet. 1: 964, 1970.

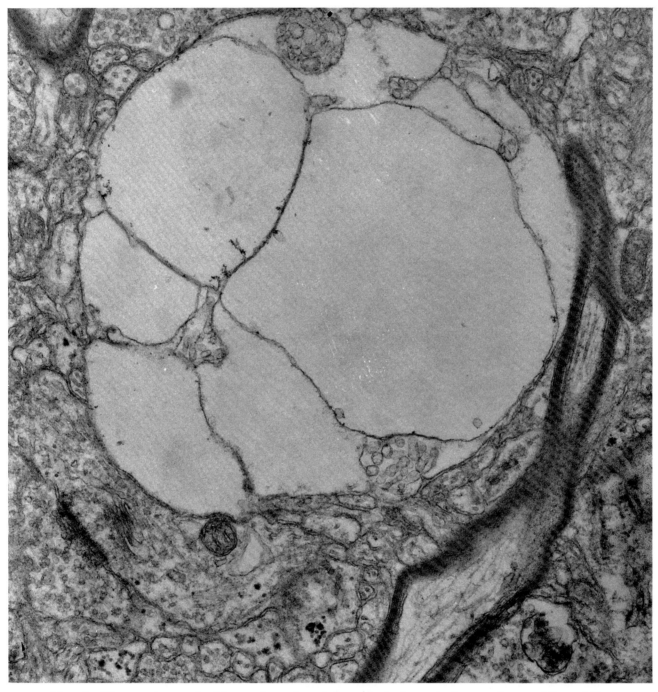

Fig. 167. Electronmicrograph of the membrane-bounded vacuoles in the cerebral cortex of a case of Creutzfeldt-Jakob's disease × 40,000

Degenerative diseases of the extrapyramidal system comprise a group of disorders in which the clinical picture is dominated by chorea, athetosis, ballismus, dystonia and parkinsonism, and in which the pathoanatomic findings predominate either in the basal ganglia, sub-thalamic nucleus and/or substantia nigra.

## HUNTINGTON'S CHOREA

Huntington's chorea is a relatively common hereditary disorder that occurs predominantly in middle age, although there are rare instances of juvenile and senile forms. It is inherited as a Mendelian single dominant autosomal gene, although there are occasional sporadic cases, presumably due to mutations. The clinical manifestations are dominated by choreo-athetoid involuntary movements, although akinetic forms may occur, and by signs of mental deterioration. The pathology is consistently one of slowly progressive degeneration of the neurons of the caudate and putamen nuclei, less often of the globus pallidus, and inconstantly and relatively mildly of the cerebral cortex. The "butterfly" shape of the lateral ventricles in pneumoencephalograms is especially noteworthy. There are no known biochemical changes other than those secondary to the degenerative process.

> *Case:* A 52-year-old man had had a history of frequent falling and inability to stand or sit since the age of forty-seven. When admitted to the hospital, he exhibited purposeless choreiform movements that interfered with all voluntary actions, including speech. The mental status was not grossly remarkable although difficult to test. The maternal great grandmother, grand-mother, mother, two sisters, and one brother died of the same disease.

The brain showed symmetrical atrophy of the caudate and putamen nuclei, and mild atrophy of the cerebral cortex, with proportionate enlargement of the lateral ventricles (Fig. 168a).

In Nissl preparations, a diffuse loss of neurons, especially of the small nerve cells (Fig. 168b), corresponded to proliferation in Holzer preparations of reactive astrocytes and of gliosis of the scattered nerve bundles (Fig. 168c).

In the cerebral cortex, the cytoarchitecture was moderately disorganized; the neurons were decreased, with the remaining nerve cells showing shrinkage and hyperchromatosis, accompanied by only mild increase in glial nuclei (Fig. 168d).

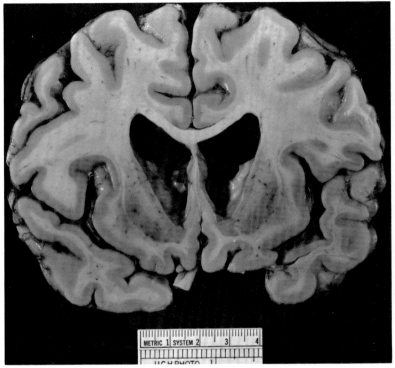

Fig. 168a. Cerebral atrophy in Huntington's chorea

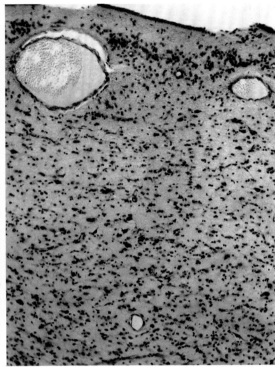

Fig. 168b. Nissl × 100

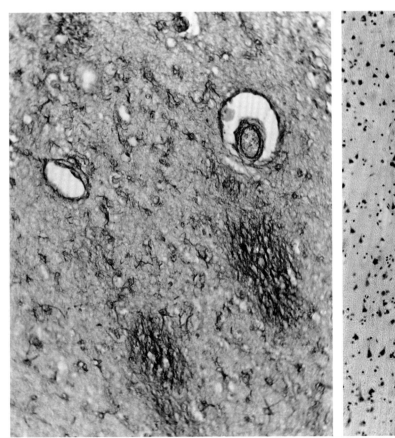

Fig. 168c. Holzer × 200

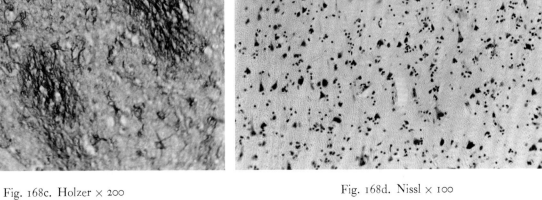

Fig. 168d. Nissl × 100

A unique disorder, characterized clinically by a syndrome of biballismus and pathologically by exclusive degeneration of the subthalamic bodies, serves to illustrate the clinical effects of a lesion in the latter location and the differential diagnosis from Huntington's chorea.

*Case;* A 36-year-old woman, whose family history, though meagre, was reportedly negative, had a two-year history of increasing disturbance of gait and movement. While walking, her legs would suddenly fly out from under her and she would fall flat to the ground. Later the upper extremities were also affected and she would constantly drop objects. As the disease progressed, she began to experience difficulty in swallowing, became more irritable and at times was incontinent. On admission, examination revealed no definite evidence of dementia. Her speech was hesitant, and there was an occasional involuntary tremor about the mouth. The most noteworthy features were gross explosive movements of the trunk, arms, and legs, which appeared suddenly in a sitting position. At times, they were described as writhing with flailing of the extremities, at others as jerking movements. The deep reflexes were hyperactive, but there were no other neurologic signs. All laboratory studies, including examination of the cerebrospinal fluid, pneumoencephalography, and electroencephalography, were negative. Her course was progressively downhill, and she died of bronchopneumonia at the age of thirty-six, four years following the onset of her illness.

The brain showed no gross abnormalities other than symmetrical atrophy and discoloration of the subthalamic bodies in the presence of normal appearance of the basal ganglia, cerebral cortex, and the size of the ventricles (Fig. 169a).

Myelin stains confirmed the marked loss of myelin confined to the subthalamic body (SB) (Fig. 169b), contrasting with the normal appearance of surrounding structures. It was reflected in the virtual disappearance of the neurons, with only a few remaining sclerotic forms (Fig. 169c).

*Reference*

Malamud, N., and N. Demmy: Degenerative Disease of the Subthalamic Bodies. J. Neuropath. and Exper. Neurol. 19: 96, 1960.

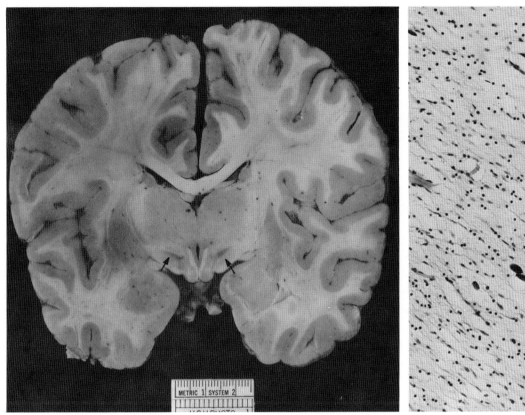

Fig. 169a. Bilateral atrophy of subthalamic bodies

Fig. 169c. Nissl × 105

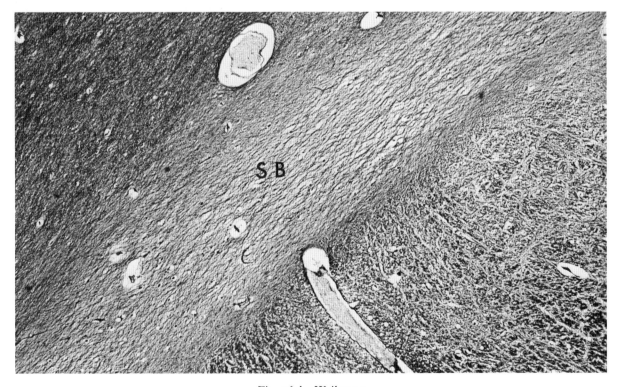

S B

Fig. 169b. Weil × 35

Parkinson's disease, as a primary degenerative form, is to be distinguished from conditions in which symptoms of parkinsonism occur in the course of other disorders, although such separation has remained ill defined. The most likely area of confusion concerns the post-encephalitic form because the history of encephalitis is often vague and because of a long latent interval before Parkinsonian symptoms appear. Recent statistics give a ratio of approximately 85% of the degenerative or idiopathic form to 15% of the postencephalitic and other rare acquired conditions.

The clinical features are characterized by an akinetic syndrome in which rigidity, loss of associated movements, and disturbances of posture are associated with a tremor at rest.

The pathologic features have increasingly focused attention on the substantia nigra as the main source of the syndrome, being often the only noteworthy lesion, although at times combined with changes in the basal ganglia. The recent formulation of parkinsonism as essentially a striatal dopamine deficiency syndrome has established a correlation between the degree of cell loss in the substantia nigra and the degree of chemical deficiency.

The histopathology of Parkinson's disease has been the subject of some controversy. On the one hand, the idiopathic form has been for many years characterized by intracytoplasmic inclusions, known as Lewy bodies (Fig. 170a), as a distinguishing feature from the post-encephalitic form in which neurofibrillary tangles of Alzheimer are commonly found (Fig. 170b). Others have disputed the claim that these findings are pathognomonic signs. Such difficulties are however understandable, being inherent in the lack of adequate historical information. Nevertheless, analysis of the findings in a large series of cases lends itself to fairly close clinicopathologic correlation, as illustrated in the accompanying Table. It can be seen that Lewy bodies were found in over 90% of cases clinically diagnosed as idiopathic, and neurofibrillary changes in 75% of cases diagnosed postencephalitic. The group showing neither change must be interpreted with caution since the demonstration of the usually sparse cellular changes require more exhaustive search than was undertaken. The group characterized as strionigral degeneration is known to lack either of the specific cellular changes.

Lewy bodies are hyaline intracytoplasmic masses, single or multiple, varying in size from 5–25 $\mu$, that may or may not be laminated and that stain positively with hematoxylin-eosin, Lendrum's phloxine-tartrazine, and a number of other methods. They are distributed largely in the melanin-bearing cells of the substantia nigra and locus caeruleus but also in the dorsal motor nucleus of the vagus and substantia innominata. They have been found on occasion in normal controls, at advanced age.

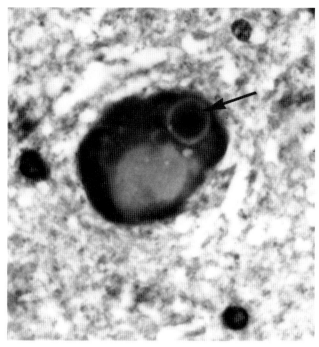

Fig. 170a. He × 900          Fig. 170b. HE × 900

TABLE. 100 CASES OF PARKINSONISM

|  |  | No. Cases | Clinical Diagnosis | Sex Distribution | |
|---|---|---|---|---|---|
| A. | Nigral Degeneration with Lewy Bodies | 46 | 43 Id. | M | 42 |
|  |  |  | 3 P.E. | F | 4 |
| B. | Nigral Degeneration with Neurofibrillary Changes | 19 | 5 Id. | M | 10 |
|  |  |  | 14 P.E. | F | 9 |
| C. | Nigral Degeneration without A or B | 26 | 12 Id. | M | 17 |
|  |  |  | 14 P.E. | F | 9 |
| D. | Striatonigral Degeneration | 9 | 8 Id. | M | 4 |
|  |  |  | 1 P.E. | F | 5 |

Id.: Idiopathic;   P.E.: Postencephalitic

## Form of Nigral Degeneration with Lewy Bodies

*Case:* A 72-year-old man gave a history of slowly progressive bilateral rigidity, paucity of movement, and left sided resting tremor that never appeared in his right extremities. His symptoms did not respond to various anti-parkinsonian drugs (prior to introduction of L-dopa therapy). He was hospitalized and underwent a right-sided chemopallidectomy using viscid alcohol. Postoperatively, he showed considerable improvement in the general rigidity and complete disappearance of the tremor in the left hand. He returned to work, and performed satisfactorily in his task as a probation officer. Follow-up examinations over a four-year period failed to demonstrate return of his most disabling symptoms on the left side, but he showed a moderate degree of rigidity and akinesia of his right extremities. He expired of an intercurrent infection.

The brain showed grossly depigmentation of the substantia nigra (Fig. 171a) and an old area of necrosis involving the globus pallidus on the right side, at the site of the previous pallidectomy, in the absence of any primary changes in the basal ganglia or other structures (Fig. 171b).

Microscopically, the significant changes were focal reduction in neurons (Fig. 171c) and the presence of Lewy bodies in the substantia nigra and locus caeruleus, characterized by eosinophilic homogeneous inclusions surrounded by halos within surviving melanin-bearing neurons (Fig. 171d).

*References*

Greenfield, J. G. and F. D. Bosanquet: The Brain-Stem Lesions in Parkinsonism. J. Neurol. Neurosurg. and Psychiat. 16: 213, 1953.

Hornykewicz, O. D. Physiologic, Biochemical and Pathological Backgrounds of Levodopa and Possibilities for the Future. Neurol. 20 (No. 12, Part 2): 1, 1970.

With the electron microscope, the fine structure of Lewy bodies consists of essentially two components. The first is a spherical core composed of a dense granular material. The second component consists of filaments of variable thickness radiating out of the core and forming a peripheral zone. Sometimes compactly arranged circular profiles intermingled with filaments may be found in concentric laminae between the core and the peripheral zone.

*Reference*

Duffy, P. O., and V. M. Tennyson. Phase and Electron Microscopic Observations of Lewy Bodies and Melanin Granula in the Substantia Nigra and Locuse Caeruleus in Parkinson's Disease. J. Neuropath. and Exper. Neurol. 26: 345, 1965.

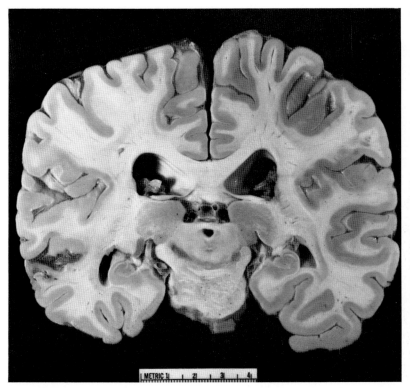

Fig. 171a. Parkinson's disease with depigmentation of substantia nigra

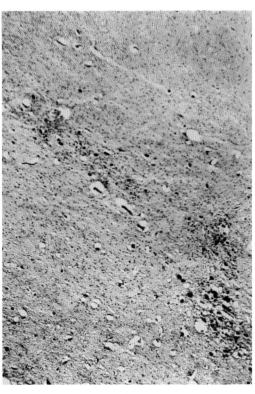

Fig. 171c. Nissl × 44

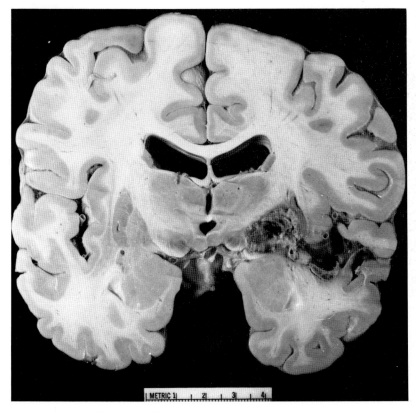

Fig. 171b. Chemopallidectomy, right side

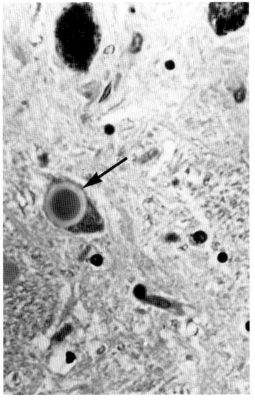

Fig. 171d. HE × 690

## Form of Striatonigral Degeneration

The striatonigral degeneration form of Parkinson's disease is a relatively uncommon condition and appears to be a multisystem disease. Clinically, although the parkinsonian symptoms are prominent, there are often other neurologic manifestations such as cerebellar tremor and ataxia, choreoathetosis, dystonia, pyramidal and pseudobulbar signs, and mental changes. The pathologic findings are most severe in the putamen where atrophy and spongy degeneration are associated with a grayish-green discoloration due to deposits of pigment in astroglia, possibly in the nature of hematin or lipofuscin encrusted with iron, and in the substantia nigra that shows depigmentation but without the specific Lewy bodies. The globus pallidus is also often involved and in addition other areas, especially the olivoponto-cerebellar system. It is thus a distinct clinicopathologic entity and is perhaps more closely related to other forms of multisystem degeneration, especially the cerebellar ataxias.

*Case:* A 61-year-old man developed at the age of fifty-three weakness of the legs and unsteadiness of gait. His condition steadily became worse until four years later when examination revealed rigidity of all extremities, a resting 3 to 5 per second tremor of the fingers, dysarthria, dysphagia, unobtainable deep or superficial reflexes, bilateral Babinski signs and hyperactive jaw jerks. It was believed that his symptoms were due to mixed extrapyramidal and pyramidal involvement, the former predominating. He was treated with various anti-parkinsonian drugs but without significant benefit. A year before his demise he was tried on L-Dopa medication which caused some improvement in the rigidity and dysphagia, however, he finally succumbed to bronchopneumonia.

The gross findings in the brain consisted of bilateral atrophy of the putamen showing grayish-green discoloration, the globus pallidus that appeared deeply brown, the substantia nigra that was depigmented, and the olivopontocerebellar system, reflected in the diffuse demyelination of the cerebellar white matter and atrophy of the brain stem (Fig. 172a).

In myelin preparations, demyelination of the putamen (Fig. 172b) was outstanding, associated with reactive gliosis that extended into the globus pallidus and with granular deposits of pigment in astroglia of the putamen (Fig. 172c).

The substantia nigra showed marked depletion of the melanin-bearing cells, accompanied by reactive gliosis (Fig. 172d).

The pontocerebellar fibers were demyelinated (Fig. 172e) as was the cerebellar white matter. The inferior olives and the olivocerebellar connections showed dense gliosis, reflecting their parenchymal degeneration (Fig. 172f).

*Reference*

Adams, R. D., L. Van Bogaert, and H. van der Ecken. Striatonigral Degeneration. J. Neuropath, and Expt Neurol. 23: 584, 1964.

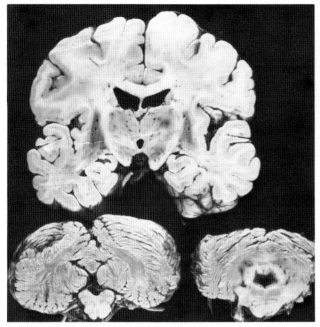

Fig. 172a. Striatonigral degeneration with olivopontocerebellar atrophy

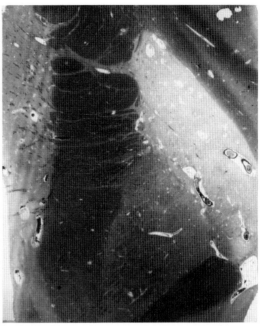

Fig. 172b. Weil stain showing demyelination of
putamen

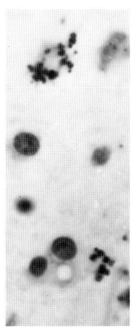

Fig. 172c. Nissl × 900

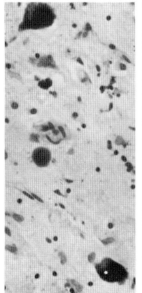

Fig. 172d. Nissl × 225

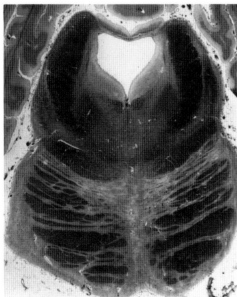

Fig. 172e. Weil stain of pons

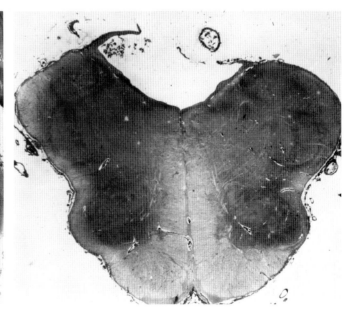

Fig. 172f. Holzer stain of medulla

The primary degenerative disorders of the cerebellum and its connections comprise a great variety of clinical and pathologic types. Schematically, they may be classified into the following clinicopathologic syndromes, allowing for transitions between them:

a) olivopontocerebellar (afferent) form; b) cerebellodentatorubrothalamic (efferent) form; and c) parenchymatous cerebellar form.

Each of these syndromes is known to occur both in children and adults, either as hereditary or sporadic disorders. Clinically, in addition to the prominent cerebellar symptoms, they are apt to show signs of involvement of the extrapyramidal system, optic atrophy, cranial nerve palsies, long tract signs and, on occasion, dementia.

### OLIVOPONTOCEREBELLAR FORM

*Case:* A 21-year-old man gradually developed disturbance in movement of his extremities. Initial examination revealed a broad-based ataxic gait, a head tremor transmitted to the body, scanning speech, heel-to-knee ataxia, and underactive deep reflexes. Later, the ataxia and dysarthria increased in severity, accompanied by coarse intention tremors of all extremities. Toward the end, purposeless movements and cogwheel rigidity supervened. The father and a younger brother of the patient were afflicted with the same disease.

The brain showed severe atrophy of the base of the pons, the cerebellum, and the inferior olives; the cerebral hemispheres appeared normal (Fig. 173a).

Holzer preparations of the pons revealed gliosis of the deep and superficial transverse fibers and of the brachium pontis, while the pyramidal tracts and the tegmentum were uninvolved (Fig. 173b). There was corresponding demyelination in myelin preparations. The inferior olives and connecting fibers through the corpus restiforme showed symmetrical gliosis (Fig. 173c).

In the cerebellum, there was diffuse gliosis of the white matter in both the folia and the central substance, but the gray matter, including the dentate nucleus, was relatively normal (Fig. 173d).

In Nissl preparations, the neurons of the pontile nuclei were replaced by fibrillary astrocytes (Fig. 173e), as were the neurons of the inferior olives.

There was also demyelinization of the posterior columns throughout the spinal cord.

In addition, there were mild to moderate signs of degeneration in the caudate nucleus, substantia nigra, subthalamic body, and medial nucleus of the thalamus. These additional changes accounted for the development of extrapyramidal signs, especially in the late stages of the disease, when they virtually masked the underlying cerebellar symptoms.

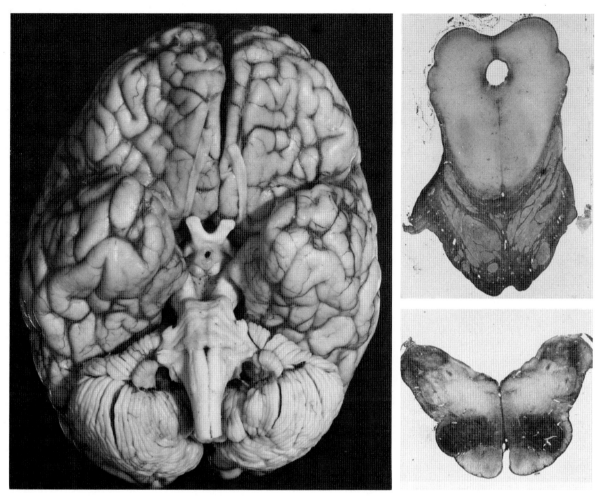

Fig. 173a. Olivopontocerebellar atrophy

Fig. 173b. Holzer stain of pons (above)

Fig. 173c. Holzer stain of medulla (below)

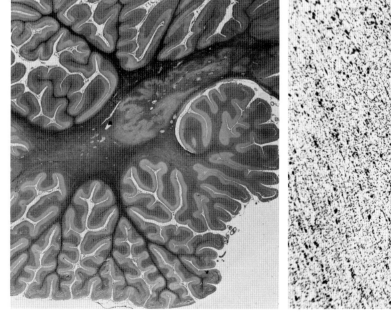

Fig. 173d. Holzer stain of cerebellum

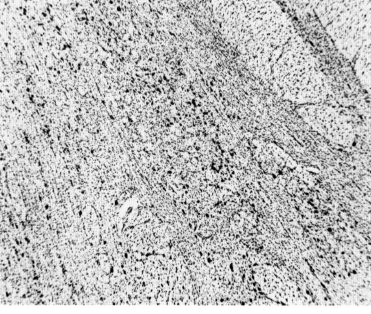

Fig. 173e. Nissl × 40

CEREBELLAR DEGENERATIVE DISORDERS (continued)

CEREBELLODENTATORUBROTHALAMIC FORM

Involvement of the efferent cerebellar system is much less common, but like the olivoponto-cerebellar form, can occur both as an hereditary and sporadic disorder, and, in either case, become associated with extrapyramidal and other signs.

> *Case:* A 7-year-old boy had a normal birth and early development, but at about sixteen months of age, he began to stumble, developed tremors of the arms, medial deviation of the left eye, and attacks of myoclonus. His condition progressed so that he was unable to speak beyond a word or two and got around only by crawling. On examination at the age of three and one-half years, the left eye was deviated medially; intention tremors were noted in the hands; there was marked ataxia on standing with tendency to fall to the left; deep reflexes were active and equal; his mental age was estimated as twenty to twenty-two months. Pneumoencephalography revealed dilatation of the fourth ventricle and of the basal cisterns consistent with cerebellar atrophy. An electroencephalogram showed generalized paroxysmal dysrhythmia of nonspecific type. Cerebrospinal fluid was normal. The further course was one of progressive deterioration. Towards the end, he became incontinent, had difficulty swallowing, the right arm was rigid, there was continuous tremor of the head, left arm and leg, and a mask-like facies was noted. He expired at the age of seven years. A maternal male cousin died of the same disease at the age of seven years (confirmed by autopsy). A detailed genetic study revealed a sex-linked recessive mode of inheritance.

The brain showed grossly diffuse atrophy of the folia of the cerebellum with no trace of the dentate nuclei, and moderate dilatation of the fourth ventricle, while the brain stem and the peduncles appeared normal (Fig. 174a).

In Holzer preparations, there was dense gliosis of the dentate nucleus, moderate gliosis of the cerebellar folia, while the cerebellar white matter was relatively normal (Fig. 174b).

At higher levels, gliosis of the brachium conjunctivum could be traced to the red nuclei that were replaced by dense gliosis (Fig. 174c), to various parts of the thalamus, including its lateral areas (Fig. 174d), and to a lesser degree to the globus pallidus, subthalamic body and optic tracts.

In corresponding Nissl preparations, loss of neurons with reactive proliferation of glia, was most severe in the dentate nucleus (Fig. 174e); in the Purkinje layer of the cerebellum, and in the red nucleus. The inferior olives were the only other structures in the brain stem that were involved, presumably secondary to the cerebellar cortical degeneration.

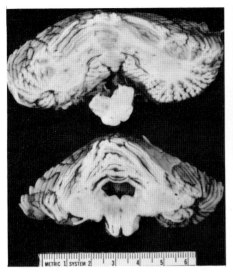

Fig. 174a. Cerebellodentate atrophy

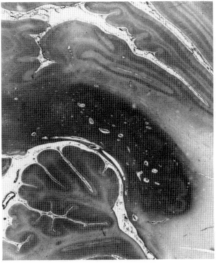

Fig. 174b. Holzer stain, region of dentate nucleus

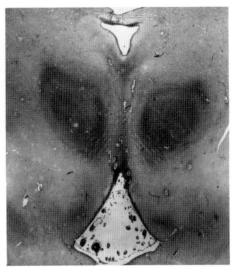

Fig. 174c. Holzer stain, region of red nucleus

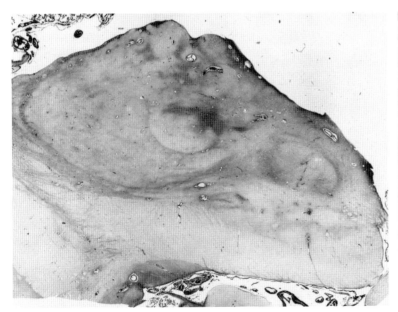

Fig. 174d. Holzer stain, region of thalamus

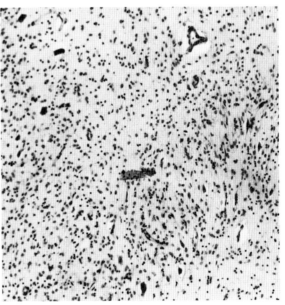

Fig. 174e. Nissl of dentate nucleus × 120

PRIMARY PARENCHYMATOUS CEREBELLAR FORM

Cases in which the principal degeneration occurs in the gray matter of the cerebellum appear to be related to a great variety of causes, some of which are primary, heredofamilial, or sporadic, while others, probably the majority, are caused by acquired nutritional, toxi-infections, anoxic, hyperthermic, and other factors.

The primary degenerative group tends to occur most often in adults past middle age and is thus often referred to as late or delayed cortical cerebellar atrophy. Because of associated degeneration of the inferior olives, whether primary or secondary, it is also termed cere-bello-olivary degeneration. As a rule, the Purkinje layer is predominantly or exclusively involved but there are rare instances in which the maximal degeneration occurs in the granular layer.

> *Case:* A 43-year-old woman had a slowly progressive seven-year history of loss of coordination, staggering, difficulty with speech, and diplopia. The patient's mother had similar symptoms and died at the age of thirty-six. Examination revealed ataxia, dysarthria, dementia, and right-sided hyperactive reflexes with a Babinski sign. Spinal fluid contained a total protein of 61 mg %. She died two years later from bowel perforation complicated by peritonitis.

The only gross abnormality in the brain was diffuse atrophy of the cerebellum that involved the hemispheres and the vermis, without evidence of atrophy of the brain stem or of the cerebral hemispheres (Fig. 175a).

Microscopically, the principal change was noted in the Purkinje layer of the cerebellum which had virtually completely disappeared, leaving behind only an occasional shrunken form, and was accompanied by proliferation of glia in the Bergmann layer, while the granular layer showed only mild rarefaction (Fig. 175b).

The only other structure involved was the inferior olive where neuronal depletion and reactive gliosis corresponded in severity to the degeneration of the Purkinje layer (Fig. 175c).

In this case, as in the other types of cerebellar degeneration, symptoms other than those referable to the cerebellum were present, such as dementia, although the underlying pathology was not always established.

*References*

Greenfield, J. G. Spinocerebellar Degenerations. Chas. C Thomas (Springfield, Ill., 1954).
Malamud, N., and P. Cohen. Unusual Form of Cerebellar Ataxia with Sex-linked Inheritance. Neurol. 8: 261–266, 1958.
Parker, H. L., and J. W. Kernohan. Parenchymatous Cortical Cerebellar Ataxia. Brain. 56: 191, 1933.

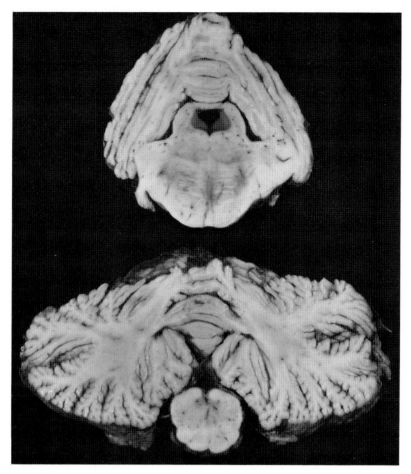

Fig. 175a. Diffuse atrophy of cerebellum

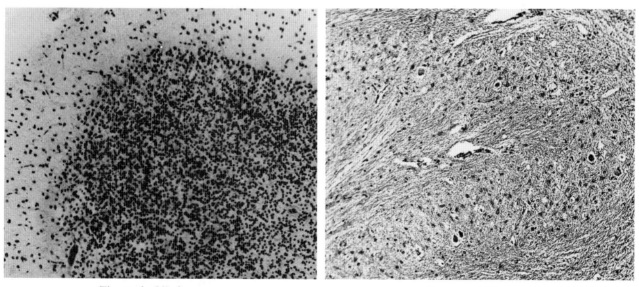

Fig. 175b. Nissl × 140

Fig. 175c. HE × 100

A progressive multisystem neurologic syndrome with either prominent cerebellar or parkinsonian manifestations, associated with orthostatic hypotension and other signs of autonomic insufficiency, was first reported by Shy and Drager. It occurs most often in the fifth to seventh decades of life. The pathologic basis for the orthostatic hypotension is generally attributed to degenerative changes in the intermediolateral horns of the spinal cord. The associated neurologic lesions are variable but the most common are either changes of olivopontocerebellar degeneration or those of parkinsonism.

*Case:* A 54-year-old man had a three-year history of heat intolerance, impotence, and gait disturbances, followed by intention tremor, dysarthria, incontinence, and irregular breathing. Examination revealed ataxia, dysarthria, nystagmus on lateral gaze, paralysis of upward gaze, intention tremor, hyperactive deep tendon reflexes with bilateral Babinskis, orthostatic fall of blood pressure of 50–60 mm Hg, dry and warm skin, irregular respirations, poor rectal sphincter tone, and mild atrophy with impairment of vibratory and position sense, chiefly in the left leg. EMG revealed denervation potentials in the lower extremities. Cardiovascular evaluation disclosed findings of severe autonomic insufficiency; respirations were characterized by brief periods of apnea. Towards the end he developed myoclonus, respiratory arrest, and expired four months following hospitalization.

The gross brain changes were depigmentation of the substantia nigra and signs of olivopontocerebellar atrophy, associated with reduction and demyelination of the cerebellar white matter (Fig. 176a). The cerebral cortex and basal ganglia were not involved in the fundamental disease process but showed evidence of acute anoxic encephalopathy related to the terminal respiratory arrest.

The principal microscopic changes were: olivopontocerebellar atrophy, consisting of demyelination of the transverse pontine fibers (Fig. 176b) associated with degeneration of the pontile nuclei; reactive gliosis to degeneration of the inferior olives (Fig. 176c) and diffuse gliosis of the white matter of the cerebellum in the absence of appreciable changes in its gray matter. In addition there was virtually complete loss of neurons in the intermediolateral horns of the spinal cord, while Clarke's column and the anterior horn cells were only mildly involved (Fig. 176d); the lateral columns of the spinal cord were moderately demyelinated.

*Reference*

Shy, G. M., and G. A. Drager. A Neurological Syndrome Associated with Orthostatic Hypotension. Arch. Neurol. 2: 511, 1960.

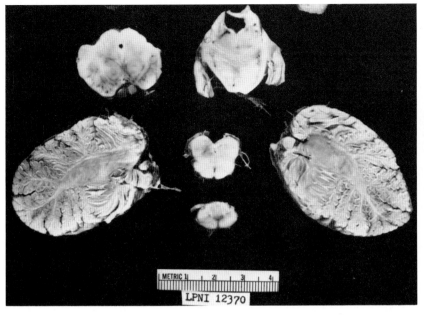
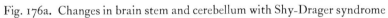

Fig. 176a. Changes in brain stem and cerebellum with Shy-Drager syndrome

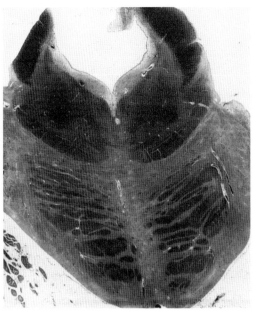

Fig. 176b. Weil stain of pons

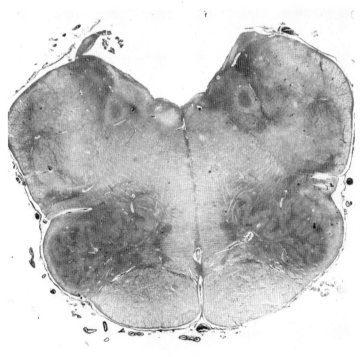

Fig. 176c. Holzer stain of medulla

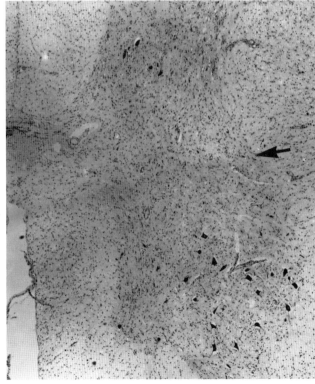

Fig. 176d. Loss of neurons in intermediolateral horns, Nissl × 25

## Neuromuscular Degenerative Disorders

Among the group of neuromyopathies, those of central nervous system origin (so-called motor neuron diseases) consist of the common sporadic form of amyotrophic lateral sclerosis, on the one hand, and the rare hereditary forms, especially that of Werdnig-Hoffmann's disease, on the other.

### Amyotrophic Lateral Sclerosis (ALS): Classic Form

The classic form of ALS is usually a disease of late middle age, occurring sporadically, in the majority of cases, without known etiologic or predisposing factors. It varies in duration from several months to a number of years, with an average of three years. Its clinical manifestations consist of signs of upper and lower motor neuron disease, bulbar and/or spinal. Clinical variants, in the past, have been distinguished as progressive spinal muscular atrophy, bulbar palsy, primary lateral sclerosis and ALS. Their pathology however links them together as one fundamental entity.

Pathologically the outstanding changes are slow degeneration of motor cells in the cerebral cortex, cranial nuclei, and anterior horn cells, along with demyelination and axonal loss of the pyramidal tracts and ventral roots, and changes of denervation atrophy in the skeletal muscles. Discrepancies in degree of change between various components of this system have led to different interpretations with respect to the primary site of the disease as to whether it is in the motor neuron and/or the pyramidal tract. The finding of additional degenerative changes in other parts of the central nervous system, though relatively mild and inconstant, has led to differences of opinion as to whether the disorder should be considered a diffuse or a system disease.

*Case:* A 60-year-old man, whose family history was negative, developed increasing weakness of the right hand associated with muscle twitching, unsteadiness of gait, and difficulty in enunciating words. When examined one and a half years later, he showed mild dysarthria, moderate atrophy and fasciculations of the right hand and arm, spasticity of the left leg, exaggerated tendon reflexes of the right upper and left lower extremities, and hyperactive jaw reflex. His condition deteriorated rapidly in the ensuing year, with development of gross dysarthria, dysphagia, hypersalivation, and dyspnea. Examination at this time revealed severe atrophy of the tongue, trapezius, and facial muscles; hyperreflexia and fasciculations in arms and legs, associated with Hoffmann and Babinski signs and ankle clonus. Electromyograms showed spiking potentials associated with fibrillations in all muscles. The patient died approximately four years following the onset of his symptoms.

The brain and spinal cord showed no gross changes.

Microscopically, there was marked diminution of Betz cells in the motor cortex (Fig. 177a), as compared with the normal appearance of this area (Fig. 177b). In the medulla the motor cells of the hypoglossal nucleus had almost completely disappeared, and there were similar changes in the nucleus ambiguus (Fig. 177c). At all levels of the spinal cord the cells of the anterior horns (arrows) were reduced to a few shrunken forms, accompanied by increase in glial elements, contrasting with the preserved neurons of Clarke's column (Fig. 177d). The depletion of the anterior horn cells was associated with chromatolysis and shrinkage of remaining neurons and with increase in reacting microglial and astroglial cells.

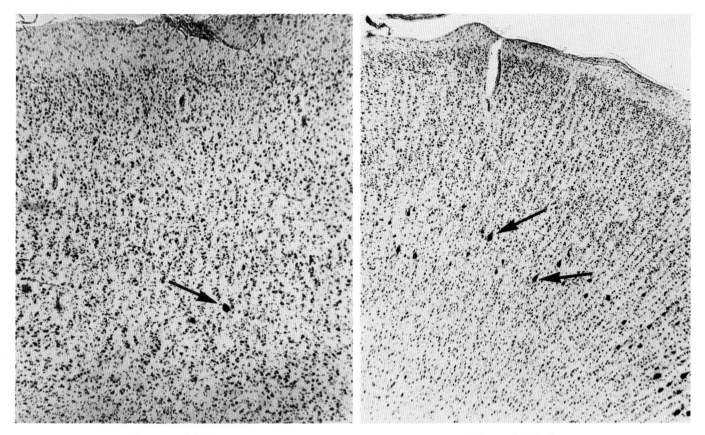

Fig. 177a. Nissl × 55

Fig. 177b. Nissl × 32

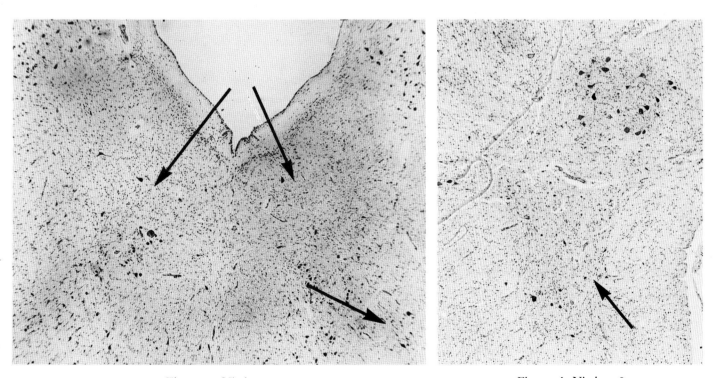

Fig. 177c. Nissl × 32

Fig. 177d. Nissl × 28

In myelin preparations the corticospinal tracts were symmetrically demyelinated through-out their course. In the spinal cord, there was severe demyelinization of the lateral and ventral corticospinal tracts, associated with mild, diffuse demyelinization of anterolateral columns, which contrasted with the normal myelin content of the dorsal columns (Fig. 178a). In the skeletal muscles, groups of normal muscle fibers alternated with groups of atrophic fibers, the latter showing loss of striations and proliferation of sarcolemmal nuclei (Fig. 178b).

### AMYOTROPHIC LATERAL SCLEROSIS (ALS): MARIANAS FORM

In recent years, a high incidence of ALS among certain native populations, in familial aggregation, of the Marianas Islands, estimated to be 100 times that of ALS in the U.S.A., has led to a series of epidemiologic, clinical, and pathologic studies with the purpose of discovering etiologic factors operating in the disease. The conclusions arrived at to date pointed to essential differences in the clinical and pathologic manifestations between the classic and Marianas forms. For, although showing pathologic similarities in the location of the neuromyopathy, the Marianas form, unlike the classic form, was characterized by the presence in neurons of neurofibrillary tangles, granulovacuolar bodies, and eosinophilic rod-like inclusions, in a characteristic mode of distribution in various parts of the central nervous system. Moreover, clinicopathologic links were established with an almost equally prevalent disease in the Marianas, characterized by a parkinsonism-dementia complex, suggesting that each may represent a portion of a continuous spectrum of degenerative disease. Although the etiology remains unknown, the Marianas form thus differs from the classic ALS.

*Case:* A 38-year-old Chamorro male developed weakness in his hands in December 1950, stiffness in both legs in August 1951, and signs of bulbar palsy in November 1952. Examination in 1957 towards the end of his life revealed that the patient was unable to move his extremities, talk, chew or swallow, breathing was labored; muscle atrophy was severe in extremities and those innervated by the motor nuclei of cranial nerves V, X and XII; the reflexes were hyperactive in the lower and absent in the upper extremities, while plantar stimulation produced no movement of the toes.

The significant pathologic changes were: severe bilateral demyelination in both lateral and ventral corticospinal tracts along with moderate, diffuse demyelination of the entire anterolateral columns (Fig. 178c); marked loss of neurons in anterior horn cells throughout the spinal cord and in nuclei of cranial nerves V, VII, IX, X and XII; and denervation atrophy of muscle fibers. All of these changes closely resembled the findings in classic ALS.

In addition, however, there were widespread neurofibrillary tangles, unaccompanied by senile plaques, throughout the central nervous system, as well as granulovacuolar bodies and rod-like inclusions confined to the hippocampus (Fig. 178d).

Electron microscopic studies confirmed that these latter changes were indistinguishable from those seen in Alzheimer's disease.

*References*

Hirano, A., N. Malamud, and L. T. Kurland. Parkinsonism-dementia Complex, an Endemic Disease on the Island of Guam. II. Pathological Features. Brain. 84: 662, 1961.
Malamud, N., A. Hirano, and L. T. Kurland. Pathoanatomic Changes in Amyotrophic Lateral Sclerosis with Special Reference to the Occurrence of Neurofibrillary Changes. Arch. Neurol. 5: 401, 1961.
Malamud, N. Neuromuscular Diseases. Pathology of the Nervous System, Vol. 1. (J. Minckler, ed.), McGraw-Hill (New York, 1968), pp. 712–724.

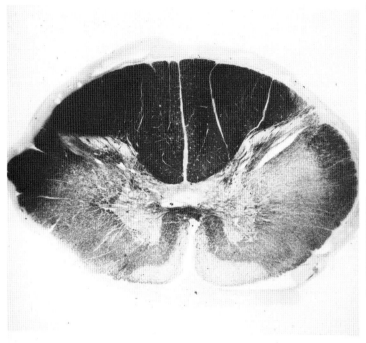

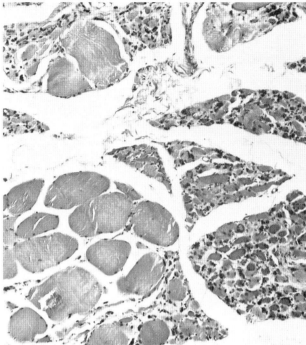

Fig. 178a. Weigert-Kulschitzky stain of spinal cord

Fig. 178b. HE × 128

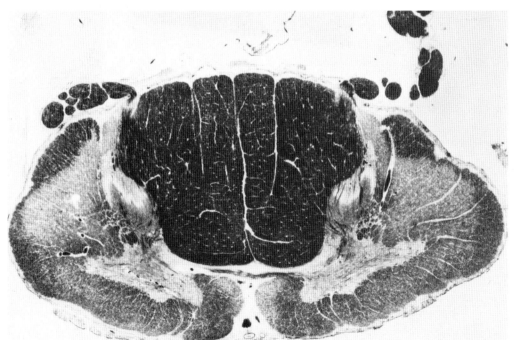

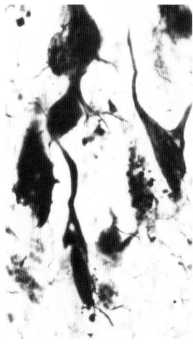

Fig. 178c. Weigert-Kulschitzky stain of spinal cord

Fig. 178d. von Braunmühl × 440

Werdnig-Hoffmann's disease is a rare familial infantile form of progressive spinal muscular atrophy due to an autosomal recessive gene. Its onset varies from birth through the first year of life and follows a rapidly progressive course to fatal termination. The clinical signs are hypotonia, flaccid paralysis, muscle atrophy, fasciculations, loss of reflexes, and bulbar signs. It should be distinguished from so-called cases of benign congenital amyotonia (Oppenheim's disease).

The pathology is one of degeneration of anterior horn cells and of motor cranial nuclei, atrophy and demyelination of peripheral nerves, and denervation atrophy of muscles. There is no evidence of upper motor neuron disease.

> *Case:* A 5-month-old, black boy whose older sister died of a similar disease, had a normal birth and early development. At the age of two months it was noted that he was unable to lift his head from a prone position. Since then all his motor activities decreased in strength and he tended to regurgitate his feedings. When admitted to the hospital at the age of four months, he exhibited absence of movement of the extremities and head, and weakness of intercostal and bulbar muscles, however, without detectable muscle atrophy or fasciculations. There were no deep tendon or Moro reflexes. A 24-hour urine specimen contained 325 mg of creatinine and 215 mg of creatine. A muscle biopsy exhibited loss of muscle striations and some increase in fat. Electromyographic studies showed very sparse normal muscle units. Constant accumulation of secretions led to pulmonary infection as the cause of death.

There were no gross changes in the central nervous system.

Microscopically, myelin stains of the spinal cord revealed no evidence of demyelination except in the atrophic ventral roots (Fig. 179a).

Nissl preparations showed marked loss of neurons in the anterior horns, contrasting with the normal appearance of the rest of the gray matter (Fig. 179b); on higher magnification the remaining motor neurons showed chromatolysis and sclerosis, accompanied by proliferation of micro- and astroglia.

In the medulla, there were only a few neurons left in the nuclei of the hypoglossus nerve (Fig. 179c); similar changes were present in the nucleus ambiguus.

In the skeletal muscles, groups of small "fetal" fibers alternated with normal fibers (Fig. 179d).

*References*

Byers, R. K., and B. O. Banker. Infantile Muscular Atrophy. Arch. Neurol. 5: 140, 1961.

Greenfield, J. G., and R. O. Stern. The Anatomical Identity of the Werdnig-Hoffmann and Oppenheim Forms of Infantile Muscular Atrophy. Brain. 50: 652, 1927.

Malamud, N. Infantile Progressive Muscular Atrophy. Pathology of the Nervous System, Vol. 1. (J. Minckler, ed.) McGraw-Hill (New York, 1968), pp. 725–730.

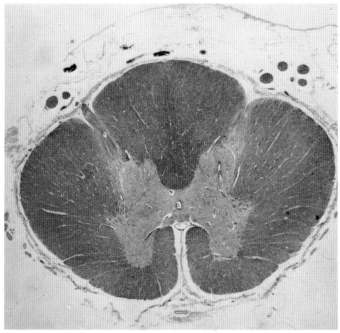

Fig. 179a. Weil stain of spinal cord

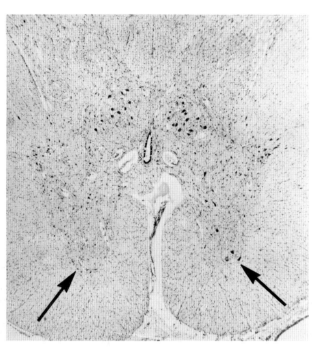

Fig. 179b. Nissl × 20

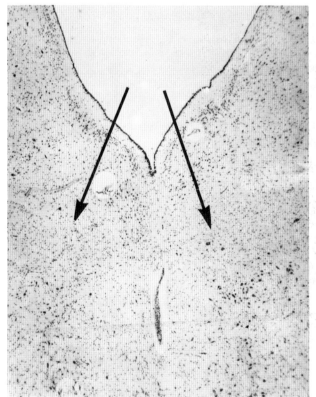

Fig. 179c. Nissl × 20

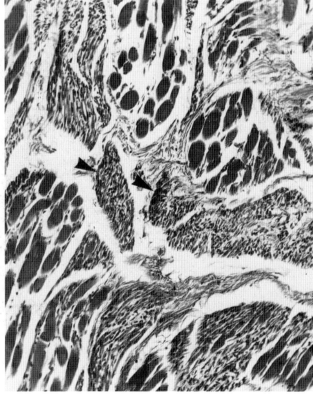

Fig. 179d. HE × 140

Werdnig-Hoffmann's disease has been the subject of a number of fine structural studies which have been confined to the examination of postmortem material.

In these studies, alterations in anterior horn cells and spinal roots were reported. Biopsies of skeletal muscle have revealed the presence of fibers of variable sizes. The smaller fibers, interpreted as atrophic, are reported to show alterations consisting of a loss or disarrangement of the myofilaments, an increase in glycogen granules, changes in the sarcoplasmic reticulum, and infolding of the plasma and nuclear membranes. These changes are interpreted as similar to those seen in other forms of neuropathy and experimental denervation.

On the other hand, it should be pointed out that many of the small fibers are remarkably well preserved and indistinguishable from normal-appearing fibers except for their size (Fig. 180). Further clarification of the significance of the small fibers is still needed. Interestingly, recently, a variation of Werdnig-Hoffmann's disease, described as small fiber disease, in which the small fibers retain both their normal histochemical and fine structural features, has been proposed. Clinically, the disease seems nonprogressive in contrast to classical Werdnig-Hoffmann's disease.

## References

Chou, S. M., and A. V. Fakadej. Ultrastructure of Chromatolytic Motoneurons and Anterior Spinal Roots in a Case of Werdnig-Hoffmann disease. J. Neuropath. and Exper. Neurol. 30: 368, 1971.

Hughes, J. T., and B. Brownell. Ultrastructure of Muscle in Werdnig-Hoffmann Disease. J. Neurol. Sci. 8: 863, 1969.

Muller, J., and W. E. DeMyer. Congenital Universal Muscular Hypoplasia. Am. J. Pathol. 63: 11a, 1972 (Abstract).

Roy, S., V. Dubowitz, and L. Wolman. Ultrastructure of Muscle in Infantile Spinal Muscular Atrophy. J. Neurol. Sci. 12: 219, 1971.

van Heelst, U. An Electron Microscopic Study of Muscle in Werdnig-Hoffmann's disease. Virch. Arch. Alt. A. Path. Anat. 351: 291, 1970.

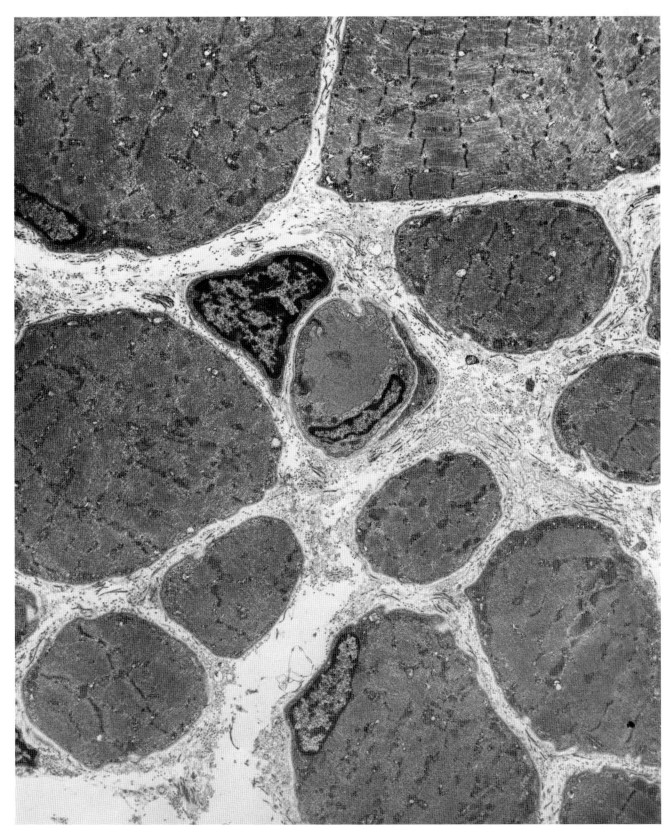

Fig. 180. An electron micrograph of cross sections of striated muscle fibers in a case of Werdnig-Hoffmann's disease × 7,000

## FRIEDREICH'S ATAXIA

Spinocerebellar degeneration or Friedreich's ataxia is probably the most common of the spinal degenerative disorders. It is a heredofamilial condition having its onset in the first or second decades of life and its clinical course is slowly progressive over several decades.

The clinical manifestations are ataxia, dysarthria, nystagmus, absent posterior column sensation, absent tendon reflexes, Babinski signs, pes cavus, kyphoscoliosis, signs of cardiac and pulmonary disorder, and at times diabetes mellitus.

The pathologic changes consist of degeneration of the neurons in Clarke's column and demyelination of dorsal columns, spinocerebellar and corticospinal tracts along with posterior roots, at times with neuronal degeneration in dorsal root ganglia, and rarely in anterior horn cells and cerebellum; the cardiac lesions are characterized by inflammation, fatty changes and fibrosis.

Variations from the classic disease may indicate a relationship to olivopontocerebellar atrophy, hereditary spastic paraplegia, Roussy-Lévy syndrome, polyneuropathy of Charcot-Marie-Tooth, and hypertrophic interstitial neuropathy.

> *Case:* A 41-year-old man had a normal birth and early development until the age of eight years when he began developing incoordination of all extremities. At the age of thirty, cardiac arrhythmia and cardiomegaly were noted. Repeated neurologic examinations revealed signs and symptoms involving the cerebellar, pyramidal, posterior column, and anterior horn cell systems. A diagnosis of Friedreich's ataxia was made. He died of bronchopneumonia complicating the myocarditis.

The principal gross changes in the central nervous system were moderate, diffuse atrophy of the cerebellum and the spinal cord.

Microscopically, myelin stains disclosed demyelination of the posterior columns, more of the gracilis than the cuneatus, the dorsal spinocerebellar more than the ventral spinocerebellar tracts, and the lateral and ventral corticospinal tracts, along with the dorsal roots (Fig. 181a).

In Nissl preparations, degeneration of the neurons of Clarke's column (CC) contrasted with mild changes in the anterior horns (A) and essentially normal appearance of the intermediolateral horns (IL) (Fig. 181b).

## HEREDITARY SPASTIC PARAPLEGIA

Hereditary Spastic Paraplegia is a familial disorder, occurring at any age, with a very chronic clinical course of stiffness and weakness, beginning in lower extremities with pyramidal tract signs but without sensory changes or ataxia.

> *Case:* A 67-year-old woman with a family history of a similar disorder in her mother, three siblings, three uncles and grandfather, developed at the age of twenty-nine progressive difficulties with her gait. Neurologic examination revealed that the upper extremities had normal strength although the tendon reflexes were exaggerated and were associated with bilateral Hoffmann's signs. The lower extremities were very weak; the knee and ankle jerks were markedly hyperactive and were associated with bilateral ankle clonus and Babinski signs. There was no definite evidence of sensory impairment in either position sense or sense of pain.

The significant neuropathologic findings were restricted to the spinal cord, in which there was symmetrical demyelination of the lateral corticospinal tracts and to a lesser degree of the fasciculus gracilis (Fig. 181c).

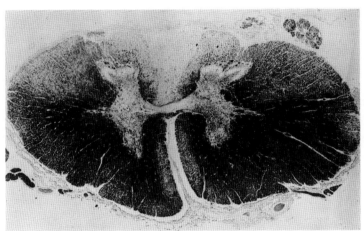

Fig. 181a. Weigert-Kulschitzky stain of spinal cord

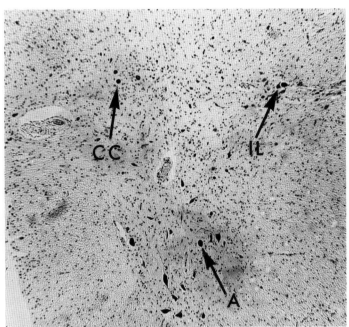

Fig. 181b. Nissl × 55

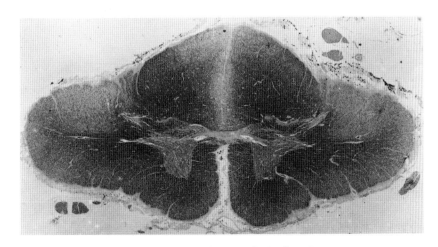

Fig. 181c. Weil stain of spinal cord

Two hereditary disorders that are characterized by primary degeneration of the peripheral nervous system and that have some features in common are Charcot-Marie-Tooth and Déjerine-Sottas diseases.

### CHARCOT-MARIE-TOOTH DISEASE

Charcot-Marie-Tooth disease, also known as peroneal muscular atrophy, is the most common of the hereditary neuropathies. It is usually characterized by dominant Mendelian inheritance, develops in the first decades of life but follows a very slow chronic course of atrophy of distal muscles that tends to spread proximally; it usually begins with peroneal muscle involvement, later involving also the upper extremities, associated with loss of tendon reflexes but only with mild distal sensory loss; there is low conduction velocity of peripheral nerves but a normal cerebrospinal fluid protein.

Pathologically, there is primarily degeneration of the peripheral nerves with secondary degeneration of dorsal roots and columns, dorsal root ganglia and of anterior horn cells. The changes in the peripheral nerves are accompanied by an excess of connective tissue, but at times resembles the hypertrophic interstitial neuropathy of Déjerine-Sottas disease. The changes in the muscles are those of denervation atrophy.

### DÉJERINE-SOTTAS DISEASE

Déjerine-Sottas disease is a rare familial disorder usually occurring in early childhood, more commonly showing recessive than dominant inheritance, characterized clinically by a progressive polyneuropathy, accompanied by palpable peripheral nerves, extremely low conduction velocity of nerves and by increased cerebrospinal fluid protein. Pathologically, it is characterized by hypertrophic, interstitial neuropathy manifested by onion bulb formation, due to lamellated proliferation of the sheath of Schwann and endoneurium and interstitial mucinoid changes.

There is reason to believe that hypertrophic interstitial neuropathy may occur in a variety of conditions, other than in the above hereditary disorders.

### CHARCOT-MARIE-TOOTH: FORM OF DEGENERATIVE NEUROPATHY

*Case:* An 87-year-old man developed at about the age of 40 clumsiness of both hands that slowly progressed to involve also the forearms, followed by a flapping gait. Examination showed atrophy of the distal musculature in all extremities, that was especially marked in calves, feet, and hands associated with absent deep tendon reflexes. Later his proximal musculature also became involved. He ultimately succumbed to an intercurrent pneumonia. The clinical diagnosis was Charcot-Marie-Tooth disease.

The significant pathologic findings were: demyelination of the posterior columns and roots (Fig. 182a) and diffuse loss of anterior horn cells (Fig. 182b) in the spinal cord, and diffuse demyelination of the peripheral nerves (Fig. 182c) accompanied by excess of collagen fibers (Fig. 182d).

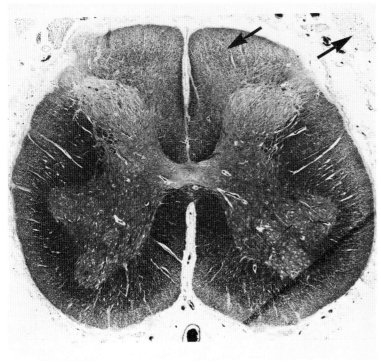

Fig. 182a. Weil stain of spinal cord

Fig. 182b. Nissl × 23

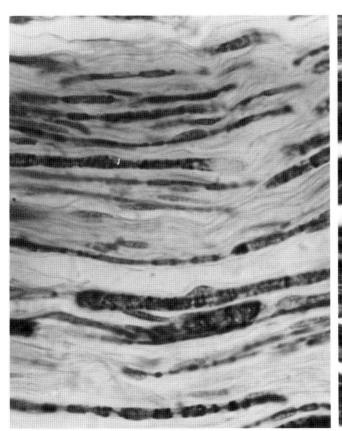

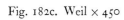
Fig. 182c. Weil × 450

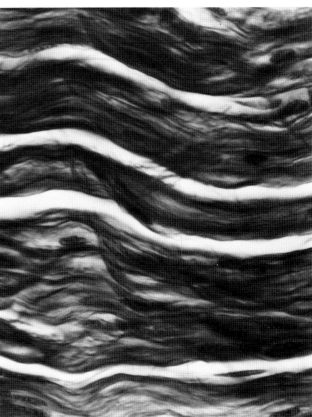

Fig. 182d. HVG × 450

*Case:* A 61-year-old woman developed at the age of 48 wasting of the calves, followed by atrophy of the forearms. On examination, there was marked atrophy of the legs, thighs, and forearms with no voluntary dorsiflexion and only slight plantar flexion of the feet, and with hypesthesias and hypalgesias of all extremities. Deep tendon reflexes showed the upper to be 2+ bilaterally; the knee and ankle jerks were 1+. She expired in 1955 of spontaneous pneumothorax due to emphysema. Clinical diagnosis was Charcot-Marie-Tooth disease.

The spinal cord showed at various levels hypertrophy of ventral and dorsal nerve roots that stood out prominently by their enlargement and demyelination amongst intact roots (arrows), while the spinal cord appeared normal (Fig. 183a). Under higher magnification, demyelination of nerve fibers was associated with proliferation of Schwann and endoneurial elements (Fig. 183b), that with connective tissue stains showed characteristic onion bulb formation consisting of concentrically lamellated collagen fibers (Fig. 183c).

*References*

Austin, J. H. Observations on the Syndrome of Hypertrophic Neuritis. Med. 35: 187, 1956.
Dyck, P. J. and E. H. Lambert. Lower Motor and Primary Sensory Neuron Diseases with Peroneal Muscular Atrophy. Arch. Neurol. 18: 603, 1968.

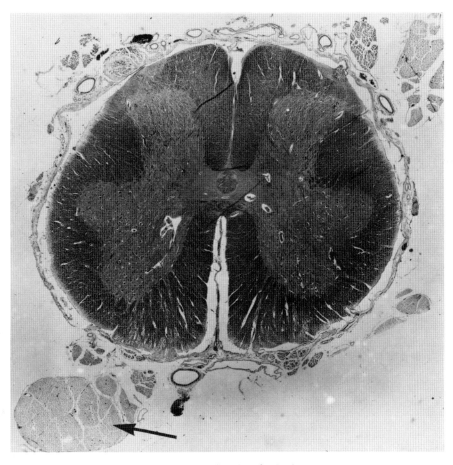

Fig. 183a. Weil stain of spinal cord

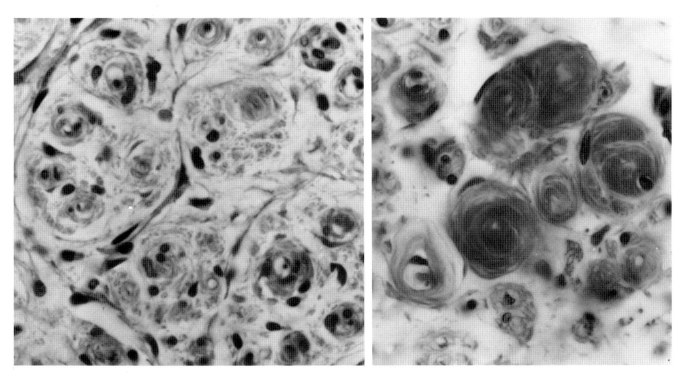

Fig. 183b. Weil × 560

Fig. 183c. HVG × 560

# IX

## *Metabolic Disorders*

Metabolic disorders comprise a group of conditions in which, according to Garrod, there is "a metabolic defect, due to absence or inactivity of a specific enzyme that in turn is dependent on the absence of the normal form of a gene."

### LIPIDOSES

Lipidoses are inherited disorders of metabolism that lead to abnormal accumulations of lipids in the cells of certain tissues and organs. Amaurotic family idiocy is the best known form of neurolipidosis.

#### AMAUROTIC FAMILY IDIOCY

A variety of forms have been included in this category: 1. congenital; 2. infantile or Tay-Sachs; 3. late Infantile or Jansky-Bielschowsky; 4. juvenile or Batten-Spielmeyer-Vogt; and 5. adult or Kufs disease. In all forms there is an autosomal recessive mode of inheritance.

##### INFANTILE FORMS (Tay-Sachs and Sandhoff's disease)

Tay-Sach's form is a disease having an onset at about the age of three to six months with progressive symptoms of psychomotor retardation, blindness, and hypotonia followed by spasticity and decerebrate rigidity. The pathognomonic clinical sign is a macular cherry-red spot. In its late phases megalencephaly is a common feature. About two-thirds of the cases occur in Jews, while the remaining are reported in non-Jews.

Biochemically, Tay-Sachs disease is considered to be a gangliosidosis, a form of sphingolipids (ceramide plus hexose) containing sialic acid of the $GM_2$ Type 1 variety, attributed to absence of the enzyme hexosaminase A. A variant occurring in non-Jews and having mild visceromegaly, is recognized as Sandhoff's disease or $GM_2$ Type 2 gangliosidosis, due to absence of hexosaminase A and B.

Pathologically, neurons of central nervous system, peripheral ganglia and retina, with their dendrites and axons, show ballooning of the cytoplasm that contains lipids accompanied by fat-laden macrophages and reactive astrocytes. Demyelination is a special feature of the infantile varieties.

*Case 1. Tay-Sachs variant:* A 2-year-old Jewish girl, an only child, began having convulsions at the age of seven months. She was committed to a State hospital at the age of eighteen months at which time she was blind, spastic, unable to sit or balance her head, and had a cherry-red spot in the region of the macula. Her course was progressively downhill.

The brain weighed 975 grams and showed mild atrophy of the cerebral convolutions and severe atrophy of the cerebellum (Fig. 184a).

Microscopically, there was universal ballooning of the nerve and glial cells; the degenerated cytoplasm had a honeycomb appearance, and the nuclei were pyknotic and eccentric (Fig. 184b).

With the Nile blue sulfate method the swollen neurons stained purplish blue (Fig. 184c) (see also Fig. 2e). With scarlet red there was only a faint yellowish staining of the lipid material in the neurons, but the macrophages stained a bright red.

372

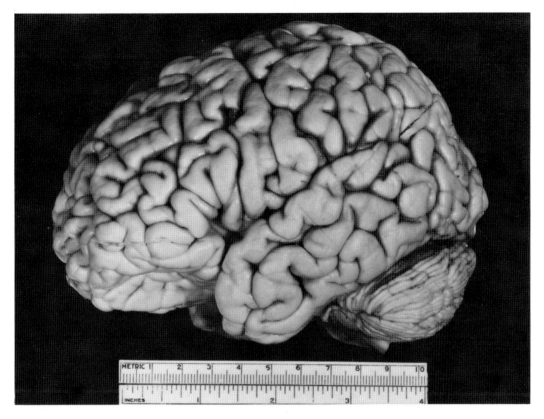

Fig. 184a.  Tay-Sachs disease

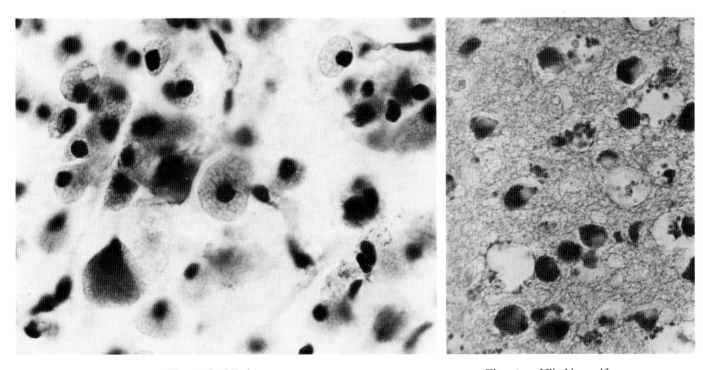

Fig. 184b.  Nissl × 750

Fig. 184c.  Nile blue sulfate × 475

## Infantile Forms (Tay-Sachs and Sandhoff's disease) (continued)

*Case 2. Sandhoff's variant:* A 4-year-old Mexican boy, an only child, began having seizures at the age of two months. Subsequent examination revealed an enlarging head and cherry-red maculae. By the age of eight months, he showed gross mental and motor retardation. A brain biopsy at the age of two years revealed marked swelling of neurons and glia that contained lipid material, staining positively with PAS, that disappeared following use of fat solvents, and was not reduced by diastase digestion, diagnostic of a neuronal glycolipid storage disorder. He was admitted to a State hospital at the age of two and one-half years where he showed unresponsiveness, bilateral corneal opacities, poor gag and swallowing reflexes, poor muscle tone, hyperactive deep tendon reflexes with Babinski signs and moderately protuberant abdomen with liver edge 1.5 cm. below the costal margin. He was now having repeated seizures that became increasingly more severe despite medication, and he succumbed to bronchopneumonia.

The brain was enlarged, weighing 1,350 grams and was found to contain excessive amounts of $GM_2$ gangliosides on chemical analysis.

Sections revealed diffuse cerebral atrophy with pallor of gray matter and grayish discoloration of white matter throughout the cerebrum and cerebellum, associated with enlargement of all ventricles (Fig. 185a).

In Nissl preparations, the neurons exhibited marked ballooning with granular cytoplasm and eccentric pyknotic nuclei (Fig. 185b). In the cerebellum, all Purkinje cells and most of the granular cells had disappeared, showing many empty balloons of their dendrites and axons and scattered macrophages that contained darkly stained lipid material. The demyelinated white matter (A) (Fig. 185c) contained large amounts of sudanophilic fat in macrophages that differed from that of the gray matter (B) where only the glia stained with oil-red O (Fig. 185d).

*References*

Menkes, J. H., J. M. Andrews, and P. A. Cancilla. The Cerebrospinal Degenerations. J. Pediat. 79: 183, 1971.
O'Brien, J. S. Ganglioside Storage Diseases. New Eng. J. Med. 284: 893–896, 1971.

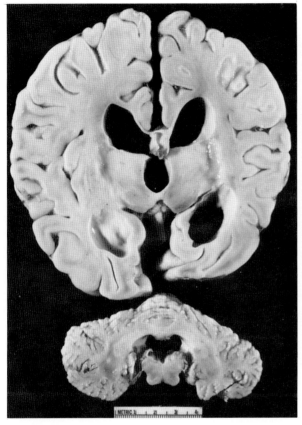

Fig. 185a. Sandhoff's variant of infantile lipidosis

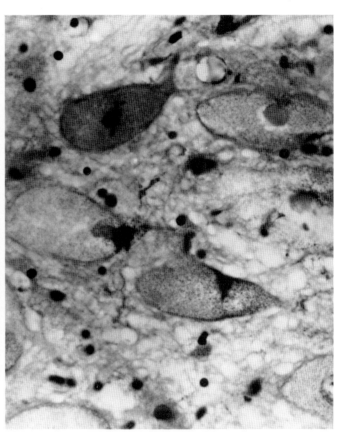

Fig. 185b. Nissl × 375

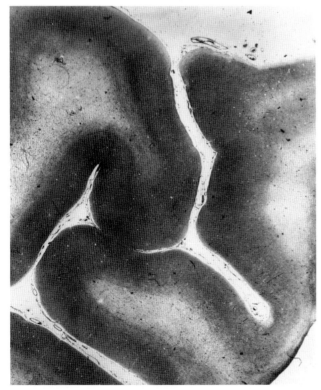

Fig. 185c. Weil stain

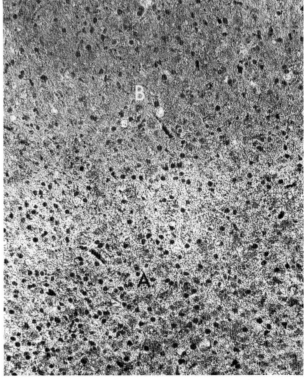

Fig. 185d. Oil Red O × 60

## Tay Sachs Disease: The Membranous Cytoplasmic Body
## in Electron Microscopy

First described by Terry in Tay-Sachs disease, where this lipid inclusion is the sole neuronal alteration, the membranous cytoplasmic body (MCB) has since been observed in a number of conditions including the mutant mink "wobbler." The MCB is formed by a series of concentric dense lamellae, each approximately 30 Å thick separated by 20 Å clear spaces (Fig. 186a). The 30 Å lamellae can split to form less dense 20 Å lamellae (arrow) (Fig. 186b). The MCB is reported to be rich in gangliosides and cholesterol.

*References*

Hirano, A. Electron Microscopy in Neuropathology. Progress in Neuropathology, Vol. I (H. M. Zimmerman, ed.). Grune and Stratton (New York, 1971), p. 1.

Hirano, A., H. M. Zimmerman, S. Levine, and G. A. Padgett. Cytoplasmic Inclusions in Chediak-Higashi and Wobbler Mink. An Electron Microscopic Study of the Nervous System. J. Neuropath. and Expt. Neurol. 30: 470, 1971.

Terry, R. D. Electron Microscopy of Selected Neurolipidoses. Handbook of Clinical Neurology, Vol. 10: Leuco-dystrophies and Poliodystrophies. (P. J. Vinken and G. W. Bruyn, eds.). American Elsevier, (New York, 1971), p. 362.

Terry, R. D., and S. R. Korey. Membranous Cytoplasmic Granules in Infantile Amaurotic Idiocy. Nature. 188: 1000, 1960.

Terry, R. D., and M. Weiss. Studies in Tay-Sachs Disease. II. Ultrastructure of the Cerebrum. J. Neuropath. and Expt. Neurol. 22: 18, 1963.

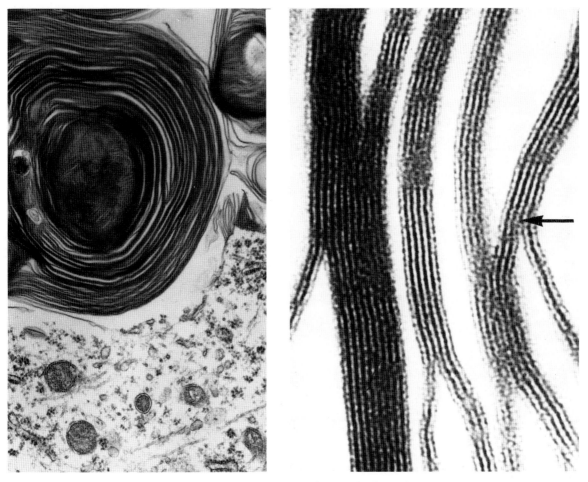

Fig. 186. Electron micrograph of a MCB in an anterior horn cell of an Aleutian mink with wobbling: a) × 12,000, b) × 360,000 (Hirano et al., J. Neuropathol. Exper. Neurol. 30: 470, 1971)

## Late Infantile Form (Jansky-Bielschowsky's Disease)

The late infantile form has its onset at about the age of two to three years, shows no racial disposition, and follows a more protracted clinical course than the infantile variety. The symptoms are progressive mental regression, seizures, pyramidal and extrapyramidal signs without retinal changes or visual symptoms except late in the disease when there may be, optic atrophy. A blood smear often shows vacuolated lymphocytes. The biochemical basis of the disease is not as yet established, although in some instances there is gangliosidosis of $GM_1$, $GM_2$, or GDIA varieties. The pathology is one of neuronal storage of lipids that are relatively insoluble in lipid solvents and that show stronger reaction to Sudan stains than the Tay-Sachs form. Membranous cytoplasmic bodies have been found in the electron microscopy of a few cases, and curvilinear bodies in others.

*Case 1:* A 7-year-old white girl with negative family history was one of twins, the other being healthy. She had a normal development until the age of two and one-half years when she became irritable and began having seizures that were either focal, akinetic or blank staring spells. The clinical findings were mental retardation, ataxia, decreased muscle tone, hypoactive deep tendon reflexes and Babinski signs. An electroencephalogram was abnormal, with moderate slowing and prominent spike and wave discharges in the right occipital region. A pneumoencephalogram revealed moderate ventricular dilatation. A rectal biopsy showed prominent ganglion cells that stained with Sudan black B. At the age of four years, a biopsy of the frontal lobe disclosed slightly swollen neurons that contained granular material staining with PAS, Sudan black, and scarlet red. Biochemically, there was marked increase in total lipid hexose, but the total ganglioside content was normal, although there was an increase in $G_{3A}$. The course was one of progressive deterioration and she expired of intercurrent pulmonary infection.

The brain weighed 730 grams and on section revealed a marked degree of diffuse atrophy of the cerebral cortex and the cerebellar folia with corresponding enlargement of the ventricles (Fig. 187a).

Microscopically, there was generalized swelling of neurons, axons and dendrites throughout the brain, the stored material staining an orange red with oil red O (Fig. 187b). Spongy degeneration and astrogliosis were seen in the atrophic areas.

The absence of consistent retinal changes in the late infantile form has often led to clinical misdiagnosis, at times to confusion with emotional disorders such as infantile autism and childhood schizophrenia, as illustrated in the following case:

*Case 2:* A 7-year-old girl had a normal birth and early development. At the age of three years, she was said to have been frightened at a Halloween party, following which she appeared fearful and anxious, thereafter becoming increasingly more seclusive, negativistic, and mute. At the age of five, she was examined in a pediatric clinic, where neurologic examination was said to be negative. The psychologist described her as showing "essentially a marked instability in her emotional reactions." She was awarded an I.Q. of 33, and was committed to a State hospital where she continued to deteriorate until her death. A younger sister was subsequently found to suffer from a similar disorder but with neurologic signs of ataxia, dysarthria, and electroencephalographic evidence of paroxysmol dysrhythmia in addition to signs of mental regression.

The brain showed a moderate degree of diffuse cortical atrophy and severe cerebellar atrophy (Fig. 187c).

Microscopically, ballooning of the neurons that contained a granular lipid material was found throughout the central nervous system (Fig. 187d).

*Reference*

Malamud, N. Heller's Disease and Childhood Schizophrenia. Am. J. Psychiat. 116: 215–218, 1959.

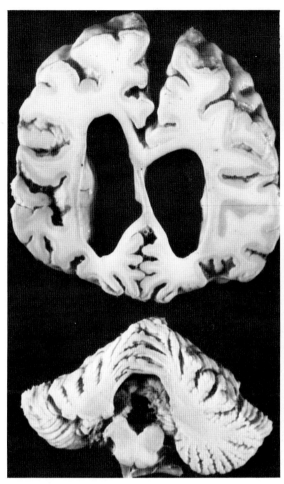

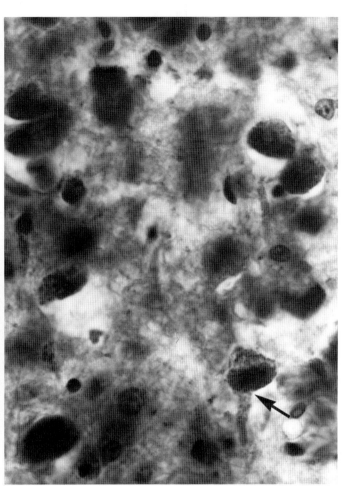

Fig. 187a. Jansky-Bielschowsky's disease

Fig. 187b. Oil Red O × 560

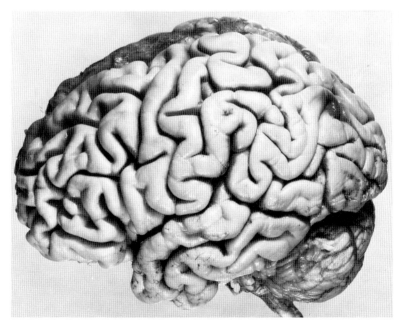

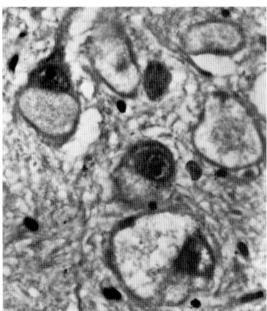

Fig. 187c. Jansky-Bielschowsky's disease

Fig. 187d. HE × 440

## Juvenile Form (Batten-Spielmeyer-Vogt's Disease)

The juvenile form of amaurotic family idiocy has its onset at about the age of five to seven years following a normal early development. It shows no particular racial predisposition. The clinical course is very slowly progressive, showing symptoms of mental and visual deterioration, ataxia, nystagmus, tremor, convulsions, and spastic quadriplegia. The cardinal diagnostic sign is retinitis pigmentosa.

Biochemical studies have failed to show consistent abnormalities, some pointing to a condition of lipofuscinosis, some to $GM_2$ gangliosidosis with partial deficiency of hexosaminase A, while others to $GM_1$ gangliosidosis with absence of galactosidase A, B, or C.

The pathology in light microscopy is similar to that of the late infantile variety. In electron microscopy, lysosome-like, multilocular, principal, and curvilinear bodies have been variously reported.

> *Case:* An 18-year-old, white male with negative family history had an onset of visual impairment at the age of five and one-half years, followed a year later by convulsions, irritability, aggressive behavior, and slurring of speech. Examination revealed optic atrophy and retinitis pigmentosa, hypoactive tendon reflexes, and signs of mental deterioration. He was admitted to a hospital at the age of ten years where he was described as retarded and hyperactive, showing a tendency to perseveration in speech and action; there were bilateral Babinski signs and a suggestion of splenohepatomegaly. Laboratory studies were essentially negative except for 61 mg % of total protein in the cerebrospinal fluid and abnormalities in the electroencephalogram. A rectal biopsy showed evidence of a lipid storage disease. Biochemically, there was a moderate increase in total gangliosides, however, not of the $GM_2$ or $GM_1$ varieties.

The brain weighed 1,000 grams and showed on section diffuse cortical atrophy of moderate degree and severe cerebellar atrophy (Fig. 188a).

Microscopically, many neurons and axons throughout the brain showed moderate ballooning and relatively mild glial reaction; the stored material stained equally with luxol-fast blue-PAS (Fig. 188b) and with oil red O.

There was also evidence of some stored material in cells of the liver and spleen that stained positively with PAS and Sudan black methods.

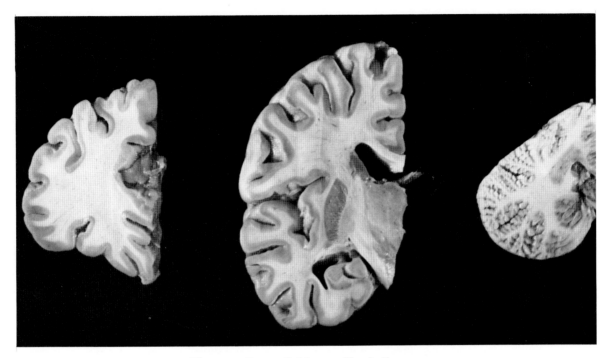

Fig. 188a. Batten-Spielmeyer-Vogt's disease

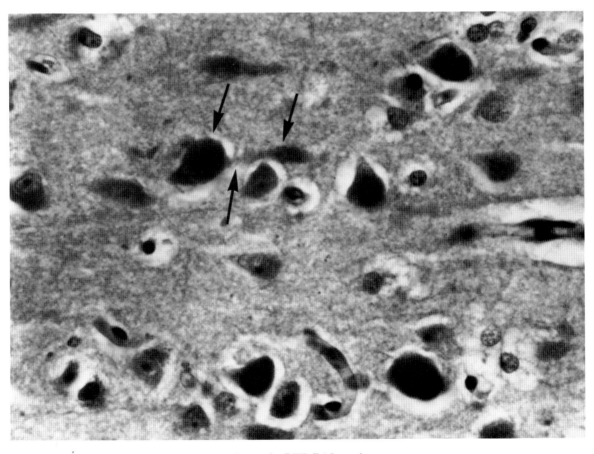

Fig. 188b. LFB-PAS × 560

Hunter-Hurler's disease, one of the most common forms of the storage diseases, is a combined mucopolysaccharidosis and lipidosis. It is inherited either as an autosomal or sex-linked recessive trait. The onset is in early childhood and the course varies greatly in duration.

The characteristic clinical findings are dwarfism, a large head with coarse hair and lips, hypertelorism, short neck, lumbar kyphosis, limitation of extension of joints, claw-like hands, corneal opacities, cardiac defects, hepatosplenomegaly, umbilical and inguinal hernias, mental retardation, deafness, and motor weakness. The diagnostic test is the demonstration of excessive excretion in the urine of certain mucopolysaccharides, especially chondroitin sulphate B and heparitin sulphate. Since these are important constituents of connective tissue, such abnormality is reflected in changes in cartilage, cornea, vascular and other tissues, including the meninges and cerebral blood vessels. At the same time an associated disturbance of lipid metabolism, in the form of an increase in gangliosides, accounts for changes in the nervous system, not unlike those of Tay-Sachs disease.

*Case:* A 3½ year-old boy, an only child, had a normal birth and early development until the age of two, when he began to develop enlargement of the head, shortening of the neck and extremities, reduced extensibility of the finger tips, kyphosis of the lumbar spine, undeveloped external genitalia, opacity of the cornea, splenohepatomegaly, and progressive mental deterioration. The duration of his illness was one and one-half years.

The brain weighed 1,300 grams, was abnormally large and somewhat malformed, and showed opaque leptomeninges (Fig. 189a). The occipital lobe on section showed thinning of the cortex and scattered minute cysts in the white matter.

Microscopically, the nerve cells throughout the central nervous system exhibited moderate ballooning with granularity and vacuolization of the cytoplasm, and eccentricity and pyknosis of the nucleus, as illustrated in stained sections of the cerebral cortex (Fig. 189b) and cerebellum, where ballooning of dendrites of Purkinje cells was especially conspicuous (Fig. 189c); the stored lipid stained with Nile blue sulfate (Fig. 189d) and PAS.

The leptomeninges and perivascular spaces showed increase in connective tissue fibers, interspersed with histiocytes, staining positively with luxol-fast blue-PAS.

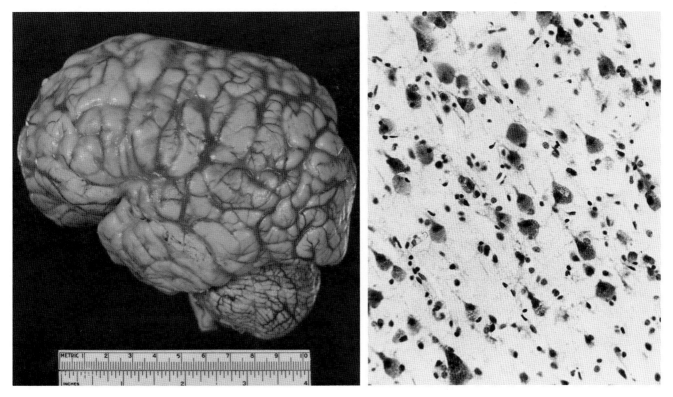

Fig. 189a. Hunter-Hurler's disease

Fig. 189b. Nissl × 240

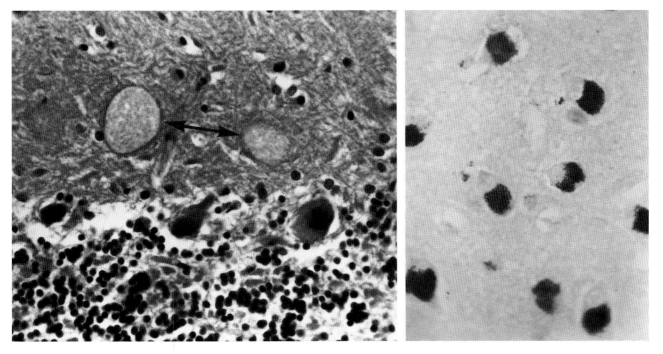

Fig. 189c. HE × 350

Fig. 189d. Nile blue sulfate × 300

In the electron microscope, the most prominent of the various pleomorphic lipid inclusions in the neurons are the so-called "zebra" bodies (Fig. 190). These membrane-bounded structures are pleomorphic and are characterized by dense lamellae 20 Å thick, separated by a 20 Å less dense space. Most frequently, the 20 Å dense lamellae are fused and form a 30 Å lamella which is even denser than the 20 Å lamellae. The electron lucent spacing remains at 20 Å so that, in well preserved bodies, a periodicity of 50 Å is apparent. These structures, however, are difficult to preserve and most commonly the 20 Å space is artefactually widened, giving rise to the striped, zebra-like appearance. Often, parts of the zebra bodies are filled with moderately dense, finely granular material and may also contain highly dense homogeneous lipid-like material. The zebra bodies have been interpreted as representing abnormal accumulations of gangliosides.

Zebra bodies are probably most numerous in gargoylism but have been reported in neurons of other human disorders, including myoclonic epilepsy, infantile Gaucher's disease, and other storage diseases. They are also found in experimental animals such as Aleutian mink with Chediak-Higashi disease accompanied by wobbling and irradiated animals. Interestingly, occasional similar structures have been reported in Schwann cells under both normal and pathologic conditions in humans and in experimental animals.

In addition to these neuronal changes, the perithelial cytoplasm displays vacuolar changes which are presumed to be related to mucopolysaccharide accumulations.

*References*

Aleu, F. P., R. D. Terry, and H. Zellweger. Electron Microscopy of Two Cerebral Biopsies in Gargoylism. J. Neuropath. and Expt. Neurol. 24: 304, 1966.

Gambetti, P., R. J. C. Levine, W. Grover., and K. Suzuki. Accumulation of Smooth Cisterns, Multivesicular Bodies and "Zebra" Bodies in Neurons. A Case of Peculiar Storage Conditions. Acta Neuropath. 18: 132, 1971.

Hirano, A., H. M. Zimmerman, S. Levine, and G. A. Padgett. Cytoplasmic Inclusions in Chediak-Higashi and Wobbler Mink. An Electron Microscopic Study of the Nervous System. J. Neuropath. and Expt. Neurol. 30: 470, 1971.

Hirano, A. Progress in Neuropathology, Vol. 1 (H. M. Zimmerman, ed.). Grune and Stratton (New York, 1971), p. 1.

Tomonage, M., and E. Sluga. Zur Ultrastruktur der 1π Granula. Acta Neuropath. 15: 56, 1970.

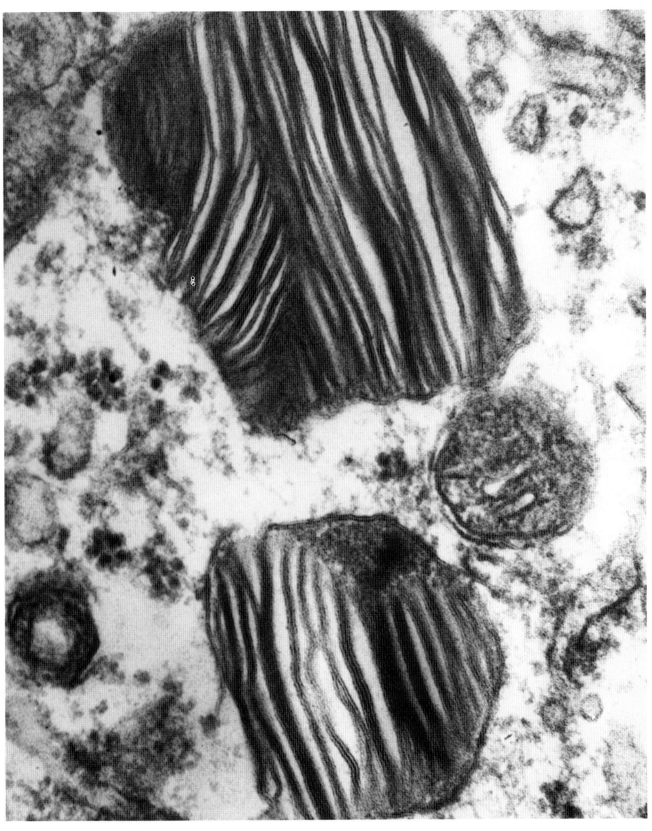

Fig. 190. An electron micrograph of a "zebra" body in an anterior horn cell of an Aleutian mink with wobbling × 150,000 (Hirano, in Progress in Neuropathology, Vol. I. (H. M. Zimmerman, ed.). Grune and Stratton (New York, 1971), p. 1.)

# LEUKODYSTROPHIES

Leukodystrophies are genetically determined errors of metabolism that are characterized by disturbances in myelin formation. Their former inclusion with the sporadic demyelinating disorders, namely, Schilder's disease and multiple sclerosis, is no longer accepted.

Some of the leukodystrophies have much in common with the lipidoses and have been classified into the following types: 1) metachromatic; 2) globoid cell or Krabbe's disease; and 3) sudanophilic. All have certain common pathologic features: diffuse and symmetrical demyelination throughout white matter with some tendency to spare the U-fibers, no myelin-axonal dissociation and accumulation of abnormal compounds that cannot be utilized in myelin anabolism. All have raised hexosamine levels.

Other forms have been considered, but not universally accepted, as leukodystrophies. These include the spongy sclerosis type (Canavan's disease); the fibrinoid type (Alexander's disease); the disorders of amino acid metabolism (phenylketonuria and maple syrup urine disease) and possibly galactosemia.

## METACHROMATIC LEUKODYSTROPHY (MLD)

MLD is a familial disorder with autosomal recessive mode of inheritance, having its onset most commonly at about the age of one year. It is characterized clinically by progressive symptoms of dementia, convulsions, ataxia, spasticity, blindness and polyneuropathy, and raised cerebrospinal fluid protein. The diagnosis is based on demonstration of metachromatic material in urinary sediment, and in peripheral nerve and brain biopsies.

Biochemically, the disease is due to a defect in the enzyme aryl sulfatase A that results in a marked increase in cerebroside sulfatides. MLD is thus considered to be sulfatide lipidosis.

Pathologically, it is characterized by diffuse demyelination. The granular deposit is found in macrophages, oligodendroglia, and Schwann cells, rarely in astrocytes. It stains brown with cresyl violet, red with toluidine blue, is PAS positive and Sudan negative.

*Case:* A 9-year-old, white boy, an only child of healthy parents and grandparents, had a normal development. After his first birthday, he gradually became spastic. At the age of four years, examination revealed spasticity, tremors, ataxia, Babinski signs, and muscle atrophy. All studies were negative with the exception of raised cerebrospinal fluid total protein that was 113 mg %. His condition showed further deterioration. He died of aspiration pneumonia at the age of nine years.

The brain weighed 1,000 grams and showed grossly extensive diffuse demyelination of the cerebral white matter with the exception of the U-fibers, the white matter appearing gray and gelatinous, while the cortex was normal; the cerebellum showed, in addition to demyelination of the white matter, severe atrophy of the folia (Fig. 191a).

In myelin stains, diffuse loss of myelin contrasted with its preservation in the U-fibers (Fig. 191b) while the corresponding Holzer preparation exhibited intense reactive gliosis (Fig. 191c).

With the cresyl violet (Hirsch-Peiffer) method, there were large deposits of granular brown material in the white matter (Fig. 191d) that were red with toluidine blue, whereas staining with oil red O was entirely negative.

*References*

Austin, J. H. Recent Studies in the Metachromatic and Globoid Forms of Diffuse Sclerosis. Ultrastructure and Metabolism of the Nervous System. ARNMD, XL, Williams and Wilkins (Baltimore, 1962), p. 189.

Austin, J. H., D. Armstrong, and L. Shearer. Metachromatic Form of Diffuse Cerebral Sclerosis, V. The Nature and Significance of Low Sulfatase Activity: A Controlled Study of Brain, Liver and Kidney in Four Patients with Metachromatic Leukodystrophy (MLD). Arch. Neurol. 13: 593, 1965.

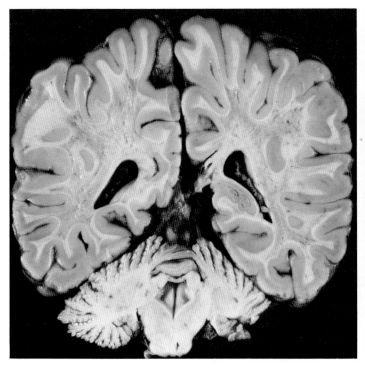

Fig. 191a. Metachromatic leukodystrophy

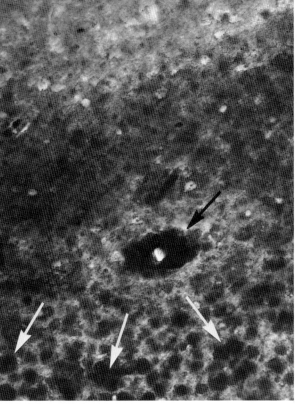

Fig. 191b. Weil stain

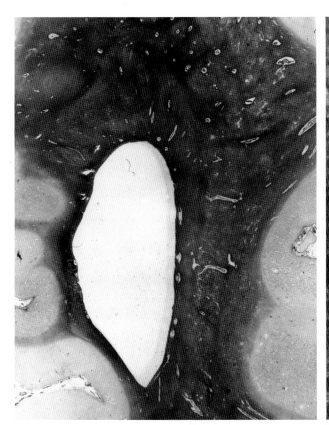

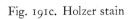

Fig. 191c. Holzer stain

Fig. 191d. Acetic-acid cresyl violet × 120

In the electron microscope, several types of inclusions have been reported. Whether all or only some of these are metachromatic is, as yet, unclear. Some inclusions display a periodic structure (Fig. 192a and b) while others do not.

*References*

Cravioto, H., J. S. O'Brien, B. H. Landing, and B. Finck. Ultrastructure of Peripheral Nerve in Metachromatic Leukodystrophy. Acta Neuropathologica 7: 111, 1966.

Gregoire, A., O. Perier, and P. Dustin, Jr. Metachromatic Leukodystrophy, an Electron Microscopic Study. J. Neuropath. and Expt. Neurol. 25: 617, 1966.

Liu, H. M. Ultrastructure of Central Nervous System Lesions in Metachromatic Leukodystrophy with Special Reference to Morphogenesis. J. Neuropath. and Expt. Neurol. 25: 624, 1968.

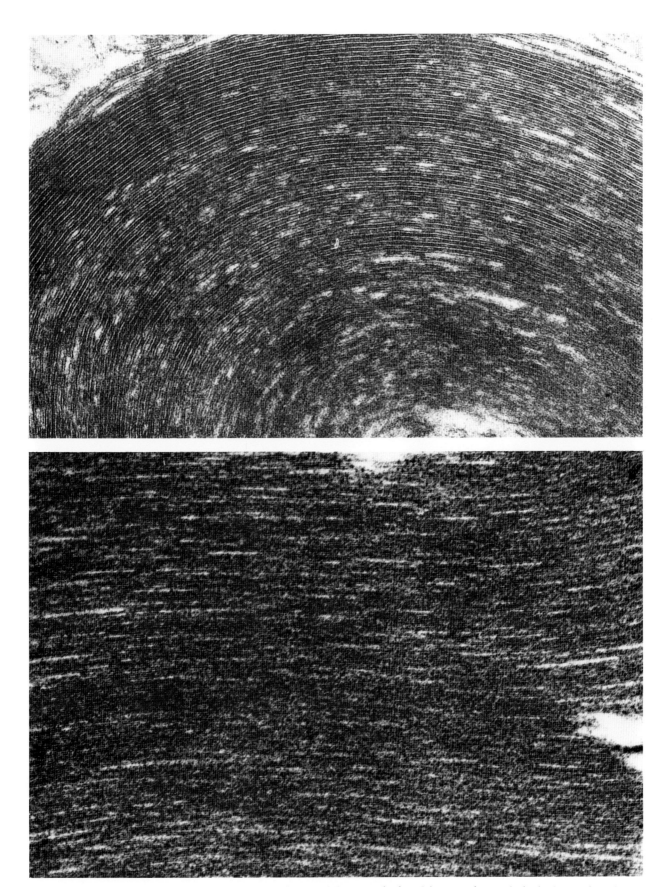

Fig. 192. Electron micrograph of a type of osmiophilic granule found in metachromatic leukodystrophy: a) × 134,000, b) × 134,000

## Globoid Cell Leukodystrophy (GLD or Krabbe's Disease)

GLD is a familial disorder having its onset at about four to six months of age. Its clinical course is relatively rapid and is characterized by progressive symptoms of mental regression, seizures, spastic quadriplegia, blindness, deafness, polyneuropathy, and raised cerebrospinal fluid protein. Diagnosis may be established by brain and nerve biopsy and by quantitative analysis of urinary sediment. Biochemically, there is an increase in nonsulfatide galacto-cerebrosides, probably due to enzyme deficiency of galactocerebroside B-galactosidase.

The pathology is one of diffuse demyelination, similar to MLD. However, the breakdown products are negative for metachromasia and sudanophilia but are PAS positive. The histologic feature is the presence of globoid multinucleated and epithelioid mononuclear cells, generally occurring in perivascular packets. The origin of these cells has been variously considered to be adventitial, microglial, oligodendroglial, and astrocytic; most likely they are adventitial cells.

In the electron microscope, the globoid cells have been reported to contain many apparently unique intracytoplasmic inclusions. These structures appear tubular in longitudinal sections and in cross-section irregularly crystalloid, their diameter ranging from 100–1,000Å.

*Case:* A female infant had a normal birth and early development until the age of five months, at which time she developed spasmodic crying followed by apathy, and mental and physical regression. When first examined at eight months she had a mental development of one or two months, and showed irregular jerking movements of the extremities, muscle wasting, spastic extremities, stiff neck, a decerebrate posture, and repeated epileptiform attacks. A pneumo-encephalogram disclosed evidence of cerebral atrophy. The course was progressively downhill, and the child died at the age of fifteen months. A younger sister was reported as having a similar neurologic disorder.

The brain showed a diffuse grayish discoloration of the cerebral and cerebellar white matter, of the optic and pyramidal tracts, of the corpus callosum, fornix, and the thalamus; the U-fibers and the cerebral cortex were spared. However, the folia of the cerebellum were atrophied (Fig. 193a).

Microscopically, the white matter contained accumulations of large mononuclear and multinucleated cells, concentrated in perivascular spaces (Fig. 193b). With the luxol fast blue-PAS method, the globoid cells stained positively with PAS while the diffuse loss of myelin was associated with proliferation of astrocytes and glial fibers (Fig. 193c). Secondary degeneration as well as repeated anoxic episodes during convulsions probably accounted for the atrophy of the cerebellar gray matter.

*References*

Suzuki, K., and W. D. Grover. Krabbe's Leukodystrophy (Globoid Cell Leukodystrophy). Arch. Neurol. 22: 385, 1970.
Suzuki, K., and Y. Suzuki. Globoid Cell Leukodystrophy (Krabbe's Disease): Deficiency of Galactocerebroside B-Galactosidase. Proc. Nat. Acad. Sci. USA. 66: 302, 1970.

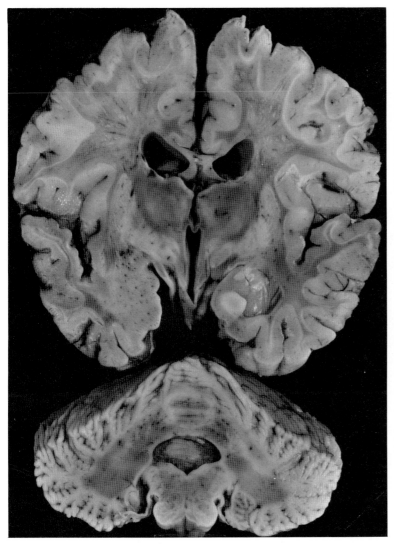

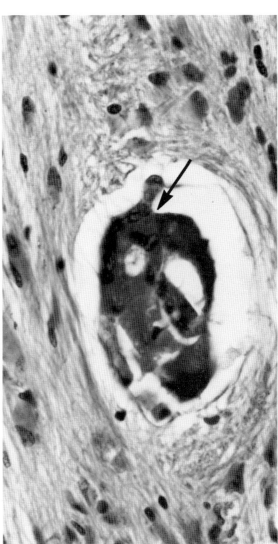

Fig. 193a. Krabbe's disease

Fig. 193b. HE × 435

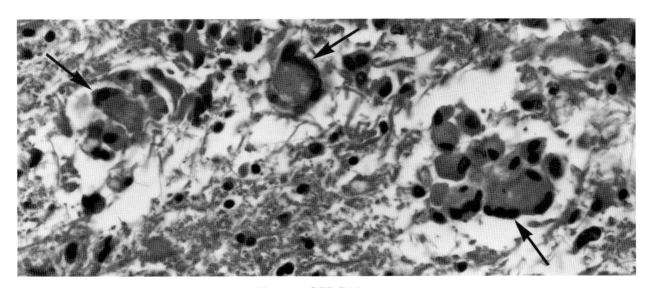

Fig. 193c. LFB-PAS × 475

There are familial forms of leukodystrophy in which the same pathologic criteria apply as in the previously described types but in which the breakdown products of myelin are sudanophilic. As such they are not readily distinguished from the sporadic demyelinating disorders, such as Schilder's disease. Their biochemical distinction is based on the demonstration of increased hexosamine levels. They have been classified into a) simple or orthochromatic type; b) Pelizaeus-Merzbacher's disease, and c) Seitelberger type.

## Pelizaeus-Merzbacher's Disease

This is a rare, familial disease, that usually has its onset in infancy but follows a very chronic course. Its mode of inheritance is sex-linked recessive, occurring only in males. Clinically, there is microcephaly and slow progression of mental deterioration and spasticity. The biochemical basis of the disorder has remained unknown.

Pathologically, a characteristic pattern of demyelination occurs in which preserved islands of myelin are left in the white matter, giving it a "tigroid" appearance. Usually only sparse sudanophilic lipid products in macrophages are found, probably because of the protracted course of the disease.

> *Case:* A 13-year-old, white boy had a normal birth and up to the age of six months his development proceeded normally. But from then on he showed increasing signs of physical and mental retardation. His body weight and height remained virtually stationary. There was marked microcephaly. He displayed no signs of intelligence or interest in his surroundings, had no sense of balance, did not learn to walk or talk and gradually developed spasticity with contractures of his lower extremities. He suffered frequently from upper respiratory infections and ultimately expired of bronchopneumonia.
>
> The family history showed that an older brother suffered from the same condition and died at the age of twenty-two years, while a sister, age fifteen, is normal.

The brain weighed 500 grams. It showed marked atrophy, restricted to the white matter of the cerebrum, accompanied by ventricular enlargement (Fig. 194a), and of brain stem and cerebellum.

In myelin stains, demyelination of the white matter was associated with scattered islands of preserved myelin (Fig. 194b), that contained sparse granules of sudanophilic lipid in demyelinated areas and in perivascular spaces (Fig. 194c).

*Reference*

Gerstl, B., N. Malamud, R. B. Hayman, and P. R. Bond. Morphological and Neurochemical Study of Pelizaeus-Merzbacher Disease. J. Neurol., Neurosurg., and Psychiat. 28: 540–547, 1965.

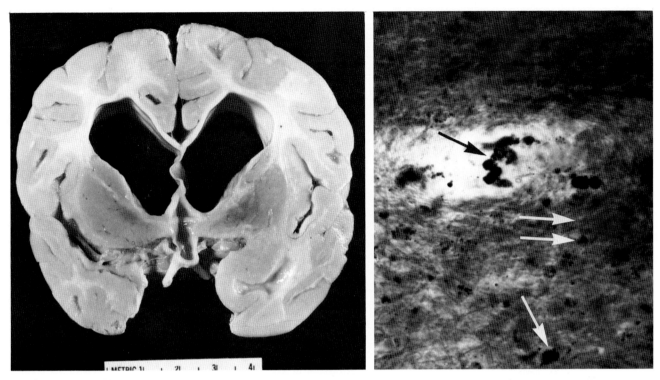

Fig. 194a. Pelizaeus-Merzbacher's disease

Fig. 194c. Oil Red O × 225

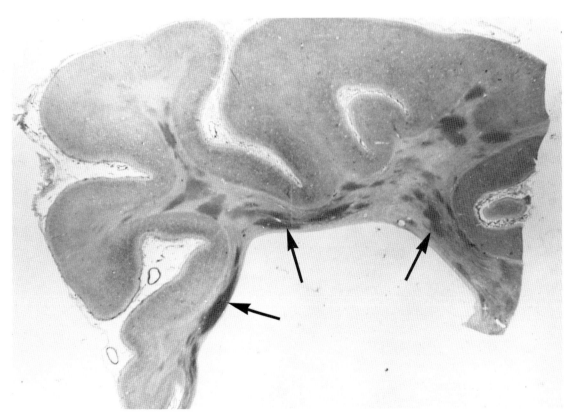

Fig. 194b. Luxol-fast blue stain

Sidman, et al., have described a murine mutant "Jimpy," which was characterized on the basis of optical microscopy as a sudanophilic leukodystrophy. The peripheral nervous system appeared essentially normal. When examined in the electron microscope, the Jimpy brain was found to contain very few intact myelin sheaths (Fig. 195). On the other hand, the axons were not actually naked. Instead, numerous axons were surrounded by thin sheaths of oligodendroglial cytoplasm. Sometimes short segments of these sheaths were fused and formed short lengths of a major dense line.

Quaking is another, similar murine mutant, which also showed a paucity of myelin formation in the central nervous system but the condition is not as severe as Jimpy. In addition to a decrease in the number of myelin sheaths, Quaking also shows bizarre, distorted configurations of the myelin geometry.

*References*

Berger, B. Quelques aspects ultrastructuraux de la substance blanche chez la souris Quaking. Brain Res. 25: 35, 1971.

Hirano, A., D. S. Sax, and H. M. Zimmerman. The Fine Structure of the Cerebella of Jimpy Mice and Their "Normal" Litter Mates. J. Neuropath. and Expt. Neurol. 28: 388, 1969.

Sidman, R. L., M. M. Dickie, and S. H. Appel. Mutant Mice (Quaking and Jimpy) with Deficient Myelination in Central Nervous System. Science. 144: 309, 1964.

Torii, J., M. Adachi, and B. W. Volk. Histochemical and Ultrastructural Studies of Inherited Leukodystrophy in Mice. J. Neuropath. and Expt. Neurol. 30: 278, 1971.

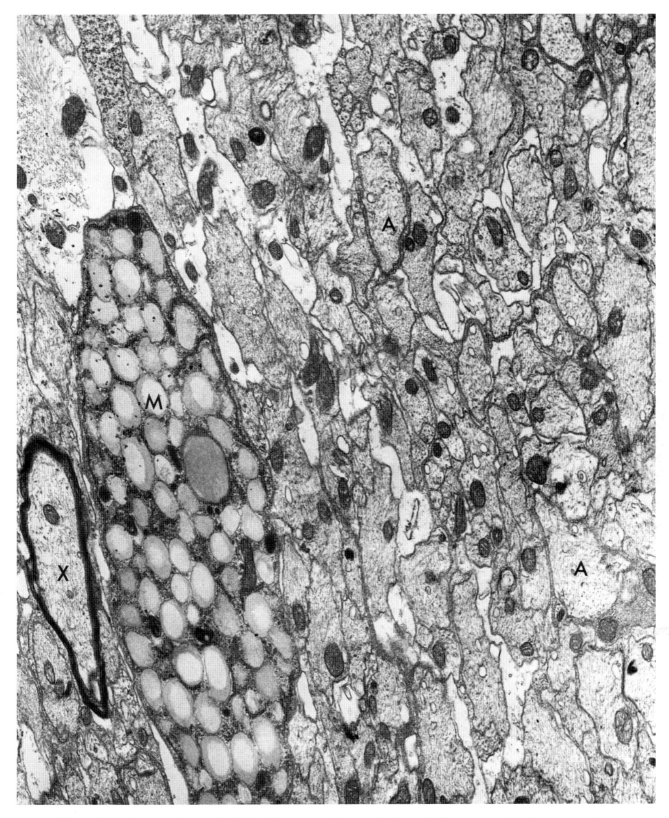

Fig. 195. An electron micrograph of the white matter of the cerebellum of a Jimpy mouse showing a macrophage (M) and a single myelinated fiber (X) adjacent to a mass of unmyelinated axons (A), × 17,000 (Hirano et al., J. Neuropathol. Exper. Neurol. 28: 388, 1969)

A rare, familial disorder, with autosomal recessive inheritance, SS occurs predominantly in Jewish children. It is characterized clinically by progressive mental retardation, macrocephaly, blindness, optic atrophy, hypotonia, spasticity, involuntary movements, seizures, and ultimate decerebrate rigidity. Death usually occurs prior to the age of three years, but on occasion there are more protracted forms.

The biochemical nature of the disease remains unknown. Its pathologic resemblance to phenylketonuria and maple syrup urine disease has led to speculation that it may be due to an accumulation of unusable amino acids that are water soluble.

Pathologically, there are two noteworthy histologic features: 1) diffuse spongy degeneration, limited to the deeper layers of the cortex and the adjacent U-fibers, and to similar border zones in the cerebellum, without evidence of macrophages and breakdown products and only mild reactive gliosis, and 2) occurrence of Alzheimer's glia of type II, represented by enlarged chromatin-poor glial nuclei without demonstrable cytoplasm.

> *Case:* A 9-year-old girl of Irish extraction, with negative family history, exhibited slow development from birth. At the age of three months, examination revealed a large head, nystagmus, esotropia and pneumoencephalographic evidence of cerebral and cerebellar atrophy. At the age of three years she was committed to a State hospital because she was severely retarded with no speech, was unable to sit or roll over in bed, had a head circumference of 50 cm, asymmetrical ears, high narrow palate, alternating esotropia and rotary nystagmus, hyperactive deep reflexes, bilaterally positive Babinskis, and a tendency to decerebrate posturing. She showed progressive deterioration and expired of bronchopneumonia.

The brain weighed 1,300 grams and showed on section diffuse atrophy and grayish discoloration of the cerebral white matter, that appeared microcystic, associated with ventricular enlargement (Fig. 196a).

Myelin stains revealed innumerable vacuoles in both gray and white matter, especially in lower layers of the cortex, and in the U-fibers where there was diffuse loss of myelin that contrasted with the better myelinated central and periventricular regions (Fig. 196b).

A higher magnification showed vacuoles of variable size in the affected gray and white matter, interspersed amongst the myelinated fibers and oligodendroglia, without any indication of breakdown products (Fig. 196c). There were scattered Alzheimer's glia in the form of large nuclei with only sparse chromatin (arrow) near the nuclear membrane (Fig. 196d).

The case illustrated a more protracted form of the disorder, characterized by decrease in the initial macrocephaly and by somewhat greater extension of the changes in the white matter than in other reported cases.

*References*

Banker, B. Q., J. T. Robertson, and M. Victor. Spongy Degeneration of the CNS in Infancy. Neurol. 14: 981, 1964.
Buchanan, D. S., and R. L. Davis. Spongy Degeneration of the Nervous System. Neurol. 15: 207, 1965.
Adachi, M., and B. W. Volk. Protracted Form of Spongy Degeneration of the CNS (van Bogaert and Bertrand Type). Neurol. 18: 1084, 1968.

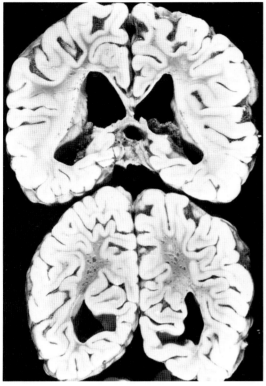

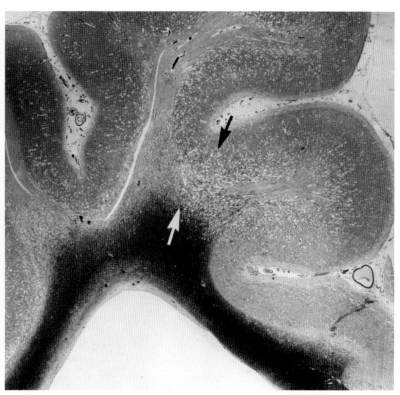

Fig. 196a. Spongy sclerosis (Canavan's disease)

Fig. 196b. LFB-PAS stain

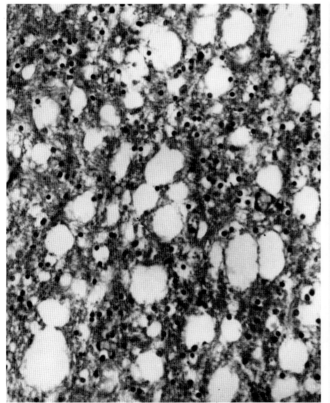

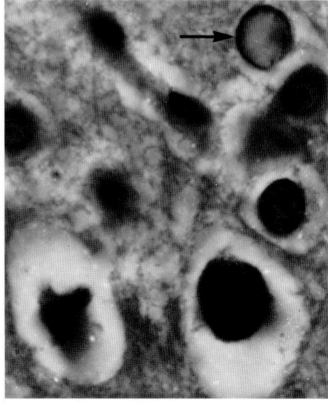

Fig. 196c. LFB-PAS × 250

Fig. 196d. HE × 600

Among the disturbances of amino acid metabolism, those of particular neuropathologic interest are phenylketonuria and maple syrup urine disease. Both are familial disorders with autosomal recessive inheritance and appear to have in common defective myelination and spongy degeneration of white matter. It has been suggested that the spongy change might be due to accumulation of polypeptides, resulting from impaired protein synthesis, stemming from the amino acid imbalance, within glial cells and so leading to impaired myelination.

## PHENYLKETONURIA (PKU)

PKU is a hereditary disease in which there is an enzymatic defect of hydroxylation of phenylalanine to tyrosine. As a result, phenylalanine accumulates in body fluids and is excreted as phenylpyruvic acid and other compounds in the urine. The prominent clinical features are mental retardation, epilepsy, hyperkinesia, dilution of hair and iris color, and eczema.

The most significant pathologic changes in the central nervous system are changes in myelin, either in the nature of defective myelination, dysmyelination and/or demyelination. A most consistent finding is spongy degeneration of the white matter that appears to develop at a slow tempo but is progressive and in late stages gives place to frank demyelination.

*Case 1:* A white male, aged eighteen years, was retarded from birth, and was committed to a hospital for the retarded because of increasing hyperactivity. A diagnosis of PKU was established on the basis of repeated urine tests. His course remained unchanged and he died of bronchopneumonia.

The brain weighed 1,100 grams, was grossly unremarkable, but microscopically showed widespread spongy state of the white matter, characterized by countless vacuoles interspersed among the myelin sheaths accompanied by only sparse fat and mild gliosis (Fig. 197a).

*Case 2:* A white male, aged thirty years, was retarded from birth and was admitted at age eight to a hospital for the retarded where he was noted to be blonde with blue eyes, underdeveloped but showing no definite neurologic abnormalities. At the age of twenty-two, he developed seizures for the first time followed by progressive spastic quadriplegia with pyramidal signs and athetosis. The electroencephalogram was abnormal, showing slow spiking activity. Several urine tests were positive for PKU. He expired of an intercurrent infection.

The brain weighed 930 grams and showed grossly bilateral diffuse demyelination of the white matter, midway between cortex and ventricles, restricted to the dorsal parts of the hemisphere (Fig. 197b).

Microscopically, large areas of demyelination were found near adjoining areas of spongy state (Fig. 197c). There were abundant deposits of sudanophilic lipid in macrophages in demyelinated areas (Fig. 197d).

The two cases thus appeared to show various stages of changes in myelin.

*References*

Benda, C. E. Developmental Disorders of Mentation and Cerebral Palsies. Grune and Stratton (New York, 1952), p. 451.
Crome, L., and C. M. B. Pare. Phenylketonuria, J. Ment. Sc. 106: 862, 1960.
Jervis, G. A. Pathology of Phenylketonuria. Phenylketonuria. Chas C. Thomas (Springfield, Ill., 1963), p. 96.
Malamud, N. Neuropathology of Phenylketonuria. J. Neuropath. and Expt. Neurol. 25: 254, 1966.
Poser, C. M., and L. van Bogaert. Neuropathological Observations in PKU. Brain. 82: 1, 1959.

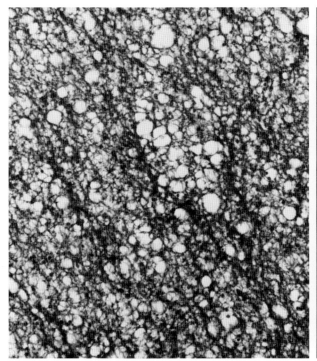

Fig. 197a. LFB-PAS × 250

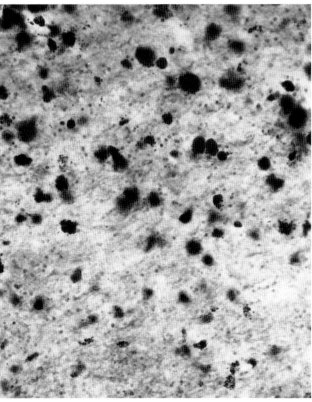

Fig. 197b. Demyelination in phenylketonuria

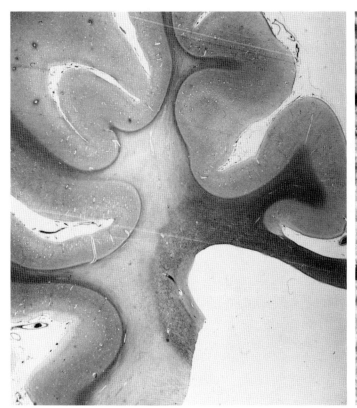

Fig. 197c. Weil stain

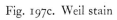

Fig. 197d. Oil Red O × 250

# DISORDERS OF GALACTOSE METABOLISM (GALACTOSEMIA)

Galactosemia is a rare familial disorder, with autosomal recessive transmission, characterized by inability to convert galactose to glucose because of deficiency of the enzyme galactose-1-phosphate uridyl transferase. The condition develops postnatally within a few days of milk ingestion and is characterized clinically by vomiting, diarrhea, hemolysis, jaundice associated with hepatomegaly, and cataracts. If not treated, there is either fatal termination or survival with cataracts and mental retardation. The pathognomonic clinical signs are elevated blood galactose and galactosuria, and demonstration of reduced enzyme in the blood. The pathogenesis is unclear but is believed to be due to the toxic effects produced by accumulation of galactitol in tissues. The effect on the nervous system is obscure, with suggestion that galactose toxicity may retard either utilization of glycogen, conjugation of bilirubin, synthesis of cerebrosides, or deficiency in ATP.

Pathologically, the hepatic lesions consist of early fatty metamorphosis followed by portal cirrhosis. The changes in the central nervous system have not been adequately investigated but on the whole have been nonspecific. In a few surviving chronic cases with mental retardation, gliosis of the white matter was reported, with or without other changes.

> *Case:** A white infant girl was the product of a full-term normal pregnancy and birth was uneventful, but on the second day she presented a feeding problem with frequent regurgitation and increasing jaundice. Total bilirubin was 21.2 mg (direct bilirubin 1.3); Coombs test was negative. Ecchymosis and purpuric spots appeared on the skin and hematologic examination indicated fragmentation hemolytic anemia, thrombocytopenia, and disseminated intravascular coagulation. Blood transfusions were administered. Liver function tests showed increasing signs of impairment. A laparotomy was then performed which revealed hepatomegaly with moderate ascites. The liver biopsy showed marked portal cirrhosis with fatty infiltration, bile stasis and pseudoacinar transformation of hepatic cells, suggestive of galactosemia. Urinalysis disclosed evidence of nonglucose reducing substances. The plasma revealed true glucose of approximately 50% and 8 mg% of nonglucose reducing substance consistent with galactosemia. Ophthalmologic examination revealed hypertelorism and bilateral nuclear lens opacities. Electrolyte imbalance, progressive edema, and increasing lethargy developed, terminating in death six weeks after onset of symptoms.

Autopsy revealed the essential findings to be marked hepatomegaly, the liver being cirrhotic with greenish-black color, and mild splenomegaly.

The brain weighed 400 grams and was not remarkable grossly.

Microscopic examination revealed some evidence of retarded myelination with virtually no myelin in the cerebral white matter (Fig. 198a). There were large numbers of macrophages in the white matter and leptomeninges containing lipid material that stained positively with oil red O (Fig. 198b) and with PAS, respectively.

This apparent sudanophilic leukodystrophy in an acute phase of the disorder may be the counterpart of the gliosis of white matter seen in chronic stages. Because of lack of biochemical information, it is however not possible to indicate its pathogenesis.

*Courtesy of N. Mortensen, M.D., St. Mary's Hospital, San Francisco.

*References*

Crome, L. A Case of Galactosemia with the Pathologic and Neuropathologic Findings. Arch. Dis. Child. 37: 415, 1962.
Haberland, C., M. Perou, E. G. Brunngraber and H. Hof. The Neuropathology of Galactosemia. A Histopathological and Biochemical Study. J. Neuropath. and Expt. Neurol. 30: 431, 1971.

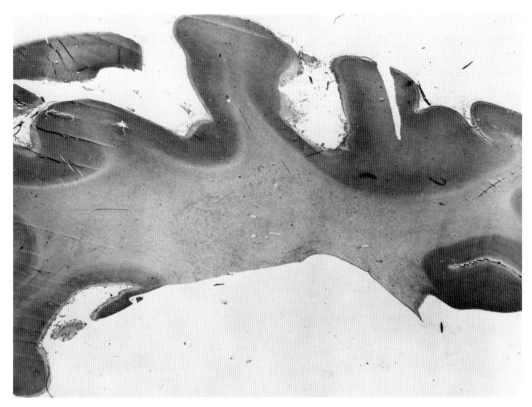

Fig. 198a. LFB-PAS stain

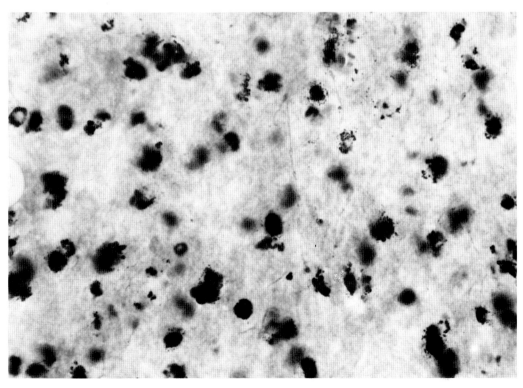

Fig. 198b. Oil Red O × 375

Wilson's disease (also known as hepatolenticular degeneration and pseudosclerosis of Westphal-Strümpell) is a familial disorder of copper metabolism, inherited as an autosomal recessive trait. It has an age range of four to forty years, although more commonly involving adolescents and young adults. The clinical symptoms vary from the more common extrapyramidal syndromes to cerebellar and pyramidal signs, and to emotional and mental changes, while symptoms of the liver cirrhosis are usually inconspicuous or absent. The diagnosis is based on the Kayser-Fleischer ring, consisting of greenish-yellow pigmentation on the periphery of the cornea, on ceruloplasmin deficiency, and on demonstration of copper in liver or muscle biopsies.

Biochemically, there is a decrease in ceruloplasmin-bound copper in the serum (less than 20 mg/100 ml), increased intestinal absorption and urinary excretion of copper, and increase in concentration of copper in various tissues, especially liver, muscle, brain and cornea. There is also amino aciduria. Chelating agents, such as Bal and penicillamine, have had a beneficial therapeutic effect in some instances.

The pathologic changes in the liver are those of a postnecrotic type of cirrhosis. In the brain, two types of changes are present: a) focal areas of spongy necrosis in the lenticular region and thalamus, lower layers of the cerebral cortex, dentate nucleus, and brain stem; and b) diffuse proliferation of abnormal astrocytes, known as Alzheimer's glia, consisting of either sparsely scattered giant cells with a hyperchromatic lobulated nucleus surrounded by a pale narrow rim of cytoplasm (Type I), or of more numerous forms having a naked chromatin-poor large nucleus without distinct cytoplasm except for a few granules (Type II); also Opalski cells, probably a variant of Type I, in which the nucleus is small and pyknotic while the cytoplasm shows signs of degeneration.

The pathogenesis of the lesions in the central nervous system has been attributed either to direct toxic action of copper or to secondary effects as a result of disturbed liver metabolism, especially since similar changes are present in other types of cirrhosis.

*Case:* An 11-year-old, white girl began having emotional difficulties at age nine and was admitted to a hospital one year later with a diagnosis of childhood schizophrenia. Later she was found to have Kayser-Fleischer corneal rings and a diagnosis of Wilson's disease was made. Examination revealed virtual unresponsiveness, marked rigidity and dystonia, with both arms and legs held in rigid extension and internal rotation, absent tendon reflexes and no pathologic reflexes. The ceruloplasmin level was 6 mg %. A liver biopsy was positive for copper. She was treated with penicillamine, 250 mg, four times daily, but there was progressive deterioration with continuing fever spikes and she expired two years following the onset of symptoms.

The liver showed a coarse multilobular cirrhosis (Fig. 199a).

The brain was not remarkable grossly with the exception of mild atrophy of the putamen and globus pallidus.

In stained preparations, a spongy type of degeneration was most pronounced in the lenticular region (Fig. 199b) that microscopically consisted of vacuolization of the nervous tissue and scattered lipid-laden macrophages (Fig. 199c). Similar lesions were found in the thalamus, dentate nucleus, and base of pons; in the latter showing a typical pattern of pontine myelinolysis.

In the same areas, and to a lesser extent elsewhere in the central nervous system, there were changes in the astrocytes, characteristic of Alzheimer's glia of Type I (Fig. 199d), Type II (Fig. 199e), and of the Opalski form (Fig. 199f).

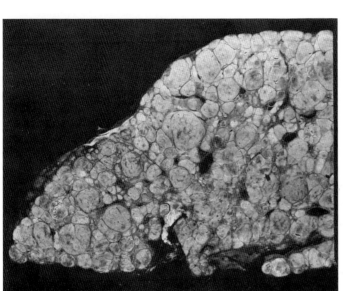

Fig. 199a. Liver cirrhosis in Wilson's disease

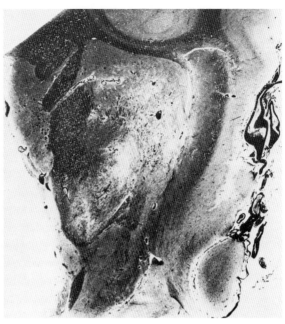

Fig. 199b. HVG stain of basal ganglia

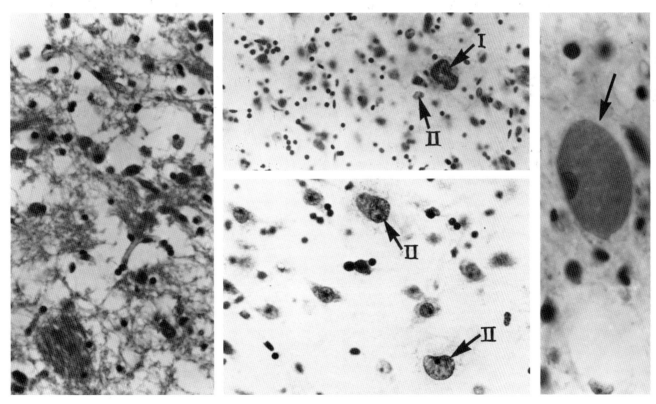

Fig. 199c. LFB-PAS × 280

Fig. 199d. Nissl × 350

Fig. 199e. Nissl × 475

Fig. 199f. Nissl × 560

HSD is a familial disorder, inherited as an autosomal recessive trait, that generally has its onset at about the end of the first decade of life and progresses slowly to death before age 30. The clinical symptoms are usually signs of an extrapyramidal syndrome, along with cerebellar signs and dementia.

Pathologically, there is a characteristic yellowish-brown pigmentation of the globus pallidus and the reticular zone of the substantia nigra, due to deposits of lipids, iron, and pseudocalcium and possibly other unknown elements. In these regions, there are degenerative changes along with prominent demyelination. In addition there is diffuse degeneration of other parts of the central nervous system, especially of the cerebellar and cerebral cortex. Another feature of the disease is the presence of axonal swellings or spheroids that are most numerous in the pigmented areas, although they may have a wider distribution.

The biochemistry of the disease remains unknown. It is not believed that it is a disorder of iron metabolism, although the pigmentary lesions occur primarily in regions normally rich in iron content. It is also noteworthy that the characteristic pigmentation has been reported in association with a great variety of other central nervous system diseases, although often without symptoms of HSD.

*Case:* A 30-year-old, white woman was admitted to a hospital with a history of normal development until age seven when increasing impairment of gait and mental changes set in. Family history was significant in that parents were second cousins and that patient's sister and brother suffered from a neurologic disease characterized by retardation and spasticity. Examination at age nine revealed inattentive and negativistic attitude; right hamstring spasm and weakness; a waddling gait; mild athetoid movements of fingers; and dysmetria of arms and legs. A few years later, there was an increase in mental deterioration and ataxia, examination revealing slurred speech, dysmetria, dyssynergia, dysdiadokokinesis, past-pointing, ataxia of gait, hyperactive reflexes, positive Babinski signs, pes cavus, and an I.Q. of 60. She was finally committed to a State hospital, where she showed a slowly progressive deterioration and expired of aspiration pneumonia.

The brain showed grossly a striking bronze discoloration of the globus pallidus (Fig. 200a) and of the substantia nigra (Fig. 200b) and diffuse atrophy of the cerebral and cerebellar cortex.

There was marked demyelination of the globus pallidus (Fig. 200c). With stains for iron (Fig. 200d) numerous granules and globules of iron pigment (A) were present in the pigmented areas, along with scattered spheroids that contained noniron pigments (B), some of which stained for lipids and for a PAS positive material. Diffuse axonal swellings (Fig. 200e) were found in these and other areas, associated with varying degrees of neuronal degeneration.

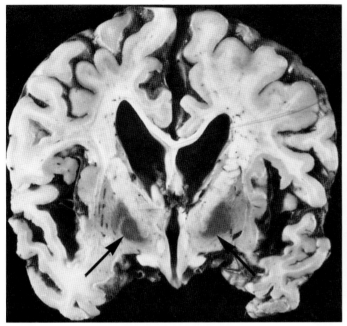

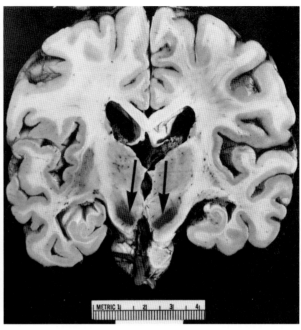

Fig. 200a. Hallervorden-Spatz disease with pigmentation of globus pallidus

Fig. 200b. Hallervorden-Spatz disease with pigmentation of substantia nigra

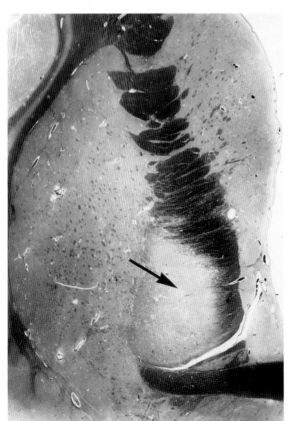

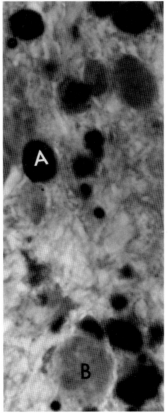

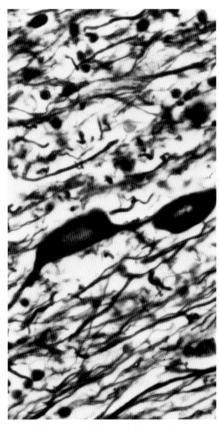

Fig. 200c. Weil stain showing demyelination of globus pallidus

Fig. 200d. Perl stain × 560

Fig. 200e. Glees stain × 560

## Hallervorden-Spatz Disease (HSD) in Electron Microscopy

In the electron microscope, the abnormally pigmented cells in HSD are found to contain a variety of inclusions embedded in a dense granular cytoplasmic matrix. Most inclusions consist of extremely dense globular (G) material (Fig. 201). In addition, some lamellated (La) structures are also present. Neither the origin nor nature of these inclusions are clearly understood.

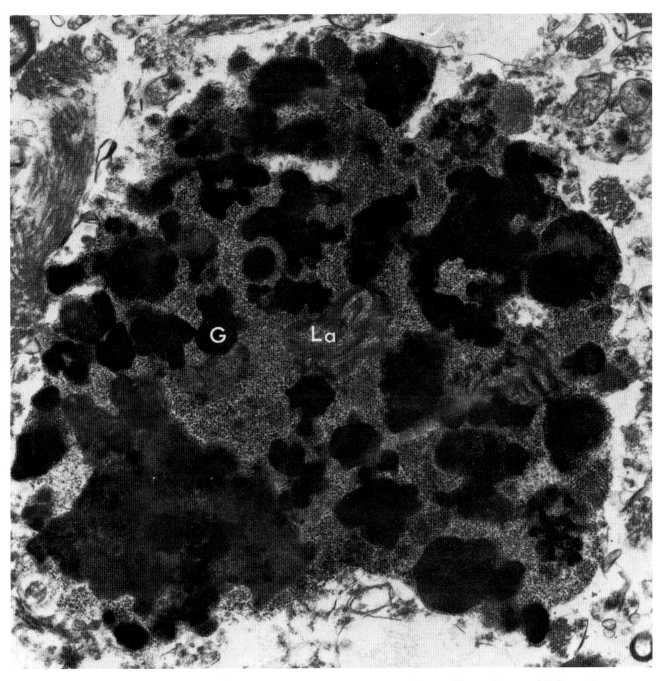

Fig. 201. Electron micrograph of an abnormally pigmented cell in the globus pallidus of a case of Hallervorden-Spatz disease × 25,000

## Infantile Neuroaxonal Dystrophy (INAD)

INAD, first described by Seitelberger in 1952, is considered to be a heredofamilial disorder, although its mode of inheritance is unknown. It has its onset in early childhood, usually before the second year of life. Its course is chronic and is manifested by symptoms of hypotonia, progressing to spasticity, with pyramidal signs, nystagmus, amaurosis, and mental retardation.

Pathologically, the principal feature is widespread occurrence of spheroids, more in gray than in white matter, affecting axons more than neurons. Although diffuse, the axonal swellings are especially numerous in the tegmentum of the medulla, posterior horns of the spinal cord, substantia nigra and globus pallidus; other findings are diffuse cerebral, cerebellar, and optic atrophy and increased lipids in basal ganglia.

In the electron microscope, the affected axons appear greatly distended due to an abnormally high number of various inclusions.

Biochemically, the axonal swellings contain proteins, lipids, and polysaccharides, and there is similar material in RE cells of the hematopoietic system. The nature of the metabolic defect remains unknown. It is noteworthy that the changes of neuroaxonal dystrophy have been observed, although in more limited degree, in a number of unrelated disorders including Hallervorden-Spatz disease, mucoviscidosis, congenital biliary atresia, the aging process and vitamin E deficiency in animals.

Opinions differ as to whether INAD is merely a form of Hallervorden-Spatz disease or a distinct entity.

*Case:* A white boy, aged three years, with negative family history, had a normal birth and early development, but at the age of five and one-half months he suddenly had four generalized seizures and was hospitalized. On examination he appeared inactive, unable to roll over or sit up, with periods of persistent screaming. There were nystagmoid movements. An electroencephalogram showed features of hypsarrhythmia. The seizures continued and he became a feeding problem, necessitating tube feeding. He was admitted at the age of three years to a State hospital, where examination disclosed complete immobility and lack of awareness of his surroundings; face was expressionless; he did not appear to see, the corneal reflexes being absent and the pupils failing to react to light. The upper and lower extremities were spastic with flexion contractures at the elbows and knees; deep tendon reflexes were hyperactive and all superficial reflexes were absent. An electroencephalogram revealed an abnormal, slow, and dysrhythmic sleep record with spike and slow wave variants and polyspike slow wave complexes. He expired one month following hospitalization.

The brain weighed 830 grams and showed evidence of diffuse cerebral, optic, and cerebellar atrophy, but without pigmentation (Fig. 202a).

The most noteworthy microscopic feature was the presence of widespread spheroids along the course of axons in the gray matter, especially numerous in the substantia nigra (Fig. 202b), globus pallidus and the nuclei gracilis and cuneatus (Fig. 202c), but also in cerebral cortex, hippocampus, thalamus, and midbrain.

The spheroids varied in size from 5-120 $\mu$, some containing central cores, and were strongly argyrophilic (Fig. 202d).

*References*

Cowen, D., and E. V. Olmstead. Infantile Neuroaxonal Dystrophy. J. Neuropath. and Expt. Neurol. 22: 175, 1963.

Indravasu, S., and R. A. Dexter. Infantile Neuroaxonal Dystrophy and Its Relationship to Hallervorden-Spatz Disease. Neurol. 18: 693, 1968.

Jellinger, K., and A. Jirasek. Neuroaxonal Dystrophy in Man: Character and Natural History. Acta Neuropath. Suppl. V, 3-16, Springer Verlag (Berlin, 1971).

Lampert, P. W. A Comparative Electron Microscopic Study of Reactive Degenerating, Regenerating, and Dystrophic Axons. J. Neuropath. and Expt. Neurol. 26: 345, 1967.

Seitelberger, F. Eine unbekannte Form von infantiler Lipoidspeicherkrankheit des Gehirns. Proc. First Internat. Congr. Neuropath. Rosenberg and Selliers Vol. 3 (Turin, 1952), p. 323.

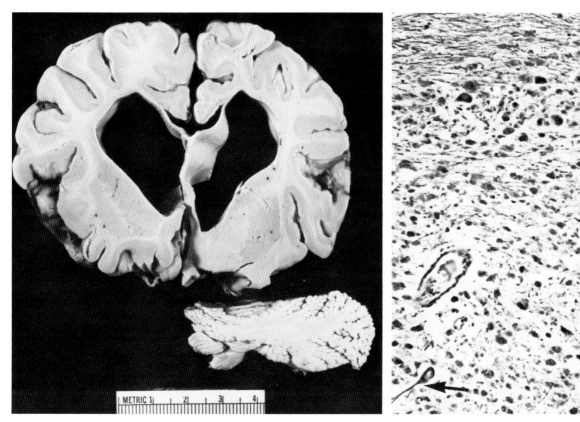

Fig. 202a. Infantile neuroaxonal dystrophy

Fig. 202b. Glees × 165

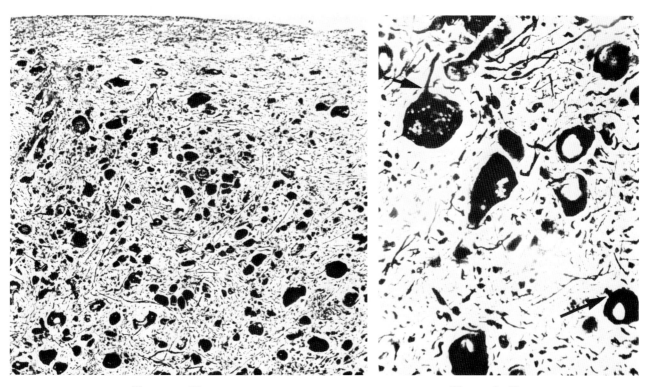

Fig. 202c. Glees × 225

Fig. 202d. Glees × 525

Primary deposition of calcium (or pseudocalcium) in the brain is encountered either in a) conditions associated with low serum calcium and high serum phosphorus, such as hypoparathyroidism and related disorders, or b) as an "idiopathic" disorder, sometimes familial, without known cause, referred to as Fahr's disease, in which the calcium appears to be super-imposed on deposition of acid mucopolysaccharides.

In either case, granular deposits of calcospherites occur in walls of blood vessels or free in the tissue and show a predilection for the basal ganglia, periventricular white matter and adjacent cortex, and cerebellum. The underlying nervous tissue is usually unaffected except in late stages. As a result, defect symptoms such as extrapyramidal signs, are relatively uncommon, and the clinical picture is dominated by symptoms of increased excitability such as tetany and convulsions. The diagnosis can be made on demonstration by x-rays of symmetrical calcification in the region of the basal ganglia.

*Case: Cerebral Calcification with Hypoparathyroidism.* A 32-year-old man began having periods of tetany and convulsions at the age of four years, at which time intracranial calcifications were demonstrated radiographically. Serum calcium was 7.6 mg % and phosphorus was 4.4 mg %. Secondary sexual characteristics were slow in developing. The seizures were controlled with intravenous calcium. The clinical diagnosis was idiopathic hypoparathyroidism. During his early twenties he developed Addison's disease. The terminal illness was caused by pulmonary infection.

General autopsy findings were primary atrophy of parathyroid glands and of adrenal cortex with secondary atrophy of testes, thyroid and pituitary glands.

Grossly, the brain showed scattered deposits of calcium that were concentrated in symmetrical parts of the caudate and putamen nuclei (Fig. 203a), the globus pallidus, thalamus, and dentate nuclei.

This was confirmed microscopically, in the form of deposits of granular material in walls of capillaries and venules with tendency to coalesce into larger masses, as evidenced in the putamen (Fig. 203b). The underlying nervous tissue showed no degenerative changes and only pseudocysts due to artefacts produced by sectioning. The material showed basophilic staining in HE and Nissl preparations, and argentophilic staining with Kossa's method for calcium.

*Case: Fahr's Disease.* A 5-year-old white girl, with negative family history and normal birth and early development, had the onset of generalized convulsions at the age of one year. Examination revealed an I.Q. of 50 but a negative neurologic status and normal electroencephalogram. When re-examined at the age of three years, there was bilateral athetosis; skull x-rays disclosed intracranial symmetric calcification, largely in the basal ganglia; the dye test for toxoplasmosis was negative; serum calcium was 9.6 mg % and phosphorus 3.6 mg %. Several months before her demise, she developed episodes of vomiting and lethargy; on re-examination there was evidence of further mental deterioration, aphonia, and extensor rigidity with bilateral positive Babinski signs. A ventriculogram disclosed what appeared to be a mass in the posterior fossa on the right side, followed by craniotomy that revealed several cysts in the right cerebellar hemisphere. Postoperatively, she developed signs of meningitis that resulted in her demise.

The brain showed grossly symmetrical deposits of calcium in central and periventricular white matter (Fig. 203c), basal ganglia, and cerebellum.

Microscopically, deposits of calcium were confirmed (Fig. 203d), that in many areas, as in the cerebellum, became associated with secondary cyst formation (Fig. 203e).

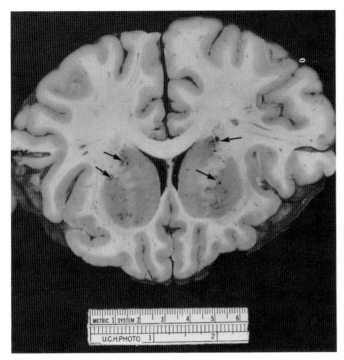

Fig. 203a. Calcification of basal ganglia in hypoparathyroidism

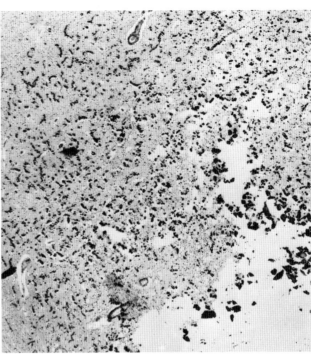

Fig. 203b. Nissl × 25

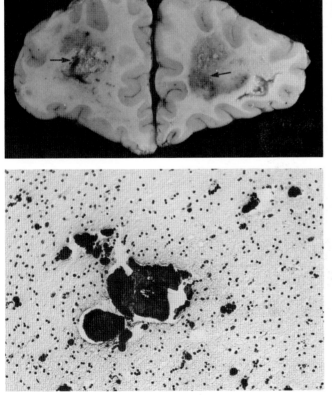

Fig. 203c. Calcification in frontal white matter of a case of
Fahr's disease (above)

Fig. 203d. Weil × 100 (below)

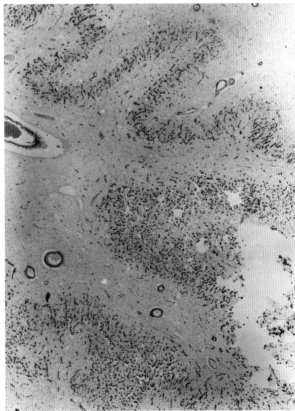

Fig. 203e. Nissl × 20

# X

## *Developmental Disorders*

Disorders of development, in a broad sense, include a great variety of conditions that have their onset pre, peri- or postnatally and form the basis for the ensuing mental retardation and/or cerebral palsy. In view of the fact that the etiologic factors often remain obscure, a pathoanatomic classification appears to be a workable basis for their separation and understanding.

The accompanying Table 1 illustrates such a classification and relative incidence in a large series of autopsied cases. This chapter will deal only with the first two groups since the metabolic and proliferative types have been discussed previously.

### Developmental Anomalies

The anomalies of the nervous system, as a group, are congenital disorders, characterized pathologically by signs of arrest or distortion of the normal fetal development, and, as a rule, lacking evidence of a destructive process.

It is possible in some instances to specify the definite stages in arrested development. These are usually gross anomalies and may be designated as specific malformations. In other instances, more subtle stigmata of arrested development justify a classification of nonspecific anomalies, whether or not they are associated clinically with Down's syndrome or other systemic anomalies.

The accompanying Table 2 includes the various types of cerebral anomalies and their incidence.

*References:*

Benda, C. E. Developmental Disorders of Mentation and Cerebral Palsies. Grune and Stratton (New York, 1952).

Crome, L. and J. Stern. The Pathology of Mental Retardation. Little Brown (Boston, 1967).

Malamud, N. Neuropathology. Mental Retardation (Stevens, H. A., and R. Heber, eds.), University of Chicago Press (Chicago, 1964), pp. 429–452.

Norman, R. M. Malformations of the Nervous System, Birth Injury and Diseases of Early Life. Neuropathology. Williams and Wilkins 2d ed. (Baltimore, 1963), pp. 324–440.

TABLE. NEUROPATHOLOGIC FINDINGS IN 2357 CASES OF

MENTAL RETARDATION AND CEREBRAL PALSY

| Type | | Number of Cases | Percent of Total |
|---|---|---|---|
| A. Developmental Anomalies | | 1,590 | 67.5 |
|     1. Specific malformations | 390 | | |
|     2. Nonspecific arrested development | 867 | | |
|     3. with Down's syndrome | 333 | | |
| B. Destructive Processes | | 598 | 25.4 |
|     1. Sequelae of perinatal trauma | 248 | | |
|     2. Sequelae of inflammatory disorders | 120 | | |
|     3. Sequelae of convulsive disorders | 53 | | |
|     4. Sequelae of icterus neonatorum | 35 | | |
|     5. Sequelae of vascular occlusion | 18 | | |
|     6. Sequelae of postnatal trauma | 8 | | |
|     7. Undetermined | 116 | | |
| C. Metabolic Disorders | | 136 | 5.7 |
| D. Proliferative (Neoplastic) Disorders | | 33 | 1.4 |
| Total | | 2,357 | 100.0 |

Table 1.

TABLE. CEREBRAL ANOMALIES IN 1,590 CASES OF MENTAL RETARDATION

| Type of Malformation | | No. of Cases |
|---|---|---|
| 1. Anomalies of convolutions (due to failures in migration) | | 150 |
|     Agyria-pachygyria | 28 | |
|     Micropolygyria | 56 | |
|     Heterotopia | 9 | |
|     Combinations | 57 | |
| 2. Holoprosencephaly (faulty cleavage of prosencephalon) (with or without arhinencephaly or microphthalmia) | | 12 |
| 3. Defects in closure of neural tube | | 40 (127*) |
|     Hydrencephaly | 13 | |
|     Porencephaly | 19 | |
|     Meningoencephalocele | 8 | |
|     Meningocele and myelomeningocele | (87*) | |
| 4. Failure in development of C.S.F. channels (hydrocephalus) | | 164 |
|     Arnold-Chiari malformation | 87 | |
|     Stenosis of aqueduct of Sylvius | 29 | |
|     Dandy-Walker syndrome | 20 | |
|     Communicating | 28 | |
| 5. Agenesis of corpus callosum** | | 15 |
| 6. Nonspecific anomalies | | 1,209 |
|     with Down's syndrome | 333 | |
|     without Down's syndrome | 876 | |
| | | 1,590 |

  * Same number of cases repeated in the category of hydrocephalus with Arnold-Chiari malformation.

  ** Only cases in which agenesis of corpus callosum was the principal
anomaly and not where it is associated with other gross malformations.

Table 2.

In the course of normal embryonic development, the brain undergoes changes in the formation of the gyri and sulci, from an initial stage of agyria or lissencephaly (Fig. 204a) through a stage of pachygyria to the mature pattern. A corresponding cellular migration takes place from the periventricular matrix (arrow) through an intermediate zone to form the cortex (Fig. 204b) at the same time as cell and layer differentiation and the formation of the white matter occurs. Disturbances in this process may result in agyria, pachygyria, micropolygyria and heterotopia, either singly or in combination.

## Agyria–Pachygyria

*Case 1:* A female infant had a premature (eighth month) breech birth, from which time she showed signs of microcephaly, idiocy, and polydactylism. She died at the age of three and one-half months.

The brain weighed 45 grams and measured 6 cm. in the antero-posterior diameter, which was approximately the same size as that of the normal fetus of three to four months. Like the latter, it showed complete agyria with only the sagittal and Sylvian fissures being developed (Fig. 204c).

*Case 2:* A female infant was born at term after a normal delivery. Her development was retarded from birth, and she presented the clinical picture of microcephalic idiocy, spastic quadriplegia, and epilepsy. She died at the age of two years.

The brain weighed 500 grams and showed symmetrical agyria of the frontal, parietal, and occipital lobes, in which only a few rudimentary sulci could be discerned (Fig. 204d).

In coronal sections, the agyric frontoparietal areas revealed an extremely wide cortex and a very narrow central core of white matter; the temporal lobes and parts of the occipital lobes, however, showed a relatively narrower cortex, though of simple pattern, with somewhat better development of white matter (Fig. 204e).

In various stains, it could be shown that an outer cortical mantle with a narrow zone of white matter beneath it, surrounded a large heterotopic mass of gray matter that extended to the walls of the ventricles.

In Nissel preparation, an unlaminated cortex, showing a columnar pattern of undifferentiated small spindle-shaped neurons, merged with the underlying heterotopic nerve cells (Fig. 204f).

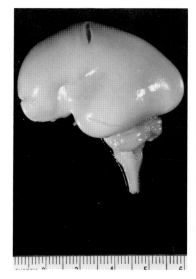

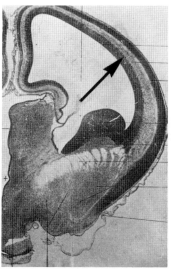

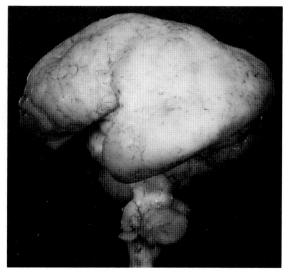

Fig. 204a. Fetal brain at 3–4 months of intrauterine development

Fig. 204b. Nissl stain of developing fetal brain

Fig. 204c. Agyria

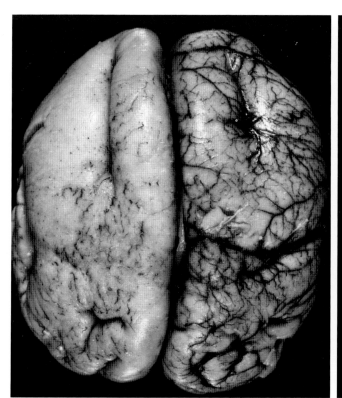

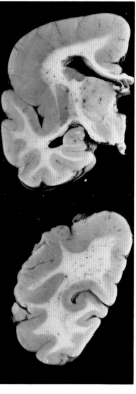

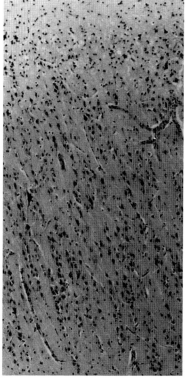

Fig. 204d. Agyria-pachygyria, external appearance

Fig. 204e. Agyria-pachygria, coronal sections

Fig. 204f. Nissl × 55

## Micropolygyria

Micropolygyria represents a more complex developmental disorder than agyria, characterized by countless small gyri and numerous yet shallow sulci, that may be generalized or focal, bilateral or rarely unilateral. Despite its complex appearance, however, the change appears to be superimposed over an underlying agyria, since like the latter there is lack of development of some of the primary fissures and sulci. It is possible that the process of migration is less uniform than in agyria.

> *Case:* A female infant, one of twins (the twin sister being normal), had an uneventful birth at term, although the pregnancy was complicated by pre-eclampsia. Convulsions and mental retardation became apparent at the age of four months. Examination revealed spastic quadriplegia, micrognathia, talipes equinovarus, and congenital laryngeal stridor. Death occurred at the age of two years.

The brain weighed 875 grams, and showed symmetrical focal micropolygyria of the central frontoparietal convolutions and absence of the Rolandic fissure (Fig. 205a).

In myelin stains, a greatly convoluted cortex (A) surrounded a narrow zone of white matter that contained scattered heterotopias (B) of gray matter that were also noted in the subependymal region of the enlarged ventricles (Fig. 205b).

Microscopically, the micropolygyric cortex lacked the normal lamination, consisting of two to three ill-defined pyramidal layers beneath a branching and deeply penetrating molecular layer associated with heterotopic nests of neurons in the underlying white matter (Fig. 205c).

In either agyria or micropolygyria, anomalies in deeper structures are rare with the exception of the cerebellum and inferior olives, where microfolia and heterotopia, respectively, are not uncommon; there is secondary agenesis of the pyramidal tracts.

Other types of malformation such as agenesis of the corpus callosum, porencephaly, etc., may coexist.

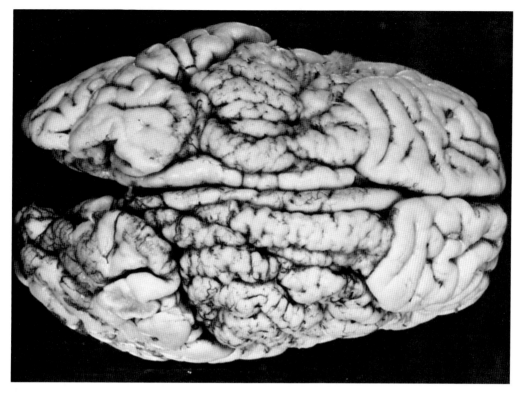

Fig. 205a. Micro-
polygyria

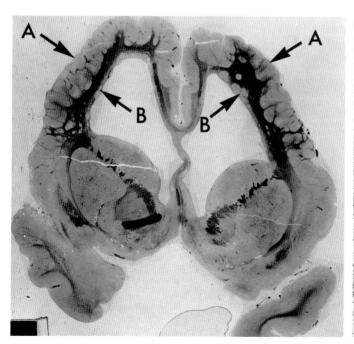

Fig. 205b. Weigert-
Kulschitzky stain in
micropolygyria

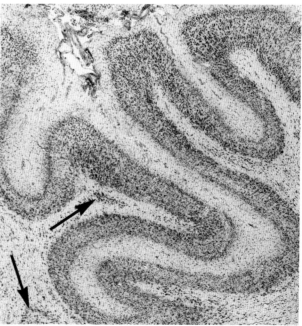

Fig. 205c. Nissl × 29

Holoprosencephaly is characterized by fusion of the cerebral hemispheres and by a single ventricle due to interference with the transformation of the embryonic single prosencephalon into the two telenecephalic structures. Generally, the fusion is partial, involving mainly the frontal lobes. Common associated features are agenesis of the olfactory pathways (arhinencephaly), microphthalmia with rudimentary optic pathways, absence of the falx cerebri, agenesis of corpus callosum and septum pellucidum, heterotopias, fusion of thalamus and absence of pyramidal tracts. There may also be extracranial anomalies in the form of median defects of face and nose and hypertelorism.

*Case:* A female infant was born at term after an uneventful pregnancy and delivery. The infant weighed four and a half pounds and had to be kept in an incubator for a week. Development was retarded from birth. When examined at the age of seven months, she showed microcephaly, idiocy, strabismus, congenital heart disease, right club foot, and anomalous external genitalia. Death occurred at the age of eight months.

The brain weighed 300 grams. It showed complete absence of olfactory bulbs and tracts; fusion of the frontal lobes; and an anomalous convolutional pattern (Fig. 206a).

A coronal section through the frontal area revealed no sign of sagittal fissure, corpus callosum and septum pellucidum, a single ventricle, and incomplete differentiation of the basal cortex, which was fused with the basal ganglia (Fig. 206b).

*Reference*

DeMyer, W., and W. Zeman. Alobar Holoprosencephaly (Arhinencephaly with Median Cleft of Lip and Palate). Confin. Neurol. 23: 1–36, 1963.

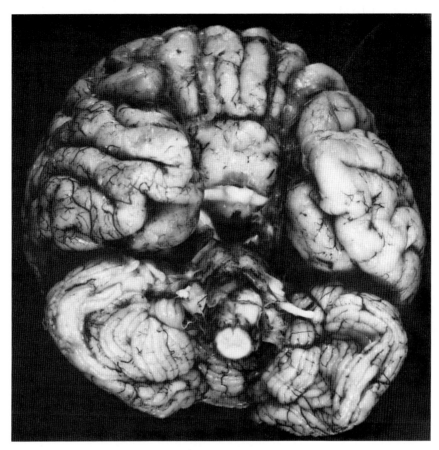

Fig. 206a. Holopros-
encephaly, external
appearance

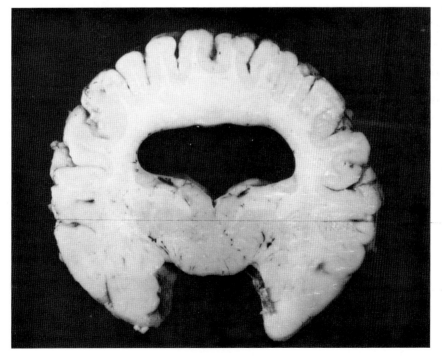

Fig. 206b. Holopros-
encephaly, coronal
section

Anomalies characterized by complete or circumscribed defects appear to be due to failure in closure of the neural tube or dysraphic states.

The most extreme example of such disorders is anencephaly in which the brain is either absent or rudimentary, associated with defect of the cranial vault and scalp, a condition that is incompatible with life. Those occurring in cases of mental retardation and cerebral palsy are hydrencephaly, porencephaly, and craniorachischisis.

## Hydrencephaly

Hydrencephaly (Fig. 207a) is characterized by absence of the major parts of the cerebral hemispheres with the exception of rudimentary basal parts of temporal and occipital lobes that along with the basal ganglia, lie in the floor of a membranous sac or dorsal cyst. The walls of the ventricles contain heterotopic nodules of gray matter, and the ependymal lining is in direct continuity with the thin roofing membrane. The latter consists of pia-arachnoid overlying a glial layer devoid of nerve cells and fibers. The brain stem and cerebellum are comparatively well formed with the exception of agenesis of the pyramidal tracts. The condition is associated with an extreme degree of microcephaly except in instances where coexistent stenosis of the aqueduct of Sylvius results in superimposed hydrocephalus.

Although hydrencephaly is considered by some to be due to impairment of circulation in the internal carotid system, it seems more likely to be a developmental disorder, closely related to the condition of porencephaly.

*Case:* A female infant, whose older sister had died shortly after birth and was described as a "monster," had a normal birth at term. The clinical features were microcephaly with failure in ossification of some areas in the frontal and parietal bones, mental retardation, spastic quadriplegia, and bilateral club feet. Death occurred at the age of three months.

Autopsy revealed many anomalies in the cardiovasculorenal system. The roofing membrane of the dorsal cyst had been removed exposing the open ventricle (A), the basal parts of the rudimentary hemispheres (B), the basal ganglia (C), while behind are small but well formed brain stem (D) and cerebellum (E) (Fig. 207b).

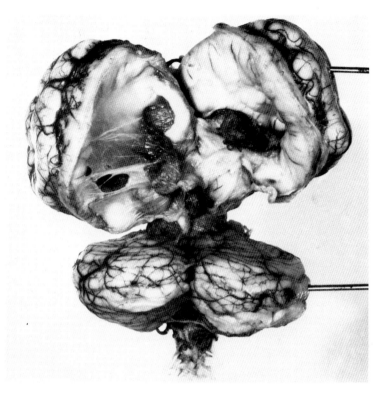

Fig. 207a. Hydren-
cephaly with roofing
membrane

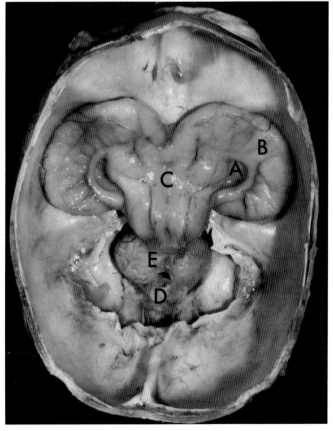

Fig. 207b. Hydren-
cephaly without roof-
ing membrane

## Porencephaly

Porencephaly (Fig. 208a) is a circumscribed defect in various locations of the cerebral hemispheres, ranging in degree from a cleft with fused lips to an open funnel-shaped gap covered by a roofing membrane. There is an uninterrupted continuity of the surface with the wall of the ventricle, the ependymal lining of the latter forming a meningo-ependymal seam with the pia-arachnoid; malformed tissue is present in the subependymal region. Symmetrical parts of the hemispheres are usually involved although often differing in the extent of the defect on the two sides.

> *Case:* A 37-year-old man had shown a spastic right hemiplegia, a mild left hemiparesis, and mental retardation from birth. The I.Q. was estimated at 41.

The brain weighed 970 grams, and contained a large cavity in the left central region and a cleft in the right central area. The funnel-shaped cavity (A) on the left contained choroid plexus (B) in its floor, was lined by ependyma and was surrounded by focal micropolygyria (C) and pachygyria (D) (Fig. 208b).

Microscopically, the ependymal lining (A) of the cavity could be traced to the surface, where it merged with the pia-arachnoid (B); numerous heterotopic masses of gray matter were found in the subependymal region (Fig. 208c).

Porencephaly has been interpreted (Yakovlev and Wadsworth) as a developmental disorder, occurring in the axis of the cerebral fissures (schizencephaly), by contrast with "pseudoporencephaly" that is acquired through circulatory or other mechanisms (encephaloclastic porencephaly).

*References*

Crome, L., and P. E. Sylvester. Hydranencephaly. Arch. Dis. Childhood. 33: 235, 1958.
Yakovlev, P. I., and R. C. Wadsworth. Schizencephalies: A Study of the Congenital Defects in the Cerebral Mantle. J. Neuropath. and Expt. Neurol. 5: 116 and 169, 1946.

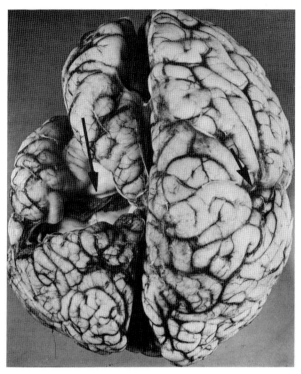

Fig. 208a. Porencephaly showing remnant of roofing membrane (above)

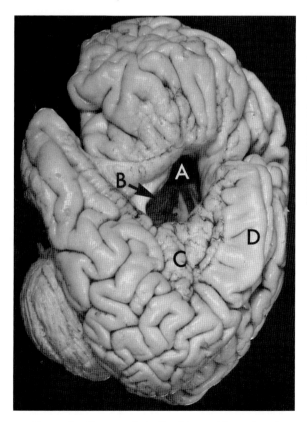

Fig. 208b. Porencephaly lined by malformed gyri (below)

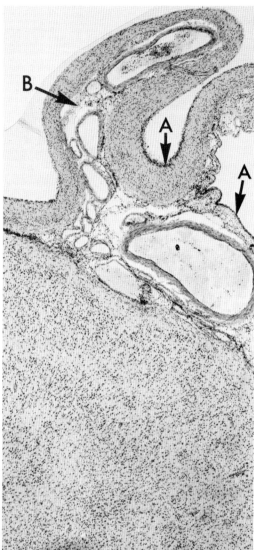

Fig. 208c. Meningoependymal seam, Nissl × 30

Midline defects in the skull or spine may result in herniation of either meninges (meningocele), brain (encephalocele) or spinal cord (myelomeningocele) into the sac.

## Meningoencephalocele (Cranium Bifidum)

Hernias of brain and/or meninges associated with skull defects occur in a variety of locations, notably occipital, frontal, and nasopharyngeal. The sac is covered by integument, to which the dura and arachnoid are adherent, and is filled with subarachnoid fluid in the case of meningocele, or with pia, malformed nervous tissue and, at times, a diverticulum of the ventricle, in the case of an encephalocele.

> *Case:* An 18-month old girl showed from birth microcephaly and an encephalocele in the occipital region, which was verified by x-rays. There were also signs of low-grade mental defect and a spastic paraplegia of the lower extremities. She died of meningitis that developed at the site of pressure erosion of the encephalocele.

The brain weighed 400 grams; it showed anomalies and flattening of the convolutions due to an internal hydrocephalus and a midline meningoencephalocele attached to the occipital region that was adherent to the scalp (Fig. 209a).

Microscopic examination of the contents of the sac revealed a mass of undifferentiated nervous tissue (A) surrounded by meninges (B) undergoing inflammatory reaction resulting from secondary infection (Fig. 209b).

## Meningocele and Myelomeningocele (Spina Bifida)

Defective fusion of the embryonal tissues in the dorsal median region results in various degrees of spinal dysraphism, from spinal bifida occulta to saclike protrusion containing meninges (meningocele) and spinal cord tissue (myelomeningocele). These anomalies are most common in the lumbosacral area, and in the case of myelomeningocele almost always complicated by hydrocephalus and Arnold-Chiari malformation.

> *Case:* A male infant was born at term. At birth spina bifida of the lumbosacral region was present, and both lower extremities were paralyzed. Later signs of progressive hydrocephalus became apparent, and there was severe mental retardation. He died at the age of two years of meningitis that developed at the site of the spinal bifida.

In the lumbosacral region a defect in the laminae of the vertebrae resulted in the formation of a sac (A) containing nerve roots, meninges, and spinal cord (B) that curved around the rostral edge of the sac (Fig. 209c).

A stained section showed the lack of fusion of the laminae in the midline, through which the spinal cord surrounded by meninges tended to protrude; the spinal cord was malformed showing incomplete separation of dorsal columns by a rudimentary dorsal septum (Fig. 209d), often accompanied by an enlarged central canal lined by ependyma, or hydromyelia.

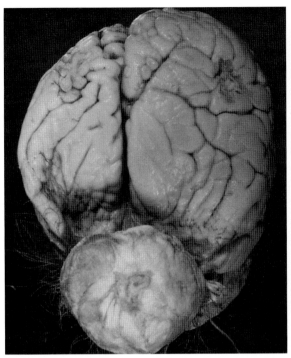

Fig. 209a. Occipital encephalocele

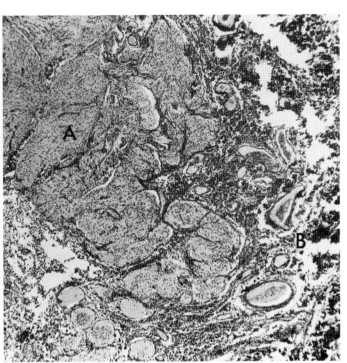

Fig. 209b. HVG × 32

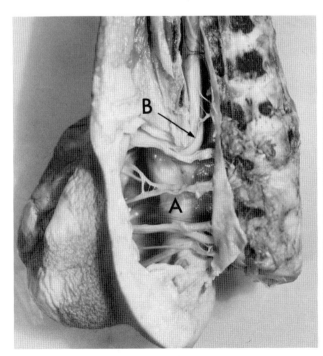

Fig. 209c. Myelomeningocele, external view

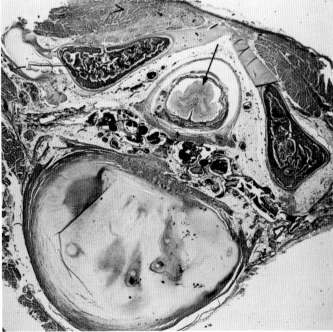

Fig. 209d. Myelomeningocele, section, HE × 20

Syringomyelia is generally regarded as a congenital malformation probably in the nature of a dysraphic state due to imperfect closure of the neural tube, although some consider it to be an embryonic central gliosis with subsequent cyst formation. It usually becomes symptomatic in middle age. It occurs most commonly in the lower cervical and upper thoracic levels of the spinal cord; when involving the medulla, it is designated as syringobulbia.

Syringomyelia usually begins as cavitation in the dorsal horn of one side (or less commonly in central parts dorsal to the central canal) and extends asymmetrically to involve both sides (Fig. 210a). A characteristic syndrome of sensory dissociation results from the early tendency to destroy the pathways subserving pain and temperature as they cross the central commissures while sparing the pathways subserving touch and sense of position at any given level. As the fluid-containing syrinx expands, increasing amounts of the surrounding gray and white matter are engulfed and undergo degeneration, giving rise to upper and lower motor neuron symptoms. The cavity is walled off by mixed glial, connective, and ependymal tissue.

The association of syringomyelia with tumors of the spinal cord is common, as illustrated in the following case:

> *Case:* A 2½-year-old boy, whose family history was negative and whose birth and early development were normal, began to have attacks of torticollis that became increasingly severe. At the age of five years he developed fever, vomiting, and difficulty in micturition. A neurologic examination revealed absent knee jerks, absent abdominal reflexes, and a Babinski sign on the right side. The findings in the cerebrospinal fluid were characteristic of Froin's syndrome. By the age of seven years he developed increasingly severe headaches, projectile vomiting, a low-grade fever, and persistent torticollis to the right. Examination disclosed thoracic kyphosis with scoliosis to the right, left hemiparesis, bilateral absence of knee jerks, absent ankle jerk on the right, and fasciculations in the muscles on the left calf. A myelogram revealed a complete block of the subarachnoid space between L-2 and L-3, and the spinal cord appeared enlarged. The total protein was 3,800 mg per 100 cc and the colloidal gold curve was 5554110000. A laminectomy was performed, revealing a cyst of the conus medullaris. The patient died postoperatively of bladder infection.

The brain showed a large cyst that almost replaced the entire medulla (Fig. 210b).

The spinal cord was diffusely enlarged throughout its length, and contained scattered intramedullary cavities, which were particularly noticeable in the conus medullaris and at the upper cervical level (Fig. 210c).

Sections through various parts of the spinal cord and medulla disclosed either diffuse tumor with secondary cavitation (A), or central syringomyelia (B) and syringobulbia (C) of the medulla, the latter causing marked compression of the surrounding restiform bodies, inferior olives, and pyramids (Fig. 210d).

The syringomyelic areas showed the irregular cavity to be lined by reactive glial and vascular tissue and partly by ependyma (Fig. 210e), whereas the neoplastic areas consisted of small fibrillary astrocytes (A) associated with cavitation (B), representing a low-grade astrocytoma (Fig. 210f).

*Reference*

Poser, C. M. The Relationship between Syringomyelia and Neoplasm. Chas. C Thomas (Springfield, Ill., 1956), American Lecture Series No. 262.

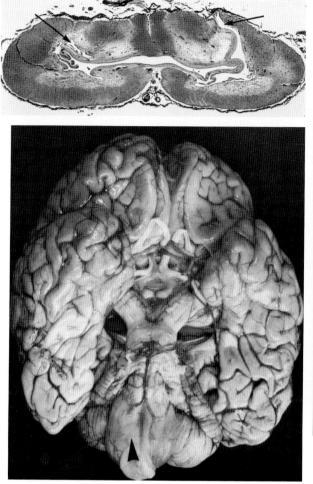

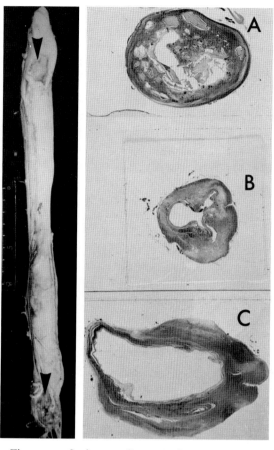

Fig. 210c. Syringomyelia and diffuse tumor of spinal cord (left)

Fig. 210d. HVG stain (right)

Fig. 210a. Syringomyelia, HVG stain (above)

Fig. 210b. Syringobulbia (below)

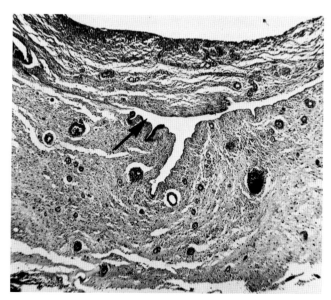

Fig. 210e. HVG × 32

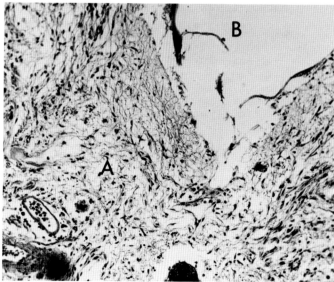

Fig. 210f. HVG × 100

A variety of disorders that manifest themselves primarily as hydrocephalus may be classified as 1) noncommunicating forms that result from stenosis or atresia of various parts of the ventricular system and its connections with the subarachnoid space, and 2) communicating forms caused by blockage of the subarachnoid spaces by an arachnoiditis or occasionally because of congenital absence of arachnoid villi. Hydrocephalus caused by excessive secretion of the cerebrospinal fluid due to hypertrophy or papilloma of the choroid plexus is a rare condition. To be excluded from this category is so-called hydrocephalus ex-vacuo, a form of ventricular dilatation caused by atrophy or hypoplasia of cerebral tissue.

The most common forms of congenital hydrocephalus are of the noncommunicating variety and may be classified into those associated with a) Arnold-Chiari malformation; b) stenosis of the aqueduct of Sylvius; and c) Dandy-Walker syndrome.

## Hydrocephalus with Arnold-Chiari Malformation

Two types of the Arnold-Chiari malformation have been distinguished:

Type I of Chiari, characterized by moderate downward displacement of the medulla into the spinal canal, covered on its dorsolateral surface by peg-like processes arising chiefly from the cerebellar tonsils (Fig. 211a). This is associated with relatively mild to moderate hydrocephalus, rarely, if ever, with myelomeningocele, and usually occurs in older children.

Type II of Chiari, characterized by marked downward displacement of the inferior vermis of the cerebellum, lower part of the medualla and fourth ventricle into the cervical spinal canal (Fig. 211b); there are signs of herniation of these structures through the foramen magnum (A), a marked degree of hydrocephalus (B), and almost invariably, an associated myelomeningocele (C). A number of other features are common in type II, such as rotation and dorsal swelling of the medulla at its junction with the spinal cord due to persistence of the embryonic cervical flexure; upward direction of the cervical nerve roots, stenosis or forking of the aqueduct of Sylvius, hydromyelia of the cervical cord, and various other cerebral anomalies. This type of malformation is usually recognized early in infancy.

The pathogenesis of the Arnold-Chiari malformation has remained controversial. The displacement has been attributed to a primary hydrocephalus, to traction produced by the mooring of the lower end of the spinal cord by the myelomeningocele, to a primary dysgenesis of the hindbrain, such as failure of development of the pontine flexure, or to an overgrowth of the formative brain.

*Case:* A 6-year-old girl was born with bilateral paraplegia due to myelomeningocele that was operated on and closed shortly after birth. Severe hydrocephalus became apparent a month later and she underwent a number of different shunting procedures. There were also other congenital anomalies, namely, bilateral hydrocephalus, congenital dislocated hips and talipes equinus. She was subject to recurrent infections that developed at the site of the surgical procedures and that led to her demise.

Coronal sections of the brain showed extensive hydrocephalus, secondary to stenosis of the aqueduct of Sylvius, and of the displaced fourth ventricle and foramina (Fig. 211c), that were surrounded by subependymal gliosis (Fig. 211d).

*References*

Peach, A. C. The Arnold-Chiari Malformation. Arch. Neurol. 12: 527–613, 1965.
Russell, D. S. Observations on the Pathology of Hydrocephalus. H.M.S.O. (London, 1949).

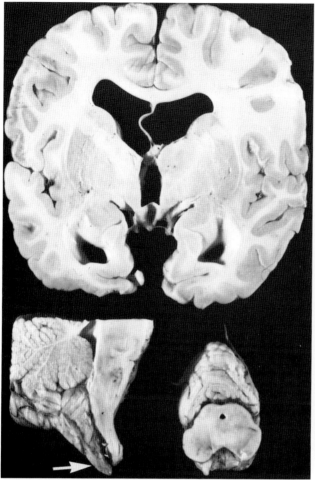

Fig. 211a. Arnold-Chiari malformation, Chiari type I

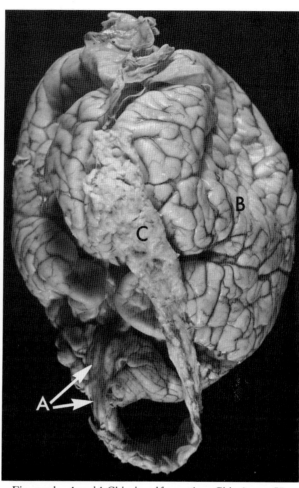

Fig. 211b. Arnold-Chiari malformation, Chiari type II, external appearance

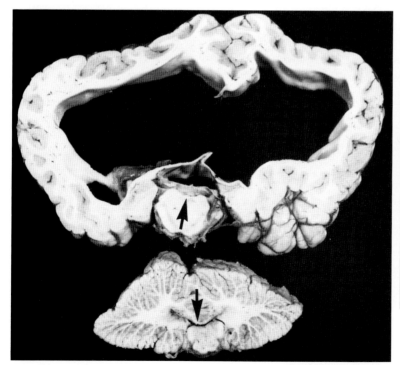

Fig. 211c. Arnold-Chiari malformation, Chiari type II, coronal section

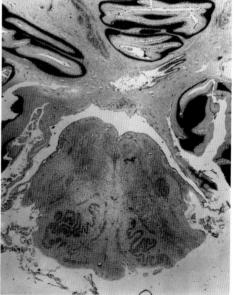

Fig. 211d. Nissl stain

## Hydrocephalus with Stenosis of Aqueduct of Sylvius

Congenital atresia or stenosis of the aqueduct of Sylvius, as a solitary anomaly, is a frequent cause of congenital hydrocephalus. It may assume a variety of forms such as simple narrowing, forking with disconnected dorsal and ventral channels, septum, or gliosis, the latter probably due to acquired intrauterine infection.

> *Case:* A 6-year-old boy had a difficult birth because of congenital hydrocephalus that was noted at birth. The head continued to enlarge and became associated with severe mental retardation.

The brain showed a marked degree of internal hydrocephalus involving symmetrically the ventricular system rostral to a stenosed aqueduct of Sylvius; all periventricular structures were severely atrophied and were disrupted postmortem (Fig. 212a).

Microscopic examination revealed marked narrowing of the entire aqueduct without signs of gliosis (Fig. 212b).

## Hydrocephalus with Dandy-Walker Syndrome

The Dandy-Walker syndrome comprises a combination of anomalies consisting of hydrocephalus, aplasia or hypoplasia of the cerebellar vermis, enlargement of the fourth ventricle and a posterior fossa cyst. The latter is covered by a greatly thinned medullary velum and tela choroidea and an inner ependymal layer, that actually represents the roof of the expanded fourth ventricle. The clinical picture is characterized by hydrocephalus, a bulging occiput, cranial nerve palsies, nystagmus, trunkal ataxia, and an elevated position of the imprint of the transverse sinuses in x-rays of the skull. There are often associated multiple cerebral and systemic anomalies.

The pathogenesis of the syndrome has been the subject of controversy as between congenital atresia of the foramina of Luschka and Magendie and persistence of the anterior membranous area in the roof of the embryonic fourth ventricle. Against the former theory is the fact that fusion of the cerebellar hemispheres to form the vermis is completed by the thirteenth week and the foramina open up only after the fourth month of fetal life.

In the following case with clinical evidence of a Dandy-Walker syndrome, the brain showed on external inspection hydrocephalus, a posterior fossa cyst, lined by a thin membrane that had been opened up postmortem to expose the enlarged fourth ventricle, and absence of the vermis (Fig. 212c).

The sections (Fig. 212d) confirmed the internal hydrocephalus, complete absence of the vermis, and narrowing of the foramina of Luschka (their patency and that of the foramen of Magendie could not be adequately determined postmortem).

*Reference*

Hart, M. N., N. Malamud, and W. G. Ellis. The Dandy-Walker Syndrome. Neurol. 22: 771, 1972.

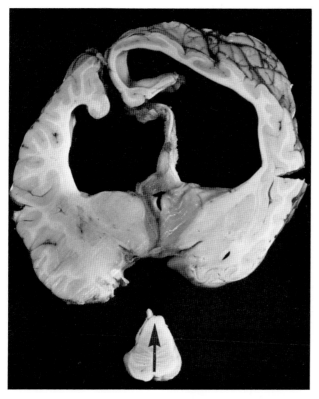

Fig. 212a. Hydrocephalus with stenosis of aqueduct of Sylvius

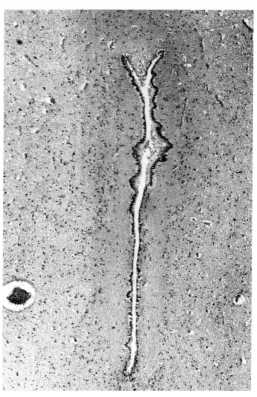

Fig. 212b. HE × 45

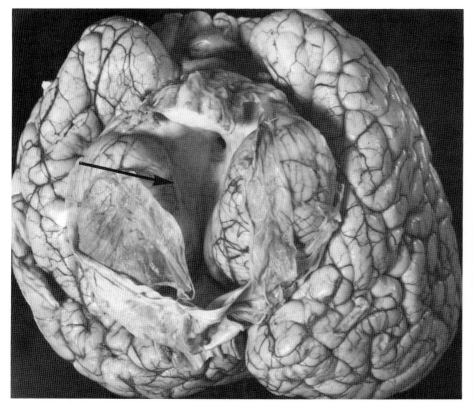

Fig. 212c. Dandy-Walker syndrome, external view

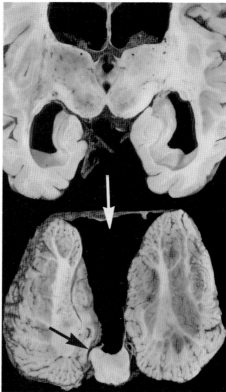

Fig. 212d. Dandy-Walker syndrome, coronal section

In the course of development, the corpus callosum along with the septum pellucidum, and the anterior and hippocampal commissures, take their origin from the upper part of the lamina terminalis and grow by expanding anteriorly and posteriorly during the twelfth to twentieth week of embryonic life (Fig. 213a).

Interference with this process may involve all or some of these structures, the most striking being an agenesis of the corpus callosum, complete or partial. It is significant that the exclusive absence of the corpus callosum is clinically asymptomatic, although, because of its frequent association with other cerebral anomalies, mental retardation and cerebral palsy are common symptoms.

> *Case:* A 10-year-old boy whose family and birth histories were negative showed retarded development from birth. He started to walk at five years and to talk at seven years. Examination revealed signs of idiocy, moderate microcephaly, and spastic quadriplegia.

The brain weighed 860 grams, and showed almost complete agenesis of the corpus callosum with only rudiments of genu and splenium (A), a small anterior commissure (B), absence of septum pellucidum, but a well-developed fornix (C); there was no clear-cut demarcation of the cingulate gyrus by a callosomarginal sulcus, and the sulci tended to radiate toward the callosal site, while the parieto-occipital and calcarine fissures failed to join (Fig. 213b).

Coronal sections disclosed a longitudinal band of fibers on the mesial walls of the laterally displaced and narrowed lateral ventricles, known as Probst's bundle, that joined the underlying fornix, while the third ventricle was displaced dorsally (Fig. 213c).

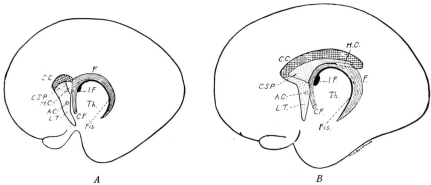

Schematic representation of the development of the septum pellucidum and telencephalic commissures: *A. C.*, Anterior commissure; *C. C.*, corpus callosum; *C. F.*, columna fornicis; *C. S. P.*, cavum septi pellucidi; *F.*, fornix; *H. C.*, hippocampal commissure; *I. F.*, interventricular foramen; *Fis.*, chorioid fissure; *L. T.*, lamina terminalis. (Based on drawings of models of the telencephalon of a four months' fetus (*A*) and of a five months' fetus (*B*) by Streeter.)

Fig. 213a. Diagram of developmental
stages of corpus callosum

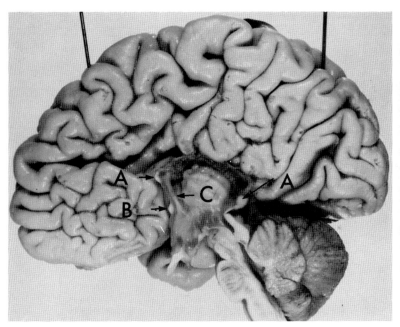

Fig. 213b. Agenesis of corpus callosum,
external view

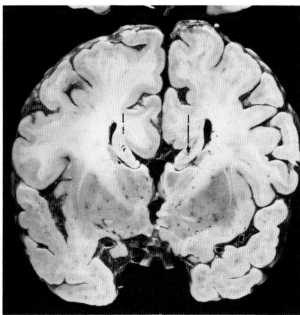

Fig. 213c. Agenesis of corpus callosum,
coronal section

The nonspecific anomalies comprise probably the largest group of cases of mental retardation and cerebral palsy that are not sufficiently characteristic to permit classification under any of the specific types previously described. This applies equally to those with and without Down's syndrome.

The anomalies are multiple, variable, and not very striking. They may consist of irregularities in sulci, variations in size of gyri, discrepancies in the relative size of the lobes, a relatively wide cortex, hypoplasia of the white matter including the corpus callosum and pyramids, hydrocephalus ex vacuo, disturbances in cytoarchitecture, and microscopic heterotopias.

The inconspicuous appearance of these anomalies is not necessarily an indication of a milder disturbance, since wide variations in the degree of mental defect are to be found in this group. Further, there is no reason to consider them as etiologically distinct from the specific malformations, since they differ from the latter only in degree but not in kind.

## Nonspecific Anomalies without Down's Syndrome

*Case:* A female infant, whose family history was negative, had a normal birth at term after an uneventful pregnancy. She never learned to walk or talk, was of low-grade intelligence, and exhibited general incoordination of voluntary movements. Death occurred at the age of three years.

The brain weighed 1,250 grams. Although the convolutional and sulcal pattern was fairly well outlined, the gyri were somewhat enlarged and simple; the frontal lobe was foreshortened, the temporal lobe was conspicuously prominent, and the occipital lobe was diminished and flat; the superior temporal gyrus was poorly outlined, and the sulci of the other temporal gyri tended to run transversely rather than longitudinally (Fig. 214a).

Coronal sections revealed a disproportionate excess of gray matter of a distinctly abnormal pattern, deep penetrations of the cortex into the white matter with consequent reduction in the latter, and hypoplasia of the corpus callosum and of the cerebral peduncles (Fig. 214b).

Microscopically, there was indistinct lamination of the cortex, with tendency to columnar rather than tangential stratification. The neurons tended to group themselves in nests, interspersed by acellular foci; there were many immature spindle-shaped cells with relatively large nuclei and scant cytoplasm (Fig. 214c).

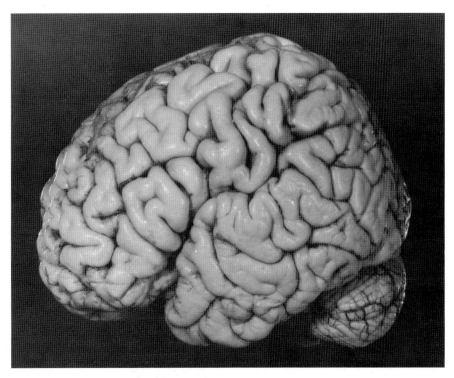

Fig. 214a. Nonspecific anomalies, external view

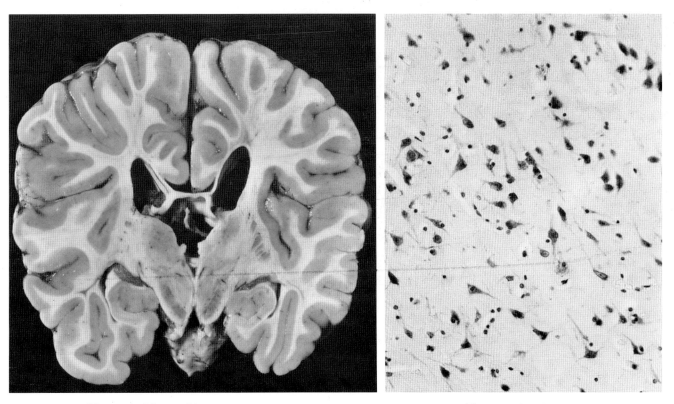

Fig. 214b. Nonspecific anomalies, coronal section

Fig. 214c. Nissl × 200

## Nonspecific Anomalies with Down's Syndrome (Mongolism)

The cerebral changes in cases of Down's syndrome are essentially similar to those in the group previously described.

> *Case:* A 25-year-old woman, whose family history was negative and birth history uneventful, showed from birth the physical features of mongolism. She was admitted at age eight to a hospital, where the I.Q. was estimated to be 32. She was diagnosed as Down's syndrome.

The brain weighed 1,272 grams; it appeared rounded because of an increase in biparietal versus anteroposterior diameters; there were many nondescript irregularities in the gyral-sulcal pattern, the convolutions being either abnormally large or small; the superior temporal gyrus was narrow; the frontal lobes were foreshortened, the occipital lobes flattened, and the cerebellum and brain stem were disproportionately small (Fig. 215a).

Coronal sections revealed an increase in the width of the cortex, deep penetrations of the gray into the white matter, and a reduced white substance (Fig. 215b).

Microscopically, the lamination of the cortex was indistinct; the nerve cells showed a tendency to cluster in groups separated by acellular areas but without evidence of gliosis; many neurons were small, round or fusiform, lacking pyramidal shape, with relative increase in size of nucleus and decrease in cytoplasm (Fig. 215c).

A number of changes, considered to be secondary, are frequently found in the brains of cases with Down's syndrome. Of these, miliary foci of gliosis to large infarcts, are attributed to the associated congenital heart disease. Minute granular deposits of calcium or pseudo-calcium in basal ganglia are common but of obscure pathogenesis (Fig. 215d).

The most consistent finding is the association with Alzheimer's disease in patients with Down's syndrome who have survived past middle age. This feature appears to be intimately related to the fundamental chromosomal abnormalities of the disorder (see p. 328).

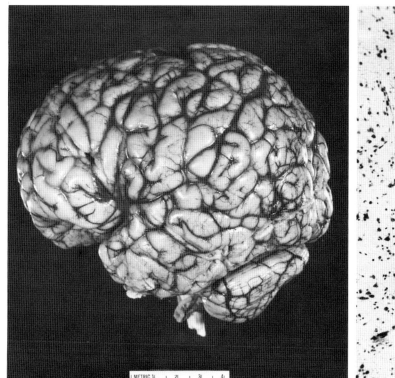

Fig. 215a. Brain in cases with Down's syndrome, external view

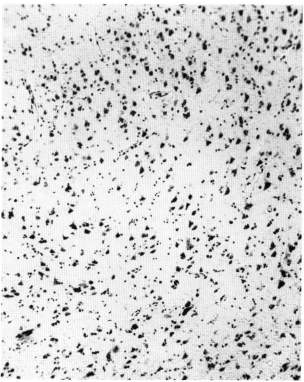

Fig. 215c. Nissl × 100

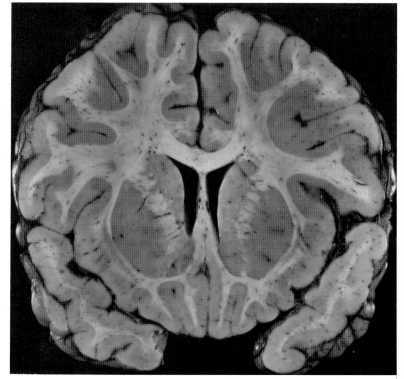

Fig. 215b. Brain in cases with Down's syndrome, coronal section

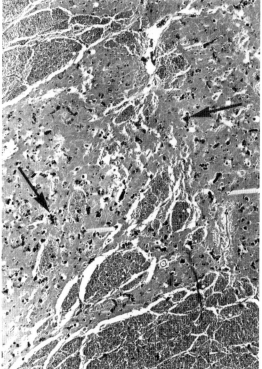

Fig. 215d. HE × 50

In the vast majority of the malformations, information with respect to etiology is still inadequate. The finding of chromosomal abnormalities in Down's syndrome is of primary importance, however, only occasionally observed in other types of malformation. The role of acquired intrauterine factors is of particular significance in the light of the findings in experimental teratology and in such human disorders as maternal cytomegalic inclusion disease and rubella.

In cytomegalic inclusion encephalitis, the teratogenic effects of the virus on the development of the brain have been quite consistent. It is noteworthy that the gross cerebral anomalies in this disorder have been associated with calcification and gliosis and are generally attributed to the occurrence of the infection early in pregnancy (see p. 98).

In maternal rubella, rare cases of gross malformation of the brain have been reported but in most instances the changes have been nonspecific arrests in development and/or microscopic vascular changes of endothelial hyperplasia, fibrosis, and calcification, associated with focal areas of degeneration.

*Case 1:* A male infant, whose mother had a skin rash (believed to be rubella) in the second month of pregnancy, showed at birth bilateral cataracts, followed by retardation of development. Examination at the age of nine months disclosed microcephaly and mental deficiency. He died of intercurrent infection at the age of thirteen months.

The principal gross findings in the brain were complete agenesis of the corpus callosum, associated with longitudinal bands of fibers on the mesial wall of either lateral ventricle, and of the septum pellucidum (Fig. 216a).

Microscopically, there were scattered foci of gliosis in the white matter of the cerebral (Fig. 216b) and cerebellar (Fig. 216c) hemispheres. Such changes resembled the residuals of perivenous encephalomyelitis seen in postnatal measles.

*Case 2:* A female infant, whose family history was negative but whose mother had German measles during the first months of pregnancy, had a normal birth at term. However, her development was retarded from birth. She began walking only at two years of age, and never learned to talk. Hospital examination revealed low-grade mental defect, spasticity with athetoid movements of all extremities, and signs of congenital heart disease.

At autopsy, the heart showed a patent ductus arteriosus. The brain weighed 1,090 grams, and was rounded; the temporal lobes were disproportionately large, while the frontal and occipital lobes appeared small and contained areas of micropolygyria at their poles (Fig. 216d).

Microscopic examination revealed relatively sparse foci of gliosis and calcification.

The two cases might represent different stages of arrested development plus degenerative effects of variable degree possibly caused by the specific virus acting at different periods of pregnancy.

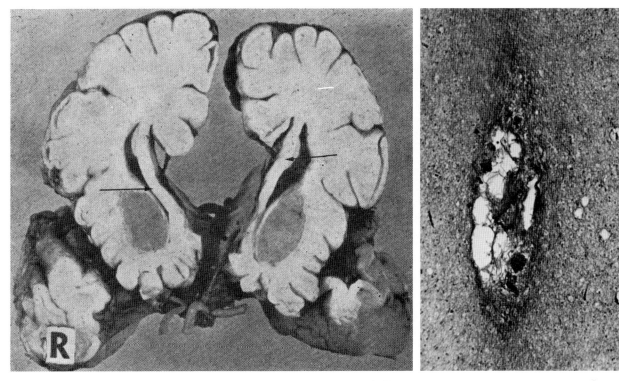

Fig. 216a. Agenesis of corpus callosum with history of maternal rubella

Fig. 216b. Holzer × 100

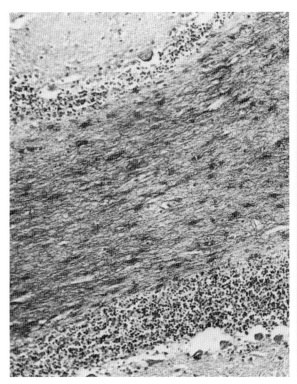

Fig. 216c. Holzer × 120

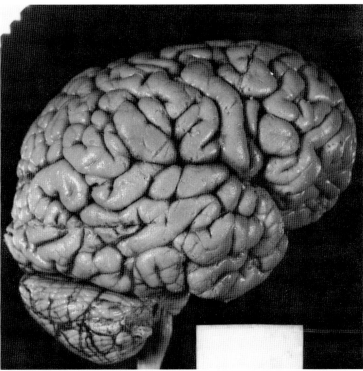

Fig. 216d. Nonspecific anomalies with history of maternal rubella

The accompanying electron micrograph illustrates an experimental model of cerebellar malformation induced by intoxication with cycasin, a toxin derived from the cycad seed, in the neonatal mouse. Animals treated in this way develop signs of cerebellar dysfunction within one week. Morphologically, the cerebellum is very small and the granule cells are almost completely absent.

Electron microscopic study confirmed the light microscopic results. Namely, granule cells and their processes, including their axons, the parallel fibers (P), were virtually absent in the cycasin-treated mice. On the other hand, the Purkinje cells remained and their dendritic spines (D) appeared normal even though they were almost always free of synaptic contact. The spines retained their postmembranous thickening and were even associated with an extracellular electron-dense material (Fig. 217).

Apparently identical results could be induced by inoculation with feline panleukopenia virus or in the murine mutation "weaver." In both cases, just as in cycasin treatment, there is an absence of granule cells and a retention of apparently intact Purkinje cell dendritic spines. Thus, three widely different etiologies, an intoxicant, an infectious agent, and a genetic defect, all can result in identical features, both clinically and morphologically.

*References*

Herndon, R. M., G. Margolis, and L. Kilham. The Synpatic Organization of the Malformed Cerebellum Induced by Perinatal Infection with the Feline Panleukopenia Virus (PLV). II. The Purkinje Cell and Its Afferents. J. Neuropath. and Expt. Neurol. 30: 557, 1971.
Hirano, A., H. M. Dembitzer, and M. Jones. An Electron Microscopic Study of Cycasin-induced Cerebellar Alterations. J. Neuropath. and Expt. Neurol. 31: 113, 1972.
Hirano, A., and H. M. Dembitzer. Cerebellar Alterations in the Weaver Mouse. J. Cell. Biol. 56: 478, 1973.

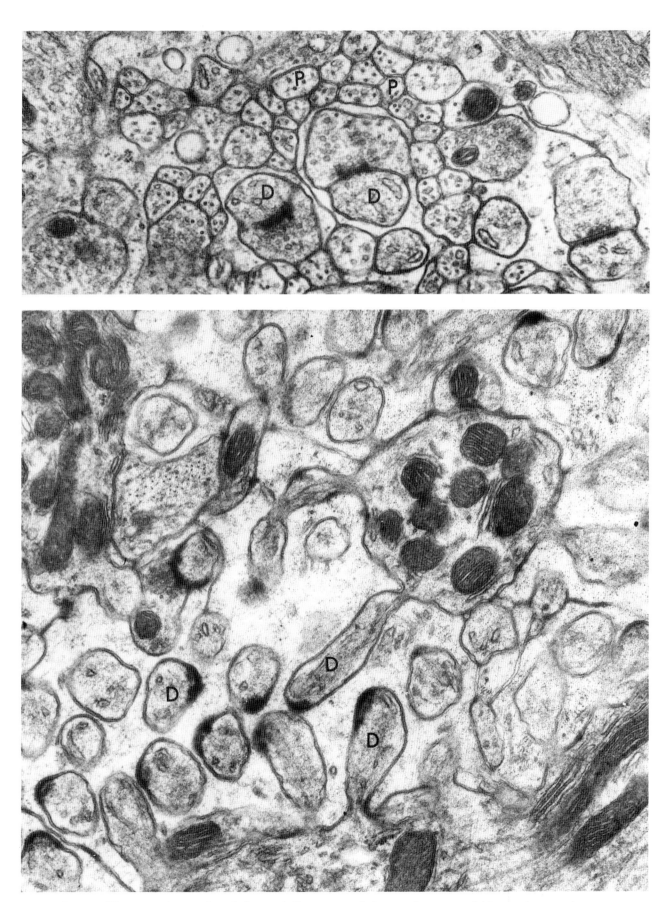

Fig. 217. Electron micrography of the cerebellar cortex of a) normal mouse and b) cycasin treated mouse
× 35,000

As listed in Table 1 on p. 413, the second most common type of disorder observed in cases of mental retardation and cerebral palsy is a group caused by a great variety of extrinsic factors. Pathoanatomically, they possess the common feature of being sequelae of a destructive process.

The lesions in this group are highly complex and heterogeneous. Since they represent end stages of disease processes, their etiology can be determined only if exact data are available about the acute stage of the illness in question. Such information is, however, often incomplete or misleading. Nevertheless, analysis of the pathology of the residual lesions can furnish some clues about their etiology, for in spite of their diversity, the pathoanatomic changes fall into distinct patterns that suggest specific modes of pathogenesis. Furthermore, the validity of such conclusions become more likely with investigations of a large series of cases, in which the same stereotyped pathologic pattern recurs in each category.

The above Table listed the various known or suspected causes, leaving a relatively small number in which the etiology remained unknown, perhaps because some of the latter may represent a complex combination of the other factors.

## SEQUELAE OF PERINATAL TRAUMA

Birth trauma in its broadest sense includes all manifestations of abnormal parturition, including circulatory and biochemical alterations, and in which mechanical trauma plays a relatively minor role.

The acute changes of hemorrhage, ischemia, and anoxia seen in the brains of stillbirths and neonates, have been widely reported in the literature but the chronic residual changes have received comparatively less attention.

In the light of the accompanying Table, which is based on correlation of clinical and pathoanatomic data, three patterns of chronic lesions may be considered as pathognomonic of sequelae of perinatal trauma: A) status marmoratus of the basal ganglia; B) sclerosis and/or cavitation of the cerebral white matter; and C) sclerotic microgyria of the cerebral cortex (Fig. 218).

*References*

Malamud, N. Sequelae of Perinatal Trauma. J. Neuropath. and Expt. Neurol. 18: 141, 1959.
Malamud, N., H. H. Itabashi, J. Castor, and H. B. Messinger. An Etiologic and Diagnostic Study of Cerebral Palsy. J. Pediat. 65: 270, 1964.

| | Number of Cases |
|---|---|
| a)  Retrospective Clinical Data | |
| Abnormalities of labor and fetal state at birth | 149 ( 75% ) |
| Normal labor and fetal abnormalities at birth | 36 ( 18% ) |
| Normal labor and normal fetal state at birth | 13 ( 7% ) |
| b)  Pathoanatomic Data | |
| Sclerosis and/or cavitation of cerebral white matter | 164 ( 83% ) |
| Status marmoratus of basal ganglia | 173 ( 88% ) |
| Sclerotic microgyria | 132 ( 62% ) |

Bilateral involvement (95%); unilateral 9 ( 5% )

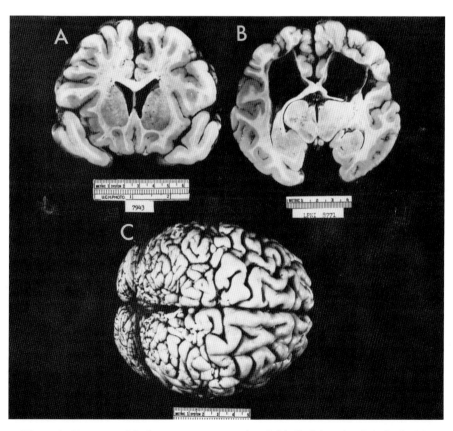

Fig. 218.  Patterns of A. Status marmoratus (top left), B. Sclerosis of cerebral white matter (top right), C. Sclerotic microgyria (bottom).

## Status Marmoratus

The condition of status marmoratus is a unique form of gliosis, accompanied by hyper-myelination, that is commonly attributed to attempted regeneration. It is rarely seen under other conditions than perinatal trauma. Its predominant involvement of basal ganglia results in an extrapyramidal syndrome. Extension of the process into adjacent areas accounts for additional symptoms of mental retardation and pyramidal tract signs.

*Case:* A 13-year-old girl with negative family history and uneventful pregnancy was born at term following a prolonged and difficult labor. Respirations were delayed although cyanosis was not present. The infant had difficulty swallowing and tube feeding was required. A cerebral hemorrhage was suspected. Seizures continued throughout the first year of life and development was retarded. She remained helpless, exhibited gross athetoid movements of all extremities, scissoring of legs and bilateral pyramidal tract signs.

The brain weighed 950 grams and on section the caudate and putamen nuclei revealed a marbled pattern consisting of ramifying white fibers arranged in bundles or networks (see Fig. 218-A).

Microscopically, the bundles consisted of a network of glial fibers that spread through the parenchyma of the caudate nucleus and putamen, as well as adjacent capsules (Fig. 219a) and further back in the thalamus (Fig. 219b), the gliosis usually being most dense in the dorsal parts, tending to fade ventrally. Within the area of gliosis there was an increase in weakly medullated fibers (Fig. 219c). In Nissl preparations there were corresponding areas of abundant glial nuclei, devoid of neurons, both in the striatum (Fig. 219d) and thalamus (Fig. 219e).

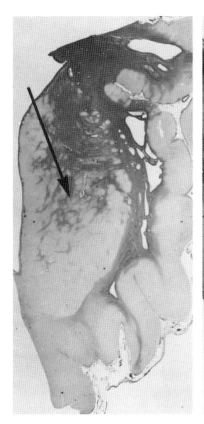

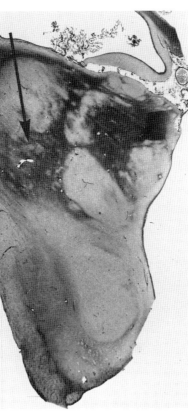

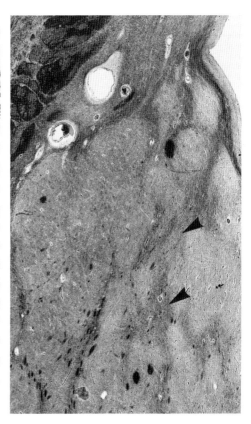

Fig. 219a. Holzer stain, region of caudate and putamen

Fig. 219b. Holzer stain, region of thalamus

Fig. 219c. Weil stain, region of thalamus

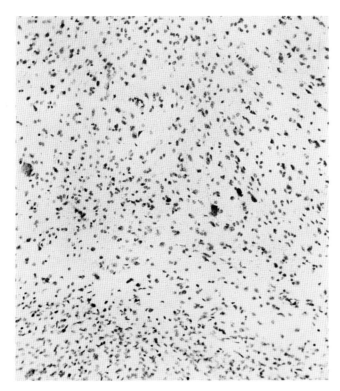

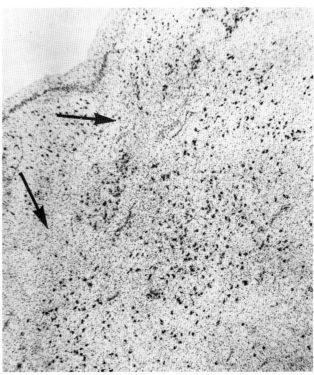

Fig. 219d. Nissl × 160

Fig. 219e. Nissl × 120

## Sclerosis-cavitation of Cerebral White Matter

*Case:* A 17-year-old boy, one of twins, was born prematurely at six and one-half months, weighing 3 lbs.; the other twin died shortly following birth. The infant was kept in an incubator for four months and was entirely helpless. Spastic quadriplegia became apparent at the age of four months. The further course was marked by profound mental retardation and contractures of the extremities.

The brain weighed 820 grams and on section revealed severe atrophy and/or cystic degeneration of the white matter, located exclusively in the dorsal parts of both hemispheres with corresponding dilatation of the ventricles (see Fig. 218b).

Microscopically, the gliosis spread diffusely throughout the dorsal white matter and extended from the ventricular wall to the cerebral cortex which it penetrated unevenly for a limited distance (Fig. 220a), with corresponding focal loss of neurons, confined to the lower layers of the cortex (Fig. 220b).

## Sclerotic Microgyria (Ulegyria)

This condition may be regarded as a further extension of the changes noted under (B). It is characterized by focal gyral atrophy and obliteration of intervening sulci, variously located in symmetrical dorsal parts of the hemispheres, more often in parieto-occipital than frontal regions (see Fig. 218-c).

Microscopically, subcortical and cortical gliosis involved primarily the regions around the troughs of sulci with relative sparing of the crests of the gyri (Fig. 220c and d). It is noteworthy that here too the pattern of gliosis tends to be marbled and is associated with hypermyelination, as in status marmoratus of the basal ganglia. The clinical manifestations of the lesions in either the white or gray matter are most commonly spastic quadriplegia, only occasionally hemiplegia, along with varying degrees of mental retardation and convulsive disorder.

As shown in the Table, the three patterns of lesions have a common clinical background and are frequently combined in various ways. In a retrospective survey, the birth histories emphasized the high incidence of abnormal labor and above all of signs of fetal distress in the majority of a series of cases.

The stereotyped lesions, despite a variety of conditions of parturitional stress, imply a common pathogenesis. Opinions differ however as to the precise mechanism; the commonly held views being either venous disturbances, especially in the Galenic venous system, impairment in arterial circulation, and cerebral anoxia. The mechanism of the lesions seen in neonatal deaths under similar conditions and their experimental reproduction may throw further light on the pathogenesis of the chronic sequelae.

*References*

Courville, C. B. Birth and Brain Damage. Published by Margaret F. Courville (Pasadena, Calif., 1971).
Malamud, N. Trauma and Mental Retardation. Physical Trauma As an Etiological Agent in Mental Retardation. Natl. Inst. Neurol. Dis. and Stroke (Bethesda, Md., 1970), pp. 35–51.
Schwartz, P. Birth Injuries of the Newborn: Morphology, Pathogenesis, Clinical Pathology and Prevention of Birth Injuries of the Newborn. Arch. Pediat. 73: 429–450, 1956.
Towbin, A. Cerebral Intraventricular Hemorrhage and Subependymal Matrix Infarction in the Fetus and Premature Newborn. Am. J. Path. 52: 121–140, 1968.

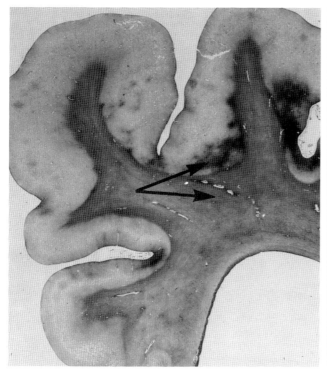

Fig. 220a. Holzer stain

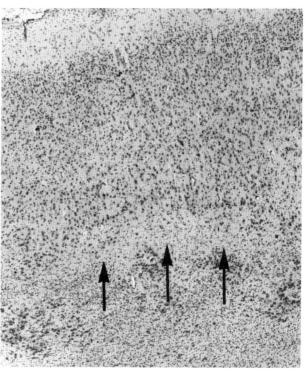

Fig. 220b. Nissl × 100

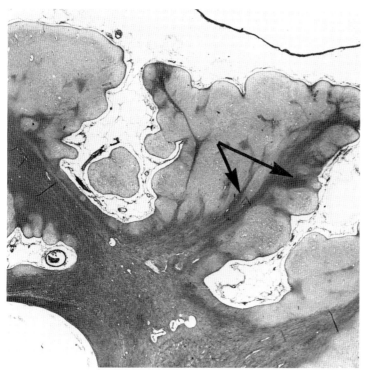

Fig. 220c. Holzer stain

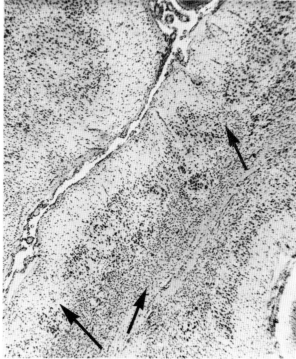

Fig. 220d. Nissl × 60

Mechanical effects of trauma induced at birth are well known as acute, usually fatal, sub-dural and subarachnoid hemorrhages brought about by tears in the falx and tentorium and laceration of adjacent venous sinuses and their tributaries. However, they are rare as chronic residuals causing mental retardation and cerebral palsy.

## Intracranial Birth Injury

*Case:* A female infant was born after a long, difficult labor and breech presentation. Oxygen was administered by cord because the baby breathed with difficulty. She regurgitated and vomited her feedings. Three weeks after birth she developed convulsions associated with fever. The spinal fluid was bloody and contained chiefly red blood cells and no organisms were demonstrated. She remained paralyzed in all her extremities, maintaining a posture of de-cerebrate rigidity, and presented a vegetative mental state. Death occurred at two and one-half years of age.

The brain showed an unusually severe degree of cerebral atrophy (A) and yellowish-brown-discolored meninges surrounded by what appeared to be an encapsulated subdural hygroma (B), filled with slightly yellowish fluid, probably representing residuals of a sub-dural hematoma (Fig. 221a).

Microscopically, the meninges and the underlying cerebral cortex were entirely replaced by fibrous glial tissue (A), within which were focal collections of hemosiderin-laden gitter cells (B) and scattered deposits of calcium without inflammatory changes (Fig. 221b).

## Spinal Cord Birth Injury

Under certain conditions of birth injury, trauma to the spinal cord may result from traction on the lower cervical and dorsal cord in breech presentations.

*Case:* A female infant was born after a double-footling breech presentation. After birth both legs showed flaccid paralysis; the left arm was spastic and flexed, and the right arm was in a splint because of fracture of the humerus. A sensory level was determined at approximately C6. There was slight improvement in the next few months, but death followed an intercurrent infection.

The spinal cord contained an atrophic segment of about 3 cm in length in the lower cervical and upper dorsal region (Fig. 221c).

In the most severely traumatized area the cord was reduced to a mere central fragment of necrotic nervous tissue (A), surrounded by a layer of gitter cells (B) and bands of collagen fibers (C) (Fig. 221d).

There was ascending and descending Wallerian degeneration of the long tracts above and below the level of transverse myelitis.

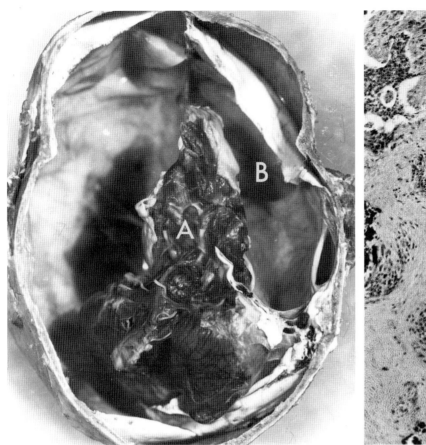

Fig. 221a. Residual changes of perinatal trauma

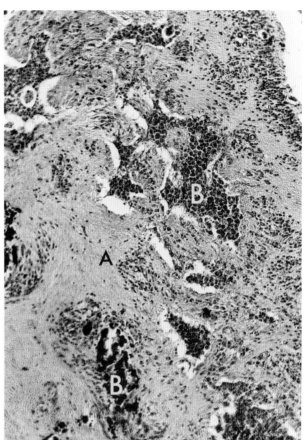

Fig. 221b. HVG × 100

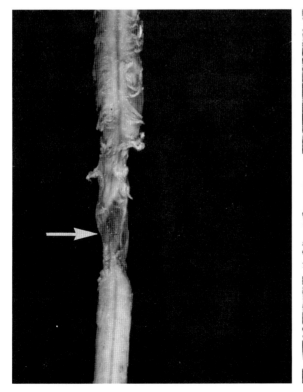

Fig. 221c. Spinal cord birth injury

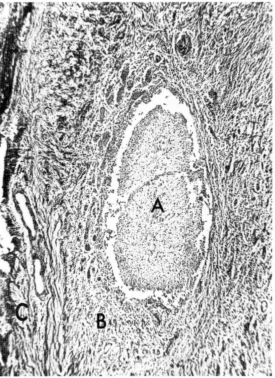

Fig. 221d. HVG × 34

Among the *sequelae of inflammatory disorders*, a great variety of conditions may result in mental retardation and cerebral palsy. The most important of these have been discussed in Chapter II.

*Sequelae of arterial and venous occlusive disease*, as well as of *postnatal trauma*, are much less common in cases of mental retardation and cerebral palsy, and do not differ in their pathology from similar conditions occurring in adults.

## SEQUELAE OF CONVULSIVE DISORDERS

A relatively large group of destructive processes are characterized by cerebral lesions that bear a close resemblance to the pathology of cerebral anoxia of adults. As such they show predominant and selective involvement of the gray matter, in the form of laminar degeneration of the cerebral cortex, sclerosis of Sommer's sector and end plate of the hippocampus, and Purkinje cell degeneration of the cerebellum. In Chapter IV, one of the conditions used to illustrate anoxic encephalopathy was epilepsy. It is of interest that a history of febrile convulsions occurring in infancy and childhood, precipitated by upper respiratory and other systemic infections, is frequently elicited in cases of mental retardation and cerebral palsy.

*Case 1:* An 11-year-old girl was the product of an uneventful pregnancy and delivery and developed normally until the age of five years. At this time the patient had a febrile seizure during which time she became semicomatose. Examination revealed irritability, forgetfulness, left hemiparesis, choreoathetoid movements of the left side of the face, bilateral visual field defects and major motor seizures, which were more marked on the left side. An electroencephalogram revealed a high voltage slow wave focus in the right hemisphere and a pneumoencephalogram showed right ventricular enlargement. Her condition continued to deteriorate and she was finally committed to a State hospital, where she succumbed to bronchopneumonia.

The brain weighed 750 grams and showed generalized atrophy of the cerebral cortex, more marked on the right side, and of the cerebellar gray matter associated with enlargement of the entire ventricular system (Fig. 222a).

*Case 2:* A 3-year-old boy with family history of diabetes had a history of normal birth and development. At the age of twenty months, after a week of fever, he became lethargic. He was admitted to a hospital where the blood glucose was found to be 400 mg %, while the spinal fluid was negative. His treatment consisted of diet and insulin medication, but a week later he had a clonic convulsion and became comatose followed by repeated convulsions during the following week. His further course was marked by mental deterioration and decerebrate rigidity necessitating commitment to the State hospital where he died of bronchopneumonia and diabetic acidosis.

In the general autopsy, the most noteworthy finding was degeneration of the islands of Langerhans.

The brain weighed 680 grams and showed marked diffuse atrophy of the cerebral cortex with enlargement of the ventricles (Fig. 222b).

In the above two cases, changes in the cerebral cortex varied from pseudolaminar degeneration, as indicated by reactive gliosis, (Fig. 222c) to cystic degeneration of the major part of the gray matter (Fig. 222d).

In both cases there was selective degeneration in the hippocampal formation and cerebellar gray matter, as in cases of anoxic encephalopathy.

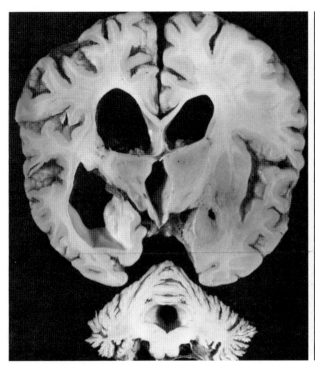

Fig. 222a. Diffuse atrophy of cerebral coftex and cerebellum, more on right side (sides reversed)

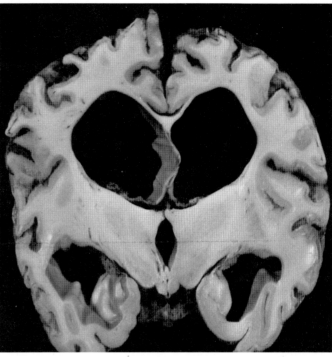

Fig. 222b. Diffuse bilateral cortical atrophy

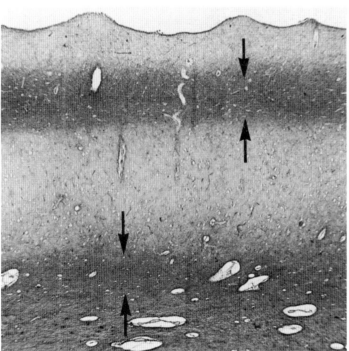

Fig. 222c. Holzer stain × 30

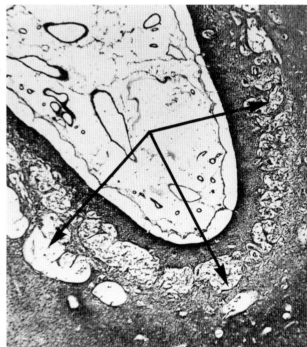

Fig. 222d. Holzer stain × 35

The condition of kernicterus (bilirubin pigmentation of the basal ganglia) takes place in the newborn, in the majority of instances on the basis of Rh incompatibility and in a minority of cases due to ABO incompatibility, neonatal sepsis, and inherited deficiency of the specific liver enzyme. During the acute stage, yellow to orange pigmentation develops in certain areas, in particular the globus pallidus, subthalamic body, reticular part of the substantia nigra, hippocampus, dentate nucleus, and parts of the medulla. In these areas, acute changes with deposition of bile pigment can be demonstrated in neurons and glia.

The pathogenesis of kernicterus is attributed to the combined effects of two factors: a) hemolysis of fetal blood due to isoimmunization by maternal anti-Rh antibodies, and b) deficiency in the liver enzyme glucuronyl transferase that causes an increase in the toxic unconjugated form of bilirubin. Twenty to forty per cent of the latter can cross the blood brain barrier and result in bilirubin encephalopathy.

The sequelae of kernicterus are characterized clinically primarily by athetoid palsy, deafness, and mental retardation. The corresponding pathologic changes, in the form of demyelination, neuronal loss, and gliosis, are consistently located in the globus pallidus, subthalamic bodies, and in the hippocampus. It is noteworthy that in the hippocampus, the dorsal cell band (H2) and the dentate gyrus are much more commonly affected than is Sommer's sector (H1), the area that is most vulnerable to anoxia.

*Case:* A 6-year-old boy, second child, the older being normal, was born at term of an Rh negative mother while father and patient were both Rh positive. Birth was normal. However, nine hours following birth, he developed jaundice and Coombs test was positive. Despite several blood transfusions, he developed convulsions and later showed evidence of mental retardation. When examined at age three years, he had no speech, showed athetoid movements, deafness, possible visual impairment, internal strabismus, and occasional seizures.

The brain weighed 1,560 grams and was externally normal but on section, revealed bilaterally symmetrical atrophy and pallor of the globus pallidus (A) and subthalamic bodies (B), (Fig. 223a).

In Holzer stains (Fig. 223b), marked gliosis was seen in both segments of the globus pallidus (A) and in the lateral part of the subthalamic body (B); there was corresponding demyelination in the two structures in myelin preparations (Fig. 223c). The hippocampal formation showed gliosis (Fig. 223d) with corresponding loss of neurons in the fascia dentata (FD), and in the H3–5 of the dentate gyrus, and in H2 of the hippocampus, whereas Sommer's sector (H1) was intact (Fig. 223e).

*References*

Haymaker, W., C. Margoles, A. Pentschew, H. Jacob, R. Lindenberg, L. S. Arroyo, U. Stochdorph, and D. Stowens. Pathology of Kernicterus and Posticteric Encephalopathy. Kernicterus and Its Importance in Cerebral Palsy. Chas. C Thomas (Springfield, Ill., 1961), pp. 21–228.

Malamud, N. Pathogenesis of Kernicterus in the Light of Its Sequelae. Kernicterus and Its Importance in Cerebral Palsy (Springfield, Ill., 1961), pp. 230–244.

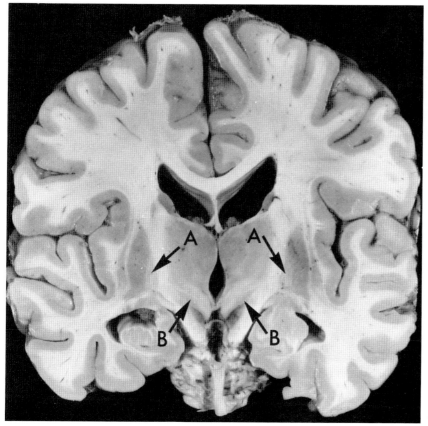

Fig. 223a. Sequelae of kernicterus, gross appearance

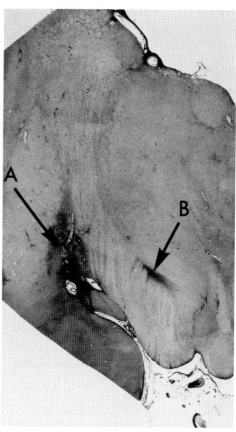

Fig. 223b. Holzer stain of basal ganglia

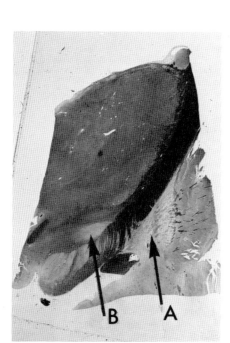

Fig. 223c. Weil stain of basal ganglia

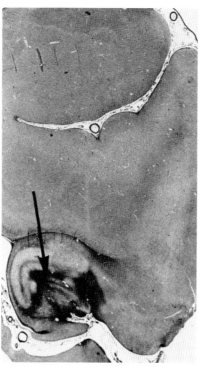

Fig. 223d. Holzer stain of hippocampal formation

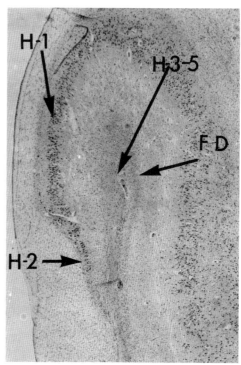

Fig. 223e. Nissl stain of hippocampal
formation × 25

# General References

1. ADAMS, R. D. and R. L. SIDMAN. Introduction to Neuropathology. McGraw-Hill, Blakiston Division (New York, 1968)
2. BAILEY, P. Intracranial Tumors. 2nd edition, Charles C.Thomas (Springfield, Ill., 1948)
3. BAILEY, P., and H. CUSHING. A Classification of Tumors of the Glioma Group on a Histogenetic Basis with a Correlated Study of Prognosis. J. B. Lippincott (Philadelphia, 1926)
4. BIGGART, J. H. Pathology of the Nervous System. 3rd edition. Livingstone (Edinburgh, 1961)
5. DUBLIN, W. B. Fundamentals of Neuropathology. 2nd edition. Charles C Thomas (Springfield, Ill., 1967)
6. GREENFIELD'S NEUROPATHOLOGY. 2nd edition. Williams and Wilkins (Baltimore, 1963)
7. KERNOHAN, J. W. and G. P. SAYRE, Tumors of the Central Nervous System. Armed Forces Institute of Pathology (Washington, D.C., 1952)
8. PETERS, G. SPEZIELLE Pathologie der Krankheiten des zentralen and peripheren Nervensystems. Georg Thieme Verlag (Stuttgart, 1951)
9. RUSSELL, D. S. and RUBINSTEIN, L. J. Pathology of Tumors of the Nervous System. 3rd edition. Williams and Wilkins (Baltimore, 1971)
10. SLAGER, U. T. Basic Neuropathology. Williams and Wilkins (Baltimore, 1970)
11. ZIMMERMAN, H. M., M. J. NETSKY and L. M. DAVIDOFF. Atlas of Tumors of the Nervous System. Lea and Febiger (Philadelphia, 1956)
12. ZÜLCH, K. J. Brain Tumors. 2nd edition. Springer (New York, 1965)
13. PATHOLOGY OF THE NERVOUS SYSTEM, (J. Minckler, ed.), 3 vols. McGraw-Hill, Blakiston Division (New York, 1968–1972)
14. NEUROPATHOLOGY, METHODS AND DIAGNOSIS, (C. G. Tedeschi, ed.) Little Brown (Boston, 1970)
15. PROGRESS IN NEUROPATHOLOGY, (H. M. Zimmerman, ed.), 2 vols. Grune and Stratton (New York, 1971–73)

# Index